Applied Linear Models with SAS

This textbook for a second course in basic statistics for undergraduates or first-year graduate students introduces linear regression models and describes other linear models including Poisson regression, logistic regression, proportional hazards regression, and nonparametric regression. Numerous examples drawn from the news and current events with an emphasis on health issues illustrate these concepts.

Assuming only a pre-calculus background, the author keeps equations to a minimum and demonstrates all computations using SAS. Most of the programs and output are displayed in a self-contained way, with an emphasis on the interpretation of the output in terms of how it relates to the motivating example. Plenty of exercises conclude every chapter. All of the datasets and SAS programs are available from the book's Web site, along with other ancillary material.

Dr. Daniel Zelterman is Professor of Epidemiology and Public Health in the Division of Biostatistics at Yale University. His application areas include work in genetics, HIV, and cancer. Before moving to Yale in 1995, he was on the faculty of the University of Minnesota and at the State University of New York at Albany. He is an elected Fellow of the American Statistical Association. He serves as associate editor of *Biometrics* and other statistical journals. He is the author of *Models for Discrete Data* (1999), *Advanced Log-Linear Models Using SAS* (2002), *Discrete Distributions: Application in the Health Sciences* (2004), and *Models for Discrete Data: 2nd Edition* (2006). In his spare time he plays the bassoon in orchestral groups and has backpacked hundreds of miles of the Appalachian Trail.

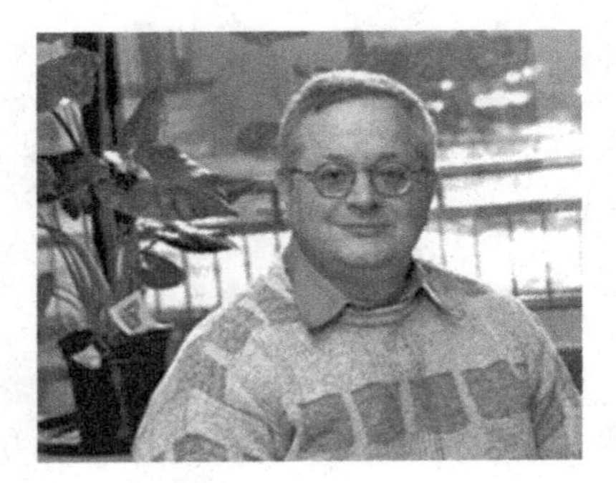

Applied Linear Models with SAS

Daniel Zelterman
Yale University

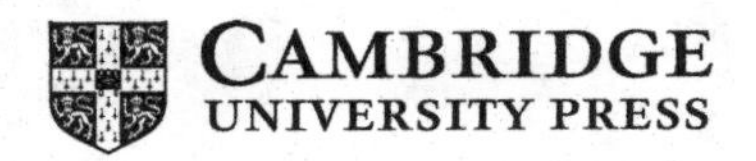

CAMBRIDGE
UNIVERSITY PRESS

University Printing House, Cambridge CB2 8BS, United Kingdom

One Liberty Plaza, 20th Floor, New York, NY 10006, USA

477 Williamstown Road, Port Melbourne, VIC 3207, Australia

314-321, 3rd Floor, Plot 3, Splendor Forum, Jasola District Centre, New Delhi - 110025, India

79 Anson Road, #06-04/06, Singapore 079906

Cambridge University Press is part of the University of Cambridge.

It furthers the University's mission by disseminating knowledge in the pursuit of education, learning and research at the highest international levels of excellence.

www.cambridge.org
Information on this title: www.cambridge.org/9780521761598

First published 2010

A catalogue record for this publication is available from the British Library

Library of Congress Cataloging in Publication data
Zelterman, Daniel.
Applied linear models with SAS / Daniel Zelterman.
p. cm.
Includes index.
ISBN 978-0-521-76159-8 (hardback)
1. Linear regression. 2. Linear models (Statistics) 3. SAS (Computer program language) I. Title.
QA278.2.Z45 2010
519.5′35–dc22 2009053487

ISBN 978-0-521-76159-8 Hardback

Copyright page continues after page xiii.

Contents

Preface

Linear models are a powerful and useful set of methods in a large number of settings. Very briefly, there is some outcome measurement that is very important to us and we want to explain variations in its values in terms of other measurements in the data. The heights of several trees can be explained in terms of the trees' ages, for example. It is not a straight line relationship, of course, but knowledge of a tree's age offers us a large amount of explanatory value. We might also want to take into account the effects of measurements on the amount of light, water, nutrients, and weather conditions experienced by each tree. Some of these measurements will have greater explanatory value than others and we may want to quantify the relative usefulness of these different measures. Even after we are given all of this information, some trees will appear to thrive and others will remain stunted, when all are subjected to identical conditions. This variability is the whole reason for statistics existing as a scientific discipline. We usually try to avoid the use of the word "prediction" because this assumes that there is a cause-and-effect relationship. A tree's age does not directly cause it to grow, for example, but rather, a cumulative process associated with many environmental factors results in increasing height and continued survival. The best estimate we can make is a statement about the behavior of the average tree under identical conditions.

Many of my students go on to work in the pharmaceutical or health-care industry after graduating with a masters degree. Consequently, the choice of examples has a decidedly health/medical bias. We expect our students to be useful to their employers the day they leave our program so there is not a lot of time to spend on advanced theory that is not directly applicable. Not all of the examples are from the health sciences. Diverse examples such as the number of lottery winners and temperatures in various US cities are part of our common knowledge. Such examples do not need a lengthy explanation for the reader to appreciate many of the aspects of the data being presented.

How is this book different? The mathematical content and notation are kept to an absolute minimum. To paraphrase the noted physicist Steven Hawking, who has written extensively for the popular audience, every equation loses half of your audience. There is really no need for formulas and their derivations in a book of this type if we rely on the computer to calculate quantities of interest. Long gone are the days of doing statistics with calculators or on the back of an envelope. Students of mathematical statistics should be able to provide the derivations of the formulas but they represent a very different audience. All of the important formulas are programmed in software so there is no need for the general user to know these.

The three important skills needed by a well-educated student of applied statistics are

1. Recognize the appropriate method needed in a given setting.
2. Have the necessary computer skills to perform the analysis.
3. Be able to interpret the output and draw conclusions in terms of the original data.

This book gives examples to introduce the reader to a variety of commonly encountered settings and provides guidance through these to complete these three goals. Not all possible situations can be described, of course, but the chosen settings include a broad survey of the type of problems the student of applied statistics is likely to run into.

What do I ask of my readers? We still need to use a lot of mathematical concepts such as the connection between a linear equation and drawing the line on $X-Y$ coordinates. There will be algebra and special functions such as square roots and logarithms. Logarithms, while we are on the subject, are always to the base e (=2.718) and not base 10.

We will also need a nodding acquaintance with the concepts of calculus. Many of us may have taken calculus in college, a long time ago, and not had much need to use it in the years since then. Perhaps we intentionally chose a course of study that avoided abstract mathematics. Even so, calculus represents an important and useful tool. The definition of the derivative of a function (What does this new function represent?) and integral (What does *this* new function represent?) are needed although we will never need to actually find a derivative or an integral. The necessary refresher to these important concepts is given in Section 1.4.

Also helpful is a previous course in statistics. The reader should be familiar with the mean and standard deviation, normal and binomial distributions, and hypothesis tests in general and the chi-squared and t-tests specifically. These important concepts are reviewed in Chapter 2 but an appreciation of these important ideas is almost a full course in itself. There is a large reliance on p-values in scientific research so it is important to know exactly what these represent.

There are a number of excellent general-purpose statistical packages available. We have chosen to illustrate our examples using SAS because of its wide acceptance and use in many industries but especially health care and pharmaceutical. Most of the examples given here are small, to emphasize interpretation and encourage practice. These datasets could be examined by most software packages. SAS, however, is capable of handling huge datasets so the skills learned here can easily be used if and when much larger projects are encountered later.

The reader should already have some familiarity with running SAS on a computer. This would include using the editor to change the program, submitting the program, and retrieving and then printing the output. There are also popular point-and-click approaches to data analysis. While these are quick and acceptable, their ease of use comes with the price of not always being able to repeat the analysis because of the lack of a printed record of the steps that were taken. Data analysis, then, should be reproducible.

We will review some of the basics of SAS but a little hand-holding will prevent some of the agonizing frustrations that can occur when first starting out. Running the computer and, more generally, doing the exercises in this book are a very necessary part of learning statistics. Just as you cannot learn to play the piano simply by reading a book, statistical expertise, and the accompanying computer skills, can only be obtained through hours of active participation in the relevant act. Again, much like the piano, the instrument is not damaged by playing a wrong note. Nobody will laugh at you if you try something truly outlandish on the computer either. Perhaps something better will come of a new look at a familiar setting. Similarly, the reader is encouraged to look at the data and try a variety of different ways of looking, plotting, modeling, transforming, and manipulating. Unlike a mathematical problem with only one correct solution (contrary to many of our preconceived notions), there is often a lot of flexibility in the way statistics can be applied to summarize a set of data. As with yet another analogy to music, there are many ways to play the same song.

rapid and can handle [illegible] datasets, so the skills learned here can easily be used [illegible] and which would never [illegible] issues encountered here.

[illegible] may have some familiarity with [illegible]. Files would include using the editor to [illegible] the program [illegible] retrieving [illegible] guiding the [illegible] popular [illegible] approaches to data analysis. While these are quick and [illegible] comes with [illegible] not always [illegible] to repeat the analysis [illegible] of a [illegible] of the steps that [illegible] analysis, then [illegible] should be recorded.

[illegible] of the basics of [illegible] with [illegible] some [illegible] that can occur when [illegible] the computer [illegible] necessary part of learning statistics, but [illegible] not [illegible] the [illegible] computers [illegible] of active participation in the [illegible] and the [illegible] is not [illegible] something truly outlandish [illegible] computer [illegible] something [illegible] look at [illegible]. [illegible] look at [illegible] of the [illegible] modeling [illegible] and manipulating. While [illegible] only [illegible] can be applied to [illegible] of data. [illegible] to play the [illegible].

Acknowledgments

Thanks to the many students and teaching assistants who have provided useful comments and suggestions to the exposition as well as the computer assignments. Also to Chang Yu, Steven Schwager, and Amelia Dziengeleski for their careful readings of early drafts of the manuscript. Lauren Cowles and her staff at Cambridge University Press provided innumerable improvements and links to useful Web sites.

The DASL (pronounced "dazzle") StatLib library maintained at Carnegie Mellon University is a great resource and provided data for many examples and exercises contained here. Ed Tufte's books on graphics have taught me to look at data more carefully. His books are highly recommended.

I am grateful to *The New York Times* for their permission to use many graphic illustrations.

Finally, thanks to my wife Linda who provided important doses of encouragement and kept me on task. This work is dedicated to her memory.

The Pennsylvania State University Department of Meteorology supplied the graphics for the weather map in Fig. 1.1.

DANIEL ZELTERMAN
Hamden, CT
August 25, 2009

The following figures are copyright *The New York Times* and used with permission: Figure 1.4 (June 23, 2007); Figure 1.6 (August 15, 2008); Figure 1.7 (August 4, 2008); Figure 1.8 (August 23, 2008); Figure 1.9 (January 8, 2009); Figure 1.10 (October 14, 2008); Figure 4.4 (April 17, 2008); Figure 6.1 (January 17, 2008); Figure 7.1 (June 13, 2007); Figure 10.3 (May 30, 2007). All rights are reserved by *The New York Times.*

Table 2.1: From J. P. Frisby and J. L. Clatworthy, "Learning to see complex random-dot stereograms," *Perception* 4(2), pp. 173–78. Copyright 1975 Pion Limited, London.

Figure 2.1: Courtesy of John Huchra.

Table 2.8: From Marcello Pagano and Kimberlee Gauvreau. *Principles of Biostatistics*, 2E. Copyright 2000 Brooks/Cole, a part of Cengage Learning, Inc. Reproduced by permission. www.cengage.com/permissions

Table 2.10: From N. Teasdale, C. Bard, J. Larue, et al., "On the cognitive penetrability of posture control," *Experimental Aging Research.* Copyright 1993 Taylor & Francis, reprinted by permission of the publisher (Taylor & Francis Group, http://www.informaworld.com).

Tables 5.1 and 6.15: From Frederick Mosteller and John W. Tukey, *Data Analysis and Regression: A Second Course in Statistics*, Table 5.1 pp. 73–74 and Table 6.15 pp. 549–51. Copyright 1977 Addison-Wesley Publishing Company, Inc. Reproduced by permission of Pearson Education, Inc.

Table 6.10: From Douglas Bates and Donald Watts, *Nonlinear Regression Analysis and Its Applications.* Copyright 2007 John Wiley and Sons, Inc. Reprinted with permission of John Wiley and Sons, Inc.

Table 6.11: From James A. Koziol and Donna A. Maxwell, "A distribution-free test for tumor-growth curve analysis with application to an animal tumor immunotherapy experiment," *Biometrics* 37, pp. 383–90. Reprinted with permission of Oxford University Press.

Table 7.1: From A. J. Dobson, *Introduction to Generalized Linear Models*, 2E. Copyright 2001 Taylor & Francis Group LLC – Books. Reproduced with permission of Taylor & Francis Group LLC – Books in the format textbook via Copyright Clearance Center.

Table 9.1: From R. G. Miller et al., *Biostatistics Casebook 318.* Copyright 1980 John Wiley and Sons, Inc. Reprinted with permission of John Wiley and Sons, Inc.

Table 10.7: From P. J. Antsaklis and K. M. Passino, *Introduction to Intelligent and Autonomous Control*, Chapter 2, pp. 27–56; Figure 2 of James S. Albus, "A Reference Model Architecture for Intelligent Systems Design." Copyright 1993 Kluwer Academic Publishers with kind permission of Springer Science and Business Media.

Table 10.11: From Pieter Joost van Wattum et al., "Patterns of response to acute Naxolone infusion in Tourette's Syndrome," *Movement Disorders* 15 (2000) pp. 1252–54. Reprinted with permission of Oxford University Press.

Table 11.2: From Jennifer Wheler et al., "Survival of patients in a phase 1 clinic," *Cancer* 115 (5), pp. 1091–99. Copyright 2009 American Cancer Society.

Table 11.4: From Thomas R. Fleming et al., "Modified Kolmogorov-Smirnov test procedures with application to arbitrarily right-censored data," *Biometrics* 36 (1980), pp. 607–25. Reprinted with permission of Oxford University Press.

Table 12.2: From Nicholas Lange et al., *Case Studies in Biometry.* Copyright 1994 John Wiley and Sons, Inc. Reprinted with permission of John Wiley and Sons, Inc.

Table 12.4: From J. M. Krall, V. A. Uthoff, and J. B. Harley. "A step-up procedure for selecting variables associated with survival," *Biometrics* 31 (1975), pp. 49–57. Reprinted with permission of Oxford University Press.

1

Introduction

We are surrounded by data. With a tap at a computer keyboard, we have access to more than we could possibly absorb in a lifetime. But is this data the same as information? How do we get from numbers to understanding? How do we identify simplifying trends – but also find exceptions to the rule? The computers that provide access to the data also provide the tools to answer these questions. Unfortunately, owning a hammer does not enable us to build a fine house. It takes experience using the tools, knowing when they are appropriate, and also knowing their limitations.

The study of statistics provides the tools to create understanding out of raw data. Expertise comes with experience, of course. We need equal amounts of theory (in the form of statistical tools), technical skills (at the computer), and critical analysis (identifying the limitations of various methods for each setting). A lack of one of these cannot be made up by the other two.

This chapter provides a review of statistics in general, along with the mathematical and statistical prerequisites that will be used in subsequent chapters. Even more broadly, the reader will be reminded of the larger picture. It is very easy to learn many statistical methods only to lose sight of the point of it all.

1.1 What Is Statistics?

In an effort to present a lot of mathematical formulas, we sometimes lose track of the central idea of the discipline. It is important to remember the big picture when we get too close to the subject.

Let us consider a vast wall that separates our lives from the place where the information resides. It is impossible to see over or around this wall, but every now and then we have the good fortune of having some pieces of data thrown over to us. On the basis of this fragmentary sampled data, we are supposed to infer the composition of the remainder on the other side. This is the aim of *statistical inference.*

The population is usually vast and infinite, whereas the sample is just a handful of numbers.

In statistical inference we infer properties of the population from the sample.

There is an enormous possibility for error, of course. If all of the left-handed people I know also have artistic ability, am I allowed to generalize this to a statement that all left-handed people are artistic? I may not know very many left-handed people. In this case I do not have much data to make my claim, and my statement should reflect a large possibility of error. Maybe most of my friends are also artists. In this case we say that the sampled data is *biased* because it contains more artists than would be found in a representative sample of the population.

The population in this example is the totality of all left-handed people. Maybe the population should be *all* people, if we also want to show that artistic ability is greater in left-handed people than in right-handed people. We can't possibly measure such a large group. Instead, we must resign ourselves to the observed or *empirical* data made up of the people we know. This is called a *convenience sample* because it is not really random and may not be representative.

Consider next the separate concepts of sample and population for numerically valued data. The sample *average* is a number that we use to infer the value of the population *mean*. The average of several numbers is itself a number that we obtain. The population mean, however, is on the other side of the imaginary wall and is not observable. In fact, the population mean is almost an unknowable quantity that could not be observed even after a lifetime of study. Fortunately, statistical inference allows us to make statements about the population mean on the basis of the sample average. Sometimes we forget that this inference is taking place and will confuse the sample statistic with the population attribute.

Statistics are functions of the sampled data. Parameters are properties of the population.

Often the sampled data comes at great expense and through personal hardship, as in the case of clinical trials of new therapies for life-threatening diseases. In a clinical trial involving cancer, for example, costs are typically many thousands of dollars per patient enrolled. Innovative therapies can easily cost ten times that amount. Sometimes the most important data consists of a single number, such as how long the patient lived, recorded only after the patient loses the fight with his or her disease.

Sometimes we attempt to collect all of the data, as in the case of a *census*. The U.S. Constitution specifically mandates that a complete census of the population be performed every ten years.[1] The writers of the Constitution knew that in order to

[1] Article 1, Section 2 reads, in part: "Representatives and direct Taxes shall be apportioned among the several States which may be included within this Union, according to their respective Numbers, which shall be

have a representative democracy and a fair tax system, we also need to know where the people live and work. The composition of the House of Representatives is based on the decennial census. Locally, communities need to know about population shifts to plan for schools and roads. Despite the importance of the census data, there continues to be controversy on how to identify and count certain segments of the population, including the homeless, prison inmates, migrant workers, college students, and foreign persons living in the country without appropriate documentation.

Statistical inference is the process of generalizing from a sample of data to the larger population. The sample average is a simple statistic that immediately comes to mind. The Student t-test is the principal method used to make inferences about the population mean on the basis of the sample average. We review this method in Section 2.5. The sample *median* is the value at which half of the sample is above and half is below. The median is discussed in Chapter 7.

> The standard deviation measures how far individual observations deviate from their average.

The sample *standard deviation* allows us to estimate the scale of variability in the population. On the basis of the normal distribution (Section 2.3), we usually expect about 68% of the population to appear within one standard deviation (above or below) of the mean. Similarly, about 95% of the population should occur within two standard deviations of the population mean.

> The standard error measures the sampling variability of the mean.

A commonly used measure related to the standard deviation is the *standard error*, also called the *standard error of the mean* and often abbreviated SEM. These two similar-sounding quantities refer to very different measures. The standard error estimates the standard deviation associated with the sample average. As the sample size increases, the standard deviation (which refers to individuals in the population) should not appreciably change. On the other hand, a large sample size is associated with a precise estimate of the population mean as a consequence of a small standard error. This relationship provides the incentive for larger sample sizes, allowing us to estimate the population mean more accurately. The relationship is

$$\text{Standard error} = \frac{\text{Standard deviation}}{\sqrt{\text{Sample size}}}$$

determined by adding to the whole Number of free Persons, including those bound to Service for a Term of Years, and excluding Indians not taxed, three fifths of all other Persons. The actual Enumeration shall be made within three Years after the first Meeting of the Congress of the United States, and within every subsequent Term of ten Years, in such Manner as they shall by Law direct."

Consider a simple example. We want to measure the heights of a group of people. There will always be tall people, and there will always be short people, so changing the sample size does not appreciably alter the standard deviation of the data. Individual variations will always be observed. If we were interested in estimating the average height, then the standard error will decrease with an increase in the sample size (at a rate of $1/\sqrt{\text{sample size}}$), motivating the use of ever-larger samples. The average will be measured with greater precision, and this precision is described in terms of the standard error. Similarly, if we want to measure the average with twice the precision, then we will need a sample size four times larger.

Another commonly used term associated with the standard deviation is *variance.* The relationship between the variance and the standard deviation is

$$\text{Variance} = (\text{Standard deviation})^2$$

The standard deviation and variance are obtained in SAS using `proc univariate`, for example. The formula appears often, and the reader should be familiar with it, even though its value will be calculated using a computer.

Given observed sample values $x_1, x_2, \ldots, x_n$, we compute the *sample variance* from

$$s^2 = \text{sample variance} = \frac{1}{n-1} \sum_i (x_i - \overline{x})^2, \tag{1.1}$$

where $\overline{x}$ is the average of the observed values.

This estimate is often denoted by the symbol s^2. Similarly, the estimated sample standard deviation s is the square root of this estimator. Intuitively, we see that (1.1) averages the squared difference between each observation and the sample average, except that the denominator is one less than the sample size. The "$n - 1$" term is the degrees of freedom for this expression and is described in Sections 2.5 and 2.7.

1.2 Statistics in the News: The Weather Map

Sometimes it is possible to be overwhelmed with too much information. The business section of the newspaper is filled with stock prices, and the sports section has a wealth of scores and data on athletic endeavors. The business section frequently has several graphs and charts illustrating trends, rates, and prices. The sports pages have yet to catch up with the business section in terms of aids for the reader.

As an excellent way to summarize and display a huge amount of information, we reproduce the U.S. weather map from October 27, 2008, in Figure 1.1. There are several levels of information depicted here, all overlaid on top of one another. First we recognize the geographic-political map indicating the shorelines and state boundaries. The large map at the top provides the details of that day's weather. The large Hs indicate the locations of high barometric pressure centers. Regions with

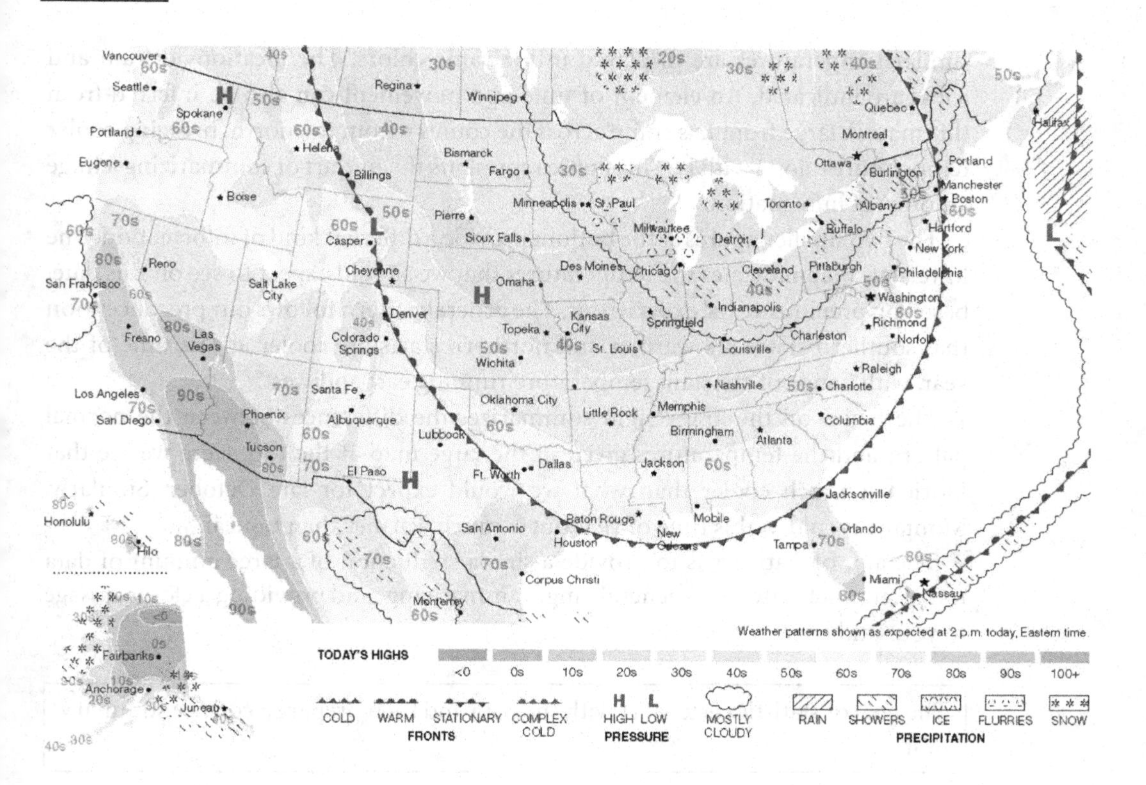

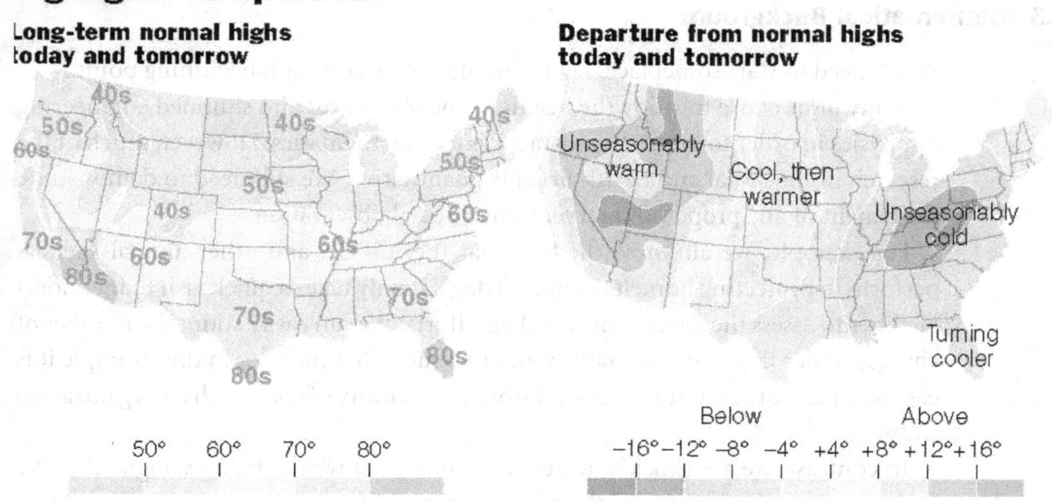

Figure 1.1 The U.S. weather map for October 27, 2008: Observed, expected, and residual data. Courtesy of Pennsylvania State University, Department of Meteorology.

similar temperatures are displayed in the same colors. The locations of rain and snow are indicated. An element of time and movement can also be inferred from this map: A large front has come across the country from the north, bringing cooler temperatures along with it. This figure represents the fine art of summarizing a huge amount of information.

The two smaller figures at the bottom provide a different kind of information. The lower-left map indicates the temperatures that we should expect to see on this date, based on previous years' experiences. The general pattern follows our preconception that southern states are warmer and northern states are cooler at this time of the year, with bands of constant temperature running east and west.

The figure on the lower right summarizes the differences between the normal pattern and the temperatures given in the large map at the top. Here we see that Florida is much cooler than what we would expect for late October. Similarly, Montana is cold at this time of year but is much warmer than typical.

The aim of statistics is to provide a similar reduction of a large amount of data into a succinct statement, generalizing, summarizing, and providing a clear message to your audience.

> The goal of statistics is to start with the data and then prepare a concise summary of it.

1.3 Mathematical Background

We all need to start someplace. Let us decide on the common beginning point.

Many of us chose to study the health or social sciences and shunned engineering or physics in order to avoid the abstract rigor of mathematics. However, much of the research in the social and health fields is quantitative. We still need to demonstrate the benefit of any proposed intervention or social observation.

For example, we all know the role that the ASPCA and other animal shelters perform in protecting homeless cats and dogs. It only takes a quick visit to their local facilities to assess the effectiveness of their efforts. We can easily count the number of charges under their care to quantify and measure what they do. In this example it is easy to separate the emotional appeal from the quantity of good such an organization supplies.

In contrast, we are shocked to see the brutality of whales being slaughtered. We are told about the majesty of their huge size and life under the sea. This is all fine and plays on our emotions. Before we send money to fund the appropriate charity, or decide to enforce global bans on whaling, we also should ask how many whales there are, and perhaps how this number has changed over the past decade. This information is much harder to get at and is outside our day-to-day experiences. We need to rely on estimates to quantify the problem. Perhaps we also need to question who is providing these estimates and whether the estimates are biased to support a certain point of view. An objective estimate of the whale population may be difficult to obtain, yet it is crucial to quantifying the problem.

As a consequence, we need to use some level of mathematics. The computer will do most of the heavy lifting for us, but we will also need to understand what is going on behind the scenes. We need to use algebra and especially linear functions. So when we write

$$y = a + bx,$$

we recall that a is referred to as the *intercept* and b is called the *slope.* We need to recognize that this equation represents a straight-line relationship and be able to graph this relationship.

We will need to use logarithms. Logarithms, or logs for short, are always to the base e = 2.718 . . . and never to base 10. The exponential function written as e^x or $\exp(x)$ is the inverse process of the logarithm. That is,

$$\log(e^x) = x$$

and

$$e^{\log x} = \exp(\log x) = x.$$

Sometimes we will use the exponential notation when the argument is not a simple expression. It is awkward to write

$$e^{a+bw+cx+dy},$$

not to mention that it is difficult to read and that publishers hate this sort of expression.

It is easier on the reader to write this last expression as

$$\exp(a + bw + cx + dy).$$

1.4 Calculus

For those who took calculus a long time ago and have not used it since, the memories may be distant, fuzzy, and perhaps unpleasant. Calculus represents a collection of important mathematical tools that will be needed from time to time in our discussion later on in this book. We will need to use several useful results that require calculus.

Fortunately, there is no need to dig out and dust off long-forgotten textbooks. The actual mechanics of calculus will be reviewed here, but there will not be a need to actually perform the mathematics involved. The reader who is fluent in the relevant mathematics may be able to fill in the details that we will gloss over.

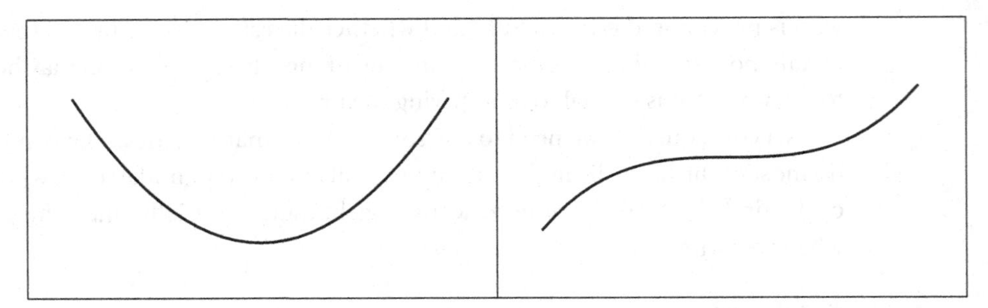

Figure 1.2 The slope is zero at the minimum of a function (left) and also at the saddle point of a function (right).

What is the point of calculus? If x and y have a straight-line relationship, we should be familiar with the concept of the *slope* of the line. When x changes by one unit, the slope is the amount of change in y.

For a nonlinear relationship, the concept of the slope remains the same, but it is a more local phenomenon. The idea of the slope depends on where in the x–y relationship your interest lies. At any point in a curve, we can still talk about the slope, but we need to talk about the slope at each point of the curve. You might think of a curve as a lot of tiny linear segments all sewn together, end to end. In this case, the concept of slope is the ratio of a small change in y to the resulting small change in x at a given point on the curve. It still makes sense to talk about the ratio of these small amounts resulting in a definition of the slope of a curved line at every point x. In calculus, the *derivative* is a measure of the (local) slope at any given point in the function.

The derivative of a function provides its slope at each point.

The derivative is useful for identifying places where nonlinear functions achieve their minimums or maximums. Intuitively, we can see that a smooth function that decreases for a while and then increases has to pass through some point where the slope is zero. Solving for the places where the derivative is zero tells us where the original function is either maximized or minimized. See Figure 1.2 for an illustration of this concept.

Some functions also exhibit *saddle points* where the derivative is also zero. A saddle point is where an increasing function flattens out before resuming its increase. We will not concern ourselves with saddle points. Similarly, a zero value of the derivative may only indicate a local minimum or maximum (that is, there are either larger maximums or smaller minimums someplace else), but we will not be concerned with these topics either. A saddle point is illustrated in Figure 1.2.

Although we will not actually obtain derivatives in this book, on occasion we will need to minimize and maximize functions. When the need arises, we will recognize

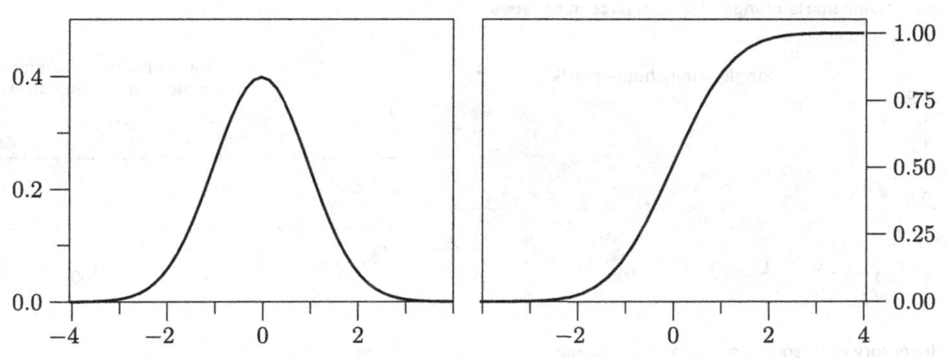

Figure 1.3 The normal density function (left) and its cumulative area (right).

the need to take a derivative and set it to zero in order to identify where the minimum occurs.

> The function achieves a maximum or minimum where the derivative is zero.

Calculus is also concerned with *integrals of functions.* Briefly, an integral gives us the area between the function and the horizontal axis. As with the derivative, we will not actually need to derive one here. Many probabilities are determined according to the area under a curved function.

> The integral of a function provides the area between the curve and the horizontal x axis.

Specifically, when we examine the normal distribution (Section 2.3), we will often draw the familiar bell-shaped curve. This curve is illustrated in Figure 1.3. For any value x on the horizontal axis, the curve on the right gives us the cumulative area under the left curve, up to x. The total area on the left is 1, and the cumulative area increases up to this value. The cumulative area under this curve is almost always of greater interest to us than the bell curve itself. Table A.1 in the appendix provides this area for us. It is very rare to see a table of the bell curve.

The area can be negative if the function is a negative number. Negative areas may seem unintuitive, but the example in the following section illustrates this concept.

1.5 Calculus in the News: New Home Sales

Home sales and building starts for new homes are both an important part of the economy. Builders will not start an expensive project unless they are reasonably sure that their investment will pay off. Home buyers will usually also purchase new furniture and carpets and will hire painters and carpenters to remodel as they move

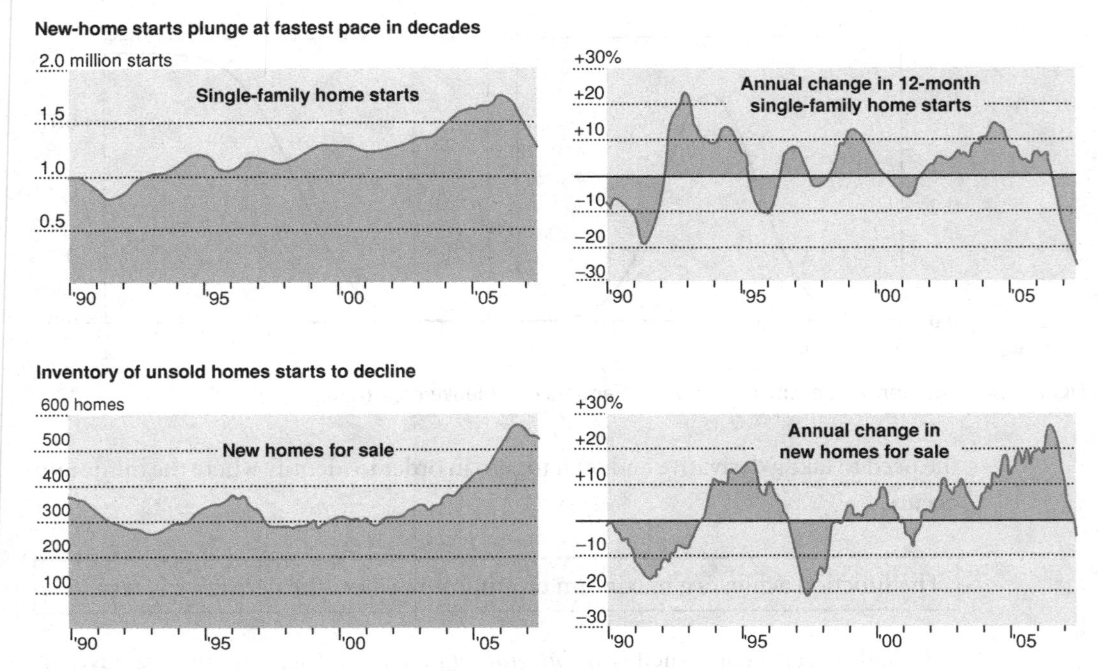

Figure 1.4 New home starts and sales. *Source: New York Times.*

in. Investors, economists, and government policy makers watch this data as a sign of the current state of the economy as well as future trends.

The graphs in Figure 1.4[2] depict new single-family home starts (upper left) and the number of new homes already on the market (lower left) over a period of a decade. There are always new homes being built and put up for sale, of course, but it is useful to know whether the trend is increasing or decreasing. The graphs on the right half of this figure show the trend more clearly in terms of the annual changes. More specifically, the graphs on the right show the slope of the line on the left at the corresponding point in time. When the figure on the left is increasing, then the figure on the right is positive. Decreasing rates on the left correspond to negative values on the right.

In words, the graphs on the right half of this figure are the derivatives of the graphs on the left half. Similarly, if we start at the values corresponding to the start of the year 1990, then the graphs on the left half are obtained by integrating the values on the right. Areas under the negative values on the right integrate to "negative areas" so that negative values on the right correspond to declining values on the left.

The times at which the derivatives on the right are zero correspond to turning points where maximums or minimums occur on the left. Remember that a zero slope is usually indicative of a change in direction. These maximums or minimums

[2] The graphs are available online at http://www.nytimes.com/2007/06/23/business/23charts.html.

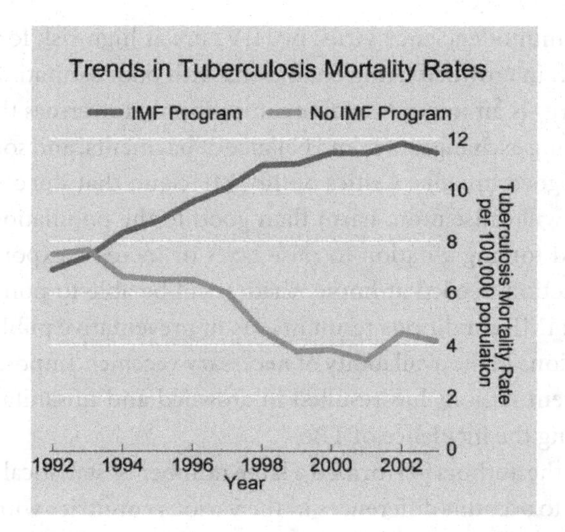

Figure 1.5 Cases of tuberculosis in Eastern Europe. *Source:* Stuckler *et al.* (2008).

may be short-lived, of course, and the underlying trend may continue after they end. The wide swings in the derivative often allow us to anticipate a change in direction of the underlying trend by a few months.

The upper headline says that there is a big decline in new home starts. But this decline is also down from the largest value in a decade. Similarly, the graph at the lower left shows a decline in the number of unsold homes on the market. Is that good for the economy because homes are selling more quickly, or bad for the economy because cautious sellers are waiting for a change in the market in order to anticipate a better price? Exercise 2.1 asks you to argue both cases: that, in the near term, the economy is improving, and also that the economy is getting worse.

1.6 Statistics in the News: IMF Loans and Tuberculosis

It is possible to learn all about statistics, computing, and data analysis and still come to an absurd conclusion. This sometimes leads to sensational headlines with often hilarious results as the story unfolds.

Figure 1.5 is reprinted from an article by Stuckler *et al.* (2008). A summary of the original article appeared in the *New York Times* on July 22, 2008.[3]

The article is about the relationship between International Monetary Fund (IMF) loans and the rate of tuberculosis (TB) in various eastern European countries. TB is an infectious disease that is spread through the air when an affected person sneezes or coughs. The disease is treated using antibiotics and is frequently fatal if left untreated. The elderly, those with diabetes, and those with a weakened immune system (such

[3] The original article is available online from *PLOS Medicine*: doi:10.1371/journal.pmed.0050143. A critique of this article appears at doi:10.1371/journal.pmed.0050162

as those with human immunodeficiency virus; or HIV) are at high risk for TB. We frequently see cases of TB in crowded living conditions with poor sanitation.

The IMF (www.imf.org) is an international organization that oversees the global monetary system, including exchange rates and balance of payments, and sometimes making loans to foreign governments. Critics of the IMF claim that the conditions imposed on these loans will cause more harm than good to the population. These conditions have included forcing a nation to raise taxes or increase exports to the exclusion of food production needed at home. Critics will be able to point to this graph and claim that the IMF conditions result in cuts in preventative public health expenditures and reductions in the availability of necessary vaccines. Imposing these conditions on the recipient nations has resulted in crowded and unsanitary living conditions, thereby raising the incidence of TB.

In the original article, the authors performed a large number of statistical analyses that attempted to take into account differences in the various countries with respect to percent of the population living in urban settings, an index of democratization, differences in per capita incomes, whether or not the country was involved in a war, and population education levels. Most of the methods used in their article will be clear to the reader by the time we complete the material in Chapter 6.

Even so, not all countries are the same. There may be large differences between the countries that these analyses fail to correct for. Are there other factors that have not been taken into account? Could factors such as the age of the population or the rate of HIV infection result in the differences in TB rates, regardless of whether or not the nation received IMF loans?

How should we treat countries that applied for IMF loans but did not qualify? Should these be considered loan recipients? Similarly, some countries may have been offered loans but ultimately refused the money. Should these countries be considered as having received loans? What about the size of the loans: Would a large loan have the same effect as a small loan if few conditions were attached to it?

Even more importantly, this is an example of an *observational study*. Why did some countries receive loans while others did not? In what ways do these countries differ? We will never be able to know the effect on TB rates if a given country that did not receive a loan had been given one, or *vice versa*. Consider Exercise 1.1 for another possible interpretation of Figure 1.5. In an observational study, the subjects (in this case, individual countries) choose their causal treatment in some nonrandom fashion. In the present example, we do not know how countries were chosen to receive loans.

We could not randomly choose the countries that were to receive loans. A *randomized study*, in contrast to an observational study, allows us to randomly assign treatments to individuals. Differences in outcomes can then be attributed solely to the random assignment. In a medical study in which patients are randomly assigned to two different treatments, for example, any underlying imbalances in the two patient groups should be minimized by chance alone. Patients bearing a trait that is unknown to us at the time of the randomization would be equally likely to appear in either of the two treatment groups, and then the trait would be averaged out when we examine the outcome. However, it is not possible to randomly give or withhold IMF loans to the various countries in the study.

One final comment on this example: Why was TB chosen to illustrate the effects of IMF loans? Of all the various disease rates that are reported, what is special about TB? Is it possible that the authors studied many different disease rates, but TB proved to be the most remarkable? We don't know how many diseases were compared between IMF loan and nonloan nations. We can intuit that if many comparisons were made, then it is virtually certain that some remarkable findings will be uncovered. One disease rate out of many must appear to have the largest difference between loan and nonloan nations.

This is the problem with *multiple comparisons*. If many comparisons are made, then the largest of these is not representative. We would need to make a correction for the number of different diseases that were studied. This topic and an appropriate adjustment for multiple comparisons are discussed again in Section 2.4.

There are many lessons that can be learned from this example. Ultimately, a study of statistical methods will provide you with a very useful set of tools. This book shows how these can be used to gain insight into underlying trends and patterns in your data. These tools, however, are only as good as the data that you provide. Of course, if you abuse the methods, it is possible to do more damage than good. You may be using the most sophisticated statistical methods available, but you are still responsible for the final conclusions that you draw.

Statistics is a useful tool, but it cannot think for you.

The same advice also holds for computers. The software can churn out numbers, but it cannot tell you whether the methods are appropriate or if the conditions for that method are valid. For other examples of statistics in action, consider the exercises at the end of this chapter. As with every chapter in this book, work out as many as you can.

1.7 Exercises

1.1 Argue that a country with a high rate of TB is more likely to receive an IMF loan. That is to say, use Figure 1.5 to claim that TB causes loans, rather than the other way around.

1.2 Do cell phones cause brain cancer? A prominent head of a cancer center sent an email to his staff urging limited use of cell phones because of a link to brain cancer. Does ownership and use of a cell phone constitute a randomized experiment or an observational study? Describe the person who is most likely to be a big user of cell phones. Is this a fair cross-section of the population?

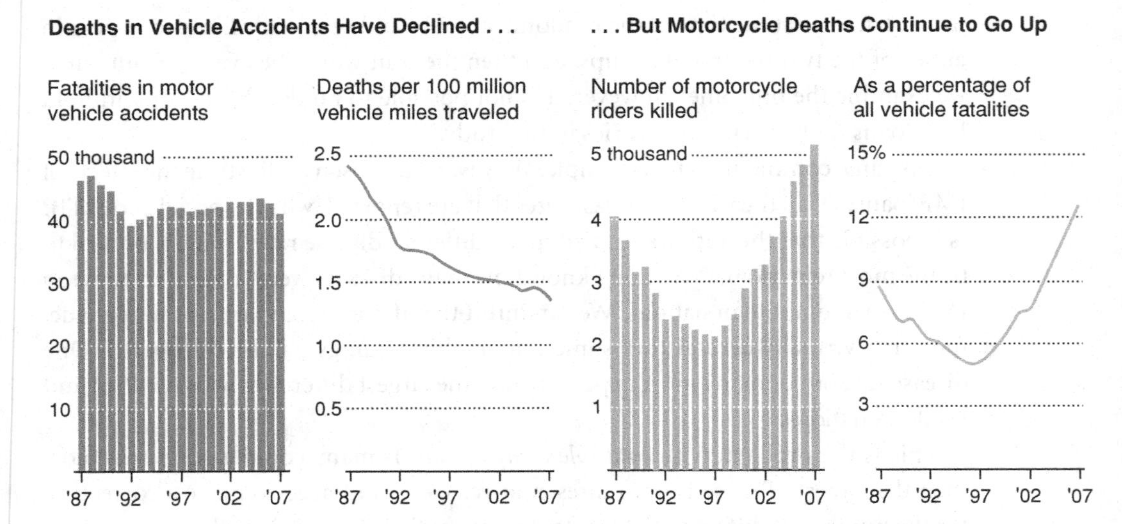

Figure 1.6 Fatality rates for autos and motorcycles. *Source: New York Times*, August 15, 2008, page A11.

1.3 Several states have passed laws to stop drivers from using cell phones. Do cell phones cause traffic accidents? Are people who own cell phones but don't use them while driving more likely to be involved in accidents?

1.4 Does consumption of soft drinks cause conjunctivitis (pink eye)? Cases of pink eye occur most often during the same months in which soft drink consumption is greatest. What do you think is going on?

1.5 A study found higher rates of obesity among ninth graders whose school is located close to a fast-food outlet.[4] In another part of the same study, pregnant women who lived near a fast-food outlet were more likely to experience a huge gain in weight. Are these experiments or observations? See if you can provide several different explanations for these findings.

1.7.1 Motorcycle Accidents

In Figure 1.6 we see that the number of motor vehicle fatalities has held steady over the two decades 1987–2007.[5] The second graph shows that the number of fatalities per miles traveled is declining. Which of these two graphs is a better indication of highway safety? Is there additional information you would need before making this conclusion? Are all travel miles the same, for example? Are there more or fewer cars on the road? Are the drivers younger or older, on average?

The two graphs on the right indicate that there has been a recent increase in fatalities involving motorcycles and that these make up an increasing percent of all accident fatalities. What additional information would you like to see? Use this graph

[4] Available online at http://www.nytimes.com/2009/03/26/health/nutrition/26obese.html.
[5] Available online at http://www.nytimes.com/2008/08/15/us/15fatal.html.

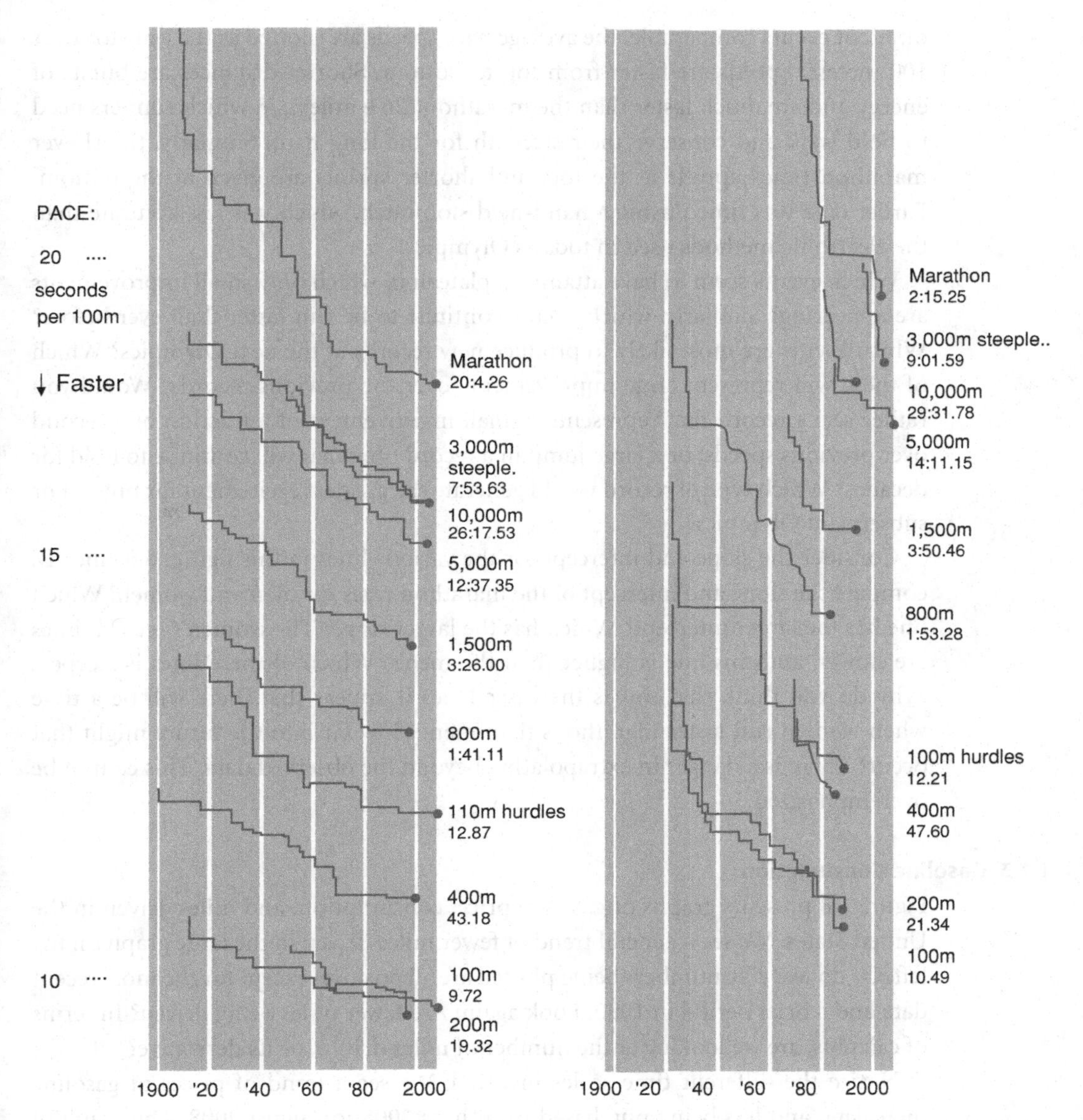

Figure 1.7 Olympic records for men and women's track events. *Source: New York Times*, August 4, 2008.

to show how inherently dangerous motorcycles are. In contrast, use this graph and argue that motorcycles are as safe as other motor vehicles. Notice how we can use the same data to make a case for both sides of this debate.

1.7.2 Olympic Records

In the modern history of the Olympics, we accumulate records as the athletes are running faster and faster than ever before. Figure 1.7 plots the times of various track events, separately for men (on the left) and women. In order to make these different events comparable, the average pace speeds are plotted as the time to cover 100 meters. Speeds are faster from top to bottom. Shorter distances are bursts of energy and are much faster than the marathon (26+ miles), in which runners need to hold back and conserve their strength for the long haul. Similarly, the slower marathon times appear at the top, and shorter sprints are given at the bottom. Earlier data was timed using a hand-held stopwatch, which was less accurate than the electronic methods used in today's Olympics.

Which events seem to have attained a plateau in which only small improvements are appearing? Similarly, which events continue to be run faster than ever before? Which events are most likely to produce new records at the next Olympics? Which of these will represent large improvements over the previous records? Would you rather see: a record that represents a small improvement of a fraction of a second over previous speeds; or a large jump in a record time that will continue to hold for decades? Which type of record would generate the greatest excitement for present or subsequent Olympics?

Consider the slope and intercept for the various lines in this figure. Specifically, compare the slope and intercept of the marathon rates for men and women. Which line has the larger intercept? Which has the larger slope? The women's record times are slower, and this line is higher than the men's. Which of these lines is steeper? Why do you think that this is the case? Does it appear that there will be a time when women run faster marathons than men? How far into the future might that occur? There is a danger in extrapolating beyond the observed data. This cannot be overemphasized.

1.7.3 Gasoline Consumption

Figure 1.8 presents graphs of gasoline price, consumption, and miles driven in the United States. We see a general trend of fewer miles driven in the large graph on the left. Or do we? The numbers being plotted are all positive, except for the most recent data and a brief period in 1990. Look again: Are fewer miles being driven? In terms of calculus, are we looking at the number of miles driven, or its derivative?

Notice the different time scales involved. We see a trend of prices of gasoline increasing and less being purchased from June 2008 to August 2008. The graph of prices is much smoother than either of the other two figures. Why do you think that this is the case? During this period, the price of gasoline runs roughly in the opposite direction from the gasoline-purchased graph. A $600 per person economic stimulus check was distributed during this period, as indicated by the shaded areas. Did this appear to have any effect?

1.7.4 Statistics in the News: China Buys U.S. Debt

Much of the U.S. debt has been purchased by foreign governments, institutions, and individuals. As the United States imports many Chinese products, China accumulates U.S. dollars. These make their way back to the United States in the form of investments

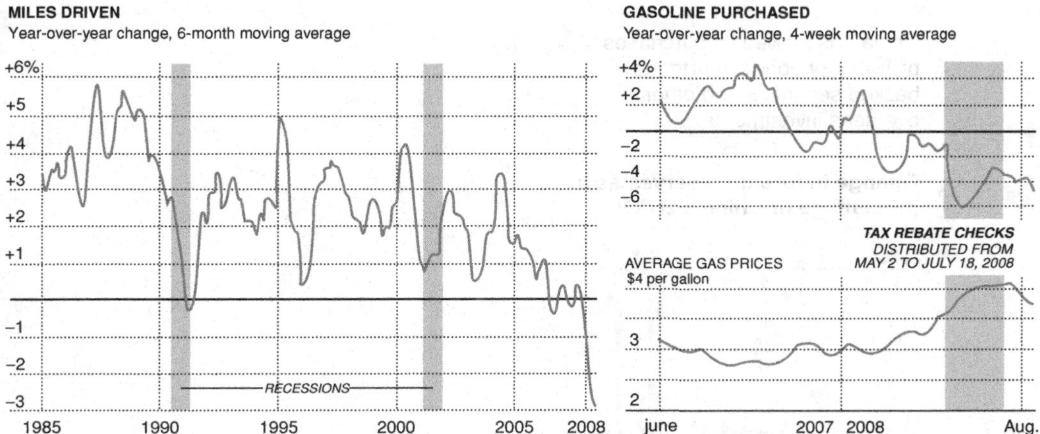

Figure 1.8 Gasoline consumption and prices. *Source: New York Times*, August 23, 2008, Page C3.

and purchases of debt in the form of bonds. The *gross domestic product* (GDP) is the total value of all goods and services produced in one year. It is a measure of the total value of the entire economy. In Figure 1.9 we see the percent of Chinese GDP that was used to purchase U.S. debt.

The heading of the graph indicates that China was buying fewer U.S. bonds as of the third quarter of 2008. Do you agree with this conclusion? The overall trend appears to be increasing over time. Notice the large amount of variability within each year and that this is also increasing over time.

Does the percent of GDP translate into dollars? The vertical scale represents the percentage of Chinese GDP that is increasing over time. How can we compare two numbers if one is a larger percentage of a smaller number? Also, the dollars are undergoing inflation, and earlier years' dollars are worth more than recent dollars.

At the time this graph appeared, interest rates returned on bonds were falling, so investors received less return on their money. Perhaps this information would be useful because there would be less incentive to buy bonds.

1.7.5 U.S. Presidents and Stock Market Returns

Since the great stock market crash of 1929, Democratic and Republican administrations have had almost the same number of years in office: six Democratic and seven Republican U.S. presidents have served almost exactly forty years each. How well have investors fared under each of these political parties? The average annual return under each president is given in Figure 1.10 as of mid-October, 2008, and we are invited to make this comparison. The figure also provides the data on a hypothetical $10,000 investment made under either Democratic or Republican presidents only.

The Hoover administration was clearly a disaster for investors, losing more than 30% per year on average. Such exceptional observations are called *outliers*. If we

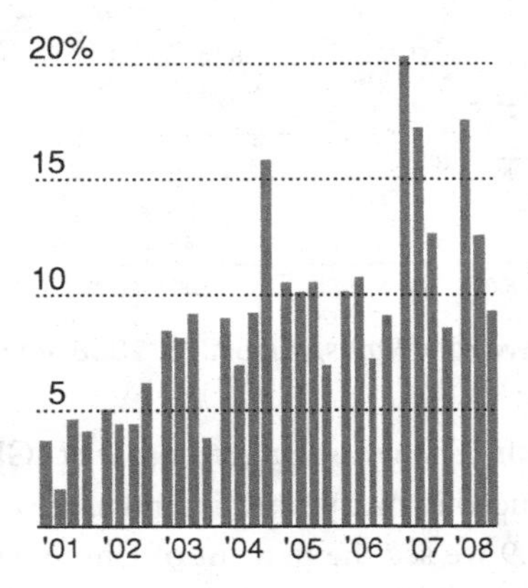
Buying Fewer Bonds
China has slowed its purchases of Treasury bonds, mortgage-backed securities and other overseas investments.
Change in foreign reserves as a percentage of China's G.D.P.
20%
15
10
5
'01 '02 '03 '04 '05 '06 '07 '08

Figure 1.9 Chinese purchases of U.S. treasury debt. *Source: New York Times*, January 8, 2009, page A14.

average the returns from all of the Republican presidential terms, the result is a meager 0.4% return per year. The $10,000 investment would have grown to $11,733 over this forty-year period. If we exclude the Hoover years, then the Republican average is 4.7%, resulting in a $51,211 return after thirty-six years. Under Democratic presidents, the average return is 8.9% per year, and the $10,000 investment would have become more than $300,000 over forty years. The figure asks us to conclude that investors experience greater rewards under Democratic presidents than under Republican presidents. But is this really the case?

Whereas it is clear that the returns under President Hoover were out of the ordinary, it also appears that only President Clinton's returns were above the Democratic average. That is, as much as Hoover was an exception on the downside, Clinton appears to be an exception on the upside.

One way to take exceptional observations into account is to examine the *median* value for each of the two political parties. (When we calculate the median for an even number of observations, as with the Democratic party, we average the two middle values.) What are the median annual returns for each of the two political parties, including the data from President Hoover? Do these lead us to the same conclusion as taking the average? Which of these two statistics do you feel is more representative for these data: the average or the median?

Recognize that there is a lot more that we could do in order to make a better comparison of the political parties. For example, an average of several different

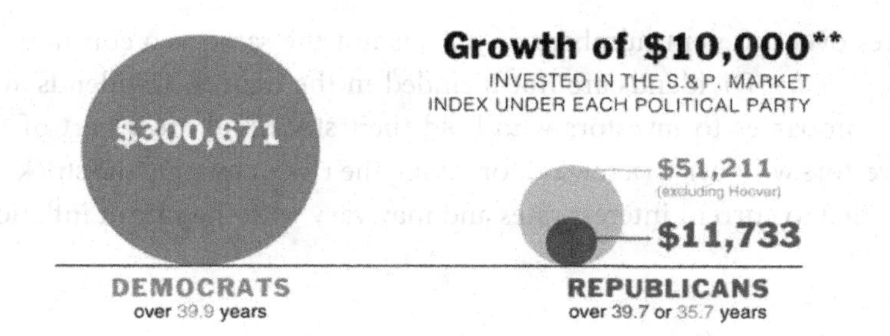

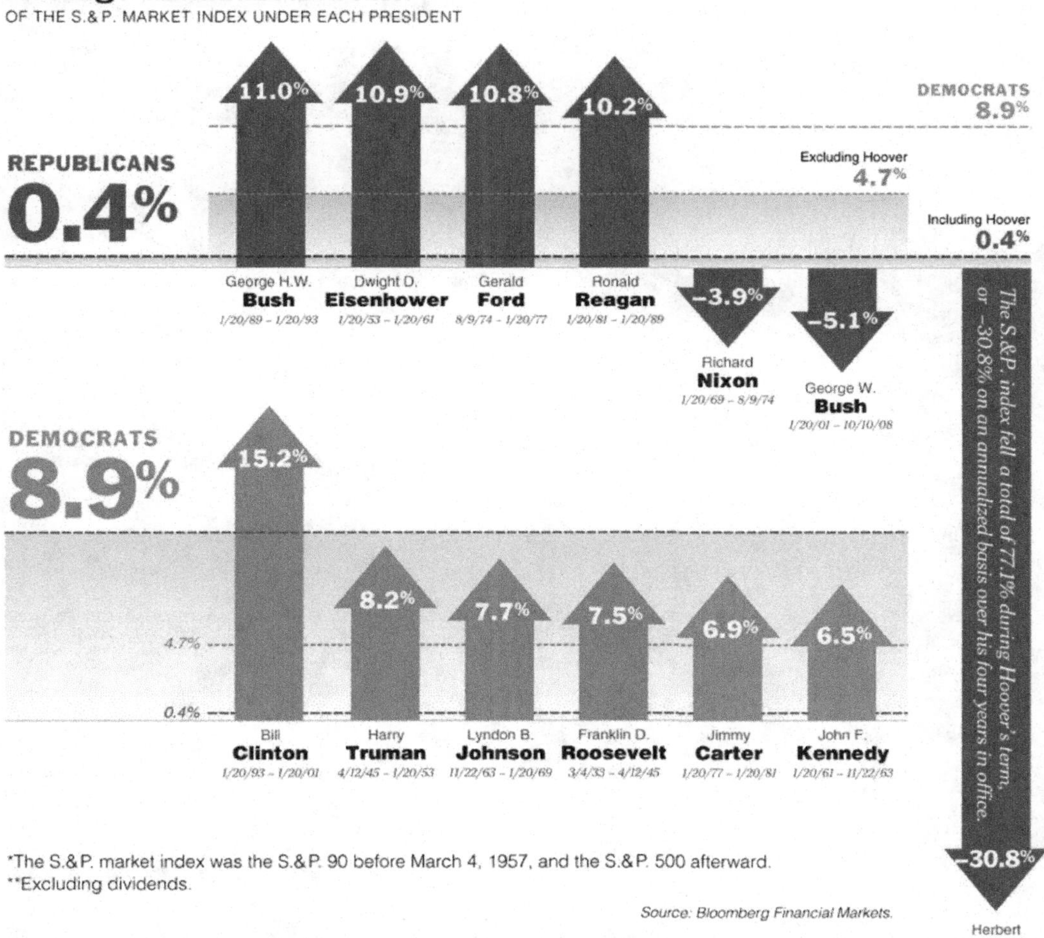

Figure 1.10 Democratic and Republican U.S. presidents and the corresponding returns in the stock market. *Source: New York Times*, October 14, 2008.

rates over different numbers of years is not the same as a constant rate over those same years. Dividends are not included in the figures. Dividends are income paid by companies to investors who hold their stock and are a part of the return that investors will earn as a reward for taking the risk of owning the stock. Dividend rates are tied to current interest rates and may vary with the rate of inflation.

2

Principles of Statistics

There is really no shortcut to taking a full introductory course to cover the basic concepts. In this section we cover the most important ideas that the reader should be familiar with. Think of this as a brief refresher to old ideas rather than the true exposure to new topics.

Historically, the development of probability predates the use of statistics by several centuries. The need for probability came about in studies of games of chance. Gamblers were then, as they are today, seeking an edge in an easy way to make a fortune. Of course, if there was a way to do so, there would be many wealthy mathematicians today. Instead, mathematicians have shown that there is no winning strategy. Card-counting at blackjack requires considerable practice and great concentration, and only then does it provide a slight edge to the player.

Statistics, on the other hand, was very much a product of the industrial revolution. Large numbers of items needed to be produced in a uniform fashion, and random variability stood in the way. Statistics became a scientific discipline in the early 1900s with the development of two important innovations: the chi-squared test, due to K. Pearson, and Student's t-test. Both of these topics are reviewed later in this chapter.

2.1 Binomial Distribution

The binomial distribution is one of the basic mathematical models for describing the behavior of a random outcome. An experiment is performed that results in one of two complementary outcomes, usually referred to as "success" or "failure." Each experimental outcome occurs independently of the others, and every experiment has the same probability of failure or success.

A toss of a coin is a good example. The coin tosses are independent of each other, and the probability of heads or tails is constant. The coin is said to be *fair* if there is an equal probability of heads and tails on each toss. A *biased* coin will favor one outcome over the other. If I toss a coin (whether fair or biased) several times, can I anticipate the numbers of head and tails that can be expected? There is no way of knowing with certainty, of course, but some outcomes will be more likely than others. The binomial distribution allows us to calculate a probability for every possible outcome.

Consider another example. Suppose I know from experience that, when driving through a certain intersection, I will have to stop for the traffic light 80% of the time. Each time I pass, whether or not I have to stop is independent of all of the previous times. The 80% rate never varies. It does not depend on the time of day, the direction that I am traveling, or the amount of traffic on the road. If I pass through this same intersection eight times in one week, how many times should I expect to have to stop for the light? What is the probability that I will have to stop exactly six times in the eight times that I pass this intersection?

The binomial model is a convenient mathematical tool to help explain these types of experiences. Let us introduce some notation. Suppose there are N independent events, where N takes on a positive integer value $1, 2, \ldots$. Each experiment either results in a success with probability p or else results in a failure with probability $1 - p$ for some value of p between 0 and 1.

> The binomial distribution provides the probability of the number of successes in N independent trials, each with the same probability p of success.

Let X denote the number of successes in N trials. The probability that X can take on the value i is

$$\Pr[X = i] = \binom{N}{i} p^i (1 - p)^{N-i} \tag{2.1}$$

for any value of $i = 0, 1, \ldots, N$.

Recall that the factorial symbol (!) is shorthand for the product of all positive integers up to that point. So we have

$$4! = 4 \times 3 \times 2 \times 1 = 24,$$

for example. (We read 4! as "four factorial.")

The binomial coefficient

$$\binom{N}{i} = \frac{N!}{i!\,(N - i)!}$$

counts all the different ordered ways in which i of the N individual experiments could have occurred. (We read this symbol as "N choose i".)

For example, $X = 2$ heads in $N = 4$ tosses of a coin could have occurred as HHTT, HTHT, HTTH, THHT, THTH, or TTHH. The six possible orders in which these occur is also obtained as

$$\binom{4}{2} = \frac{4!}{2!\,2!} = 6.$$

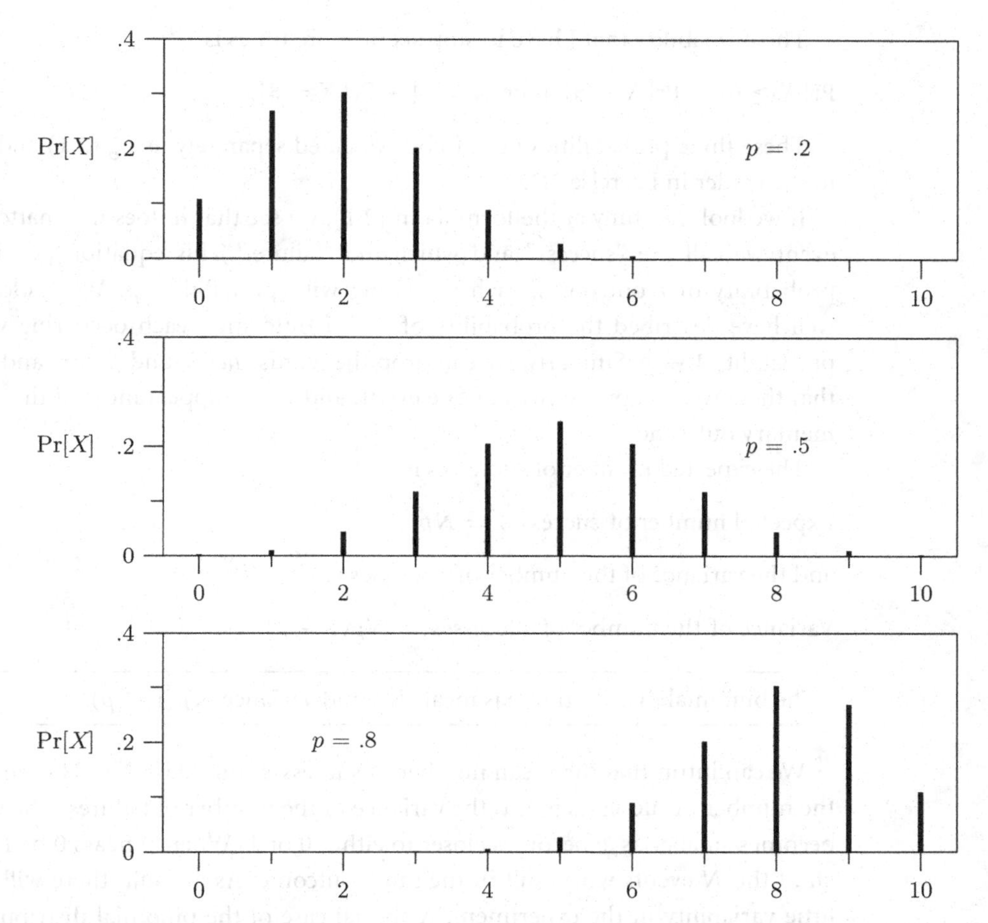

Figure 2.1 The binomial distribution of X is illustrated for $N = 10$ with parameters $p = 0.2, 0.5$, and 0.8.

A plot of the probabilities in (2.1) is given in Figure 2.1 for $N = 10$, values of $p = .2$, $.5$, and $.8$, and all values of $i = 0, 1, \ldots, 10$. When $p = .2$, we see that the distribution favors smaller numbers of events so that seven or more successes is very unlikely. When $p = .8$, we see a "mirror image," and three or fewer success are rarely expected to occur. The model with $p = .5$ in the center is symmetric. This symmetric shape is beginning to look like a normal or bell curve. The normal distribution is discussed in Section 2.3.

> When N is large and p is not too close to either 0 or 1, the binomial model is approximated by the normal distribution.

Returning to the example of eight trips past the intersection, the probability that I have to stop six times is

$$\Pr[X = 6] = \binom{8}{6} (0.8)^6 (0.2)^2 = 28 \times 0.0105 = 0.2936.$$

The probability that I have to stop six or more times is

$$\Pr[X \geq 6] = \Pr[X = 6] + \Pr[X = 7] + \Pr[X = 8].$$

These three probabilities need to be evaluated separately using (2.1) and are left to the reader in Exercise 2.2.

If we look carefully at the formula in (2.1), we see that it does not matter which event we call the "success" and which the "failure." This equation provides the probability of i outcomes, each occurring with probability p. We could just as well have described the probability of $N - i$ outcomes, each occurring with the probability $1 - p$. Similarly, we can drop the words *success* and *failure* and just say that there were i appearances of one event, and $N - i$ appearances of the complementary outcome.

The expected number of successes is

$$\text{Expected number of successes} = Np \tag{2.2}$$

and the variance of the number of successes is

$$\text{Variance of the number of successes} = Np(1 - p). \tag{2.3}$$

The binomial distribution has mean Np and variance $Np(1 - p)$.

We can intuit that the mean number of successes should be Np. The variance of the number of successes is also the variance of the number of failures. The variance becomes smaller as p becomes closer to either 0 or 1. When p nears 0 or 1, almost all of the N events will result in the same outcome. As a result, there will be very little variability in the experiment. A special case of the binomial distribution for large values of N and small values of p is discussed in Chapter 10 on the Poisson distribution.

When we conduct a binomial experiment and observe the number of successes x, then we usually estimate p by x/N or the empirical fraction of observed successes. We must be careful to distinguish between the unobservable probability p and its estimated value. For this reason, we usually denote the estimate as $\widehat{p}$, where the caret signifies an estimate of the unknown quantity. We read the expression $\widehat{p}$ as "p hat."

The mean of $\widehat{p}$ is equal to p, so we say that $\widehat{p}$ is *unbiased* for p. The standard deviation of $\widehat{p}$ is equal to $\sqrt{p(1 - p)/N}$. It is common practice to replace the ps in this expression by $\widehat{p}$ itself, resulting in an estimated standard deviation. (We recall from Section 1.1 that the standard deviation is the square root of the variance.)

Our uncertainty associated with the unknown parameter p can be expressed either in terms of its estimated standard deviation

$$\sqrt{\frac{\widehat{p}(1 - \widehat{p})}{N}}$$

or else in terms of a *confidence interval.*

A 95% confidence interval for the binomial p parameter is

$$\left(\widehat{p} - 1.96\sqrt{\frac{\widehat{p}(1-\widehat{p})}{N}}, \quad \widehat{p} + 1.96\sqrt{\frac{\widehat{p}(1-\widehat{p})}{N}}\right).$$

A confidence interval, in general, expresses our uncertainty about the true parameter value in terms of an interval that combines the sampling error and the idea of repeating the basic experiment. In the present case, if we repeated the binomial experiment many times and N was always the same large number, then we would find that the distribution of all of the $\widehat{p}$s would look approximately like the normal or bell curve. (More details on the normal distribution are given in Section 2.3.)

Because 95% of the normal curve is contained between the mean minus 1.96 standard deviations and the mean plus 1.96 standard deviations, it follows that the true value of the parameter p would be contained in this interval 95% of the time. This is a fairly long list of assumptions because we (1) have only one sample, not many, and (2) the value of N is not necessarily large in most cases. Nevertheless, the confidence interval for p given here is a well-accepted way to express our uncertainty about this parameter.

2.2 Confidence Intervals and the Hubble Constant

Einstein's mathematics gave theoretical evidence that the universe is expanding, but it wasn't until 1929 that Edwin Hubble[1] provided the empirical evidence for this. Even more remarkable was the claim that the farther galaxies were from us, the faster they were moving away. The current estimate is that objects 3.3 million light years farther away are moving 74 kilometers per second faster. The exact rate, called the Hubble Constant, is important to cosmologists: so much depends on it. Will the universe keep expanding following the Big Bang, or will it reach a maximum and then come back together again because of gravity? Cosmologists now say that the Hubble quantity is not really constant, because gravity will slow the expansion but dark energy will speed it up over long periods of time.

Over time there have been different estimates as scientists use increasingly sophisticated methods. There were also a few estimates before Hubble's in 1929. The estimates of the Hubble constant, along with their corresponding confidence intervals, are plotted in Figure 2.2. Notice that the earlier measurements had larger confidence intervals, and these did not always overlap one another. More recently, increasingly precise instruments have been used, and these provide smaller confidence intervals. The present estimates all fall in the range of 50 to 100. This figure shows the history of the Hubble constant and demonstrates how a consensus is being reached.

[1] Edwin Hubble (1898–1953), American astronomer. The Hubble Space Telescope carried into orbit in 1990 was named after him.

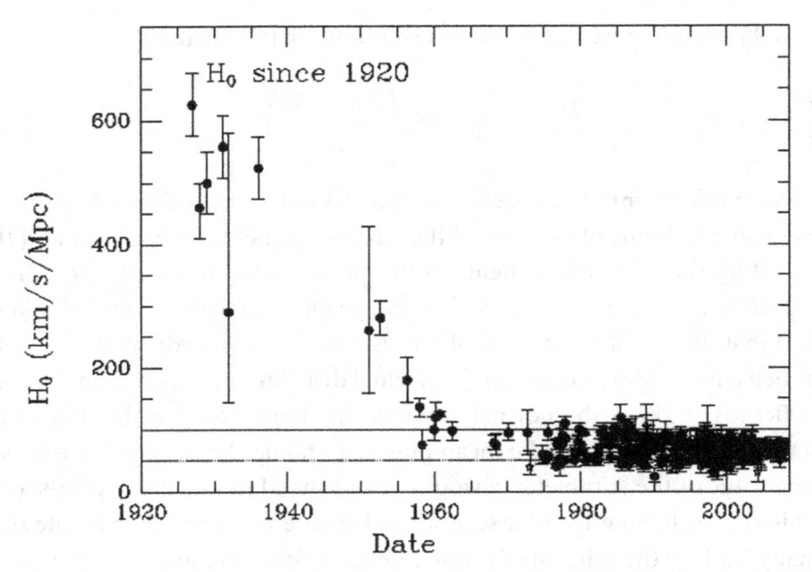

Figure 2.2 Measurements of the Hubble constant over time. *Source:* John Huchra and the Harvard-Smithsonian Center for Astrophysics.

Two statistical methods can be used to examine data such as these. Both are beyond the scope of this book but can be explained briefly here. The first of these methods is called *meta-analysis.* Meta-analysis seeks to combine different sources of information in order to obtain a single estimate. In the present example, different experimental methods were used to estimate the Hubble constant, and these are based on different sources of empirical data. Some of these are clearly less precise than others but still have some value in obtaining the final estimate. We might give some measurements more weight than others in our combined estimate, for example.

A second useful method for data such as these is *Bayesian statistics.* A statistician employing Bayesian methods would express uncertainty about the Hubble constant in terms of a statistical distribution with a mean and a standard deviation. As more data is obtained, Bayesian methods show how to update this uncertainty, resulting in another statistical distribution. In this manner, the Bayesian approach demonstrates how we can improve on our knowledge of the Hubble constant by incorporating all of the prior knowledge and data that has been accumulated to date.

2.3 Normal Distribution

The normal distribution is central to a lot of statistics. It is often referred to as the "bell curve" because of its shape. Its origins date back to de Moivre,[2] who used it in 1734 to approximate the binomial distribution. Today it is more often associated

[2] Abraham de Moivre (1667–1754). Mathematician and probabilist, born in France and later moved to London.

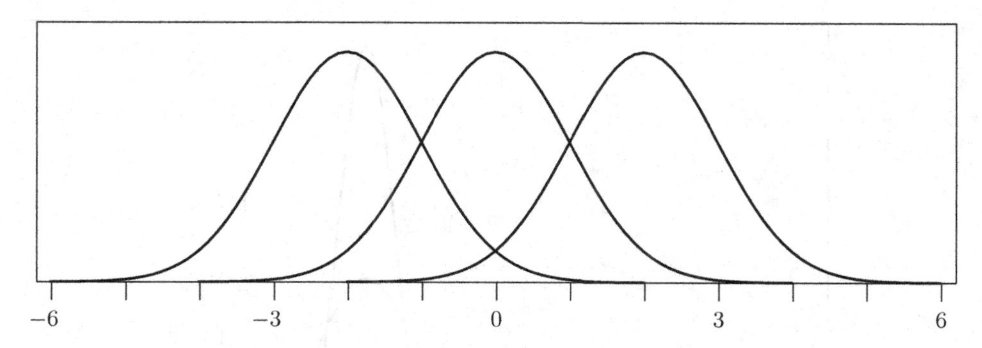

Figure 2.3 The normal distribution for means equal to −2, 0, and +2, all with a standard deviation of 1.

with the work of Gauss[3] about a century later. It is frequently referred to as the Gaussian distribution. The normal distribution is characterized by its mean and standard deviation. When we change the mean, Figure 2.3 shows that the same shape is moved right and left. When we change the standard deviation, Figure 2.4 shows that it is either stretched or squeezed along the horizontal axis. The area under the normal curve is always equal to 1, so when the curve is squeezed, it must also rise in order to maintain the same area.

Notice, then, an important difference in the way the normal model is used. In the binomial distribution (Section 2.1), we can talk about the probability of a discrete event such as getting stopped at a traffic light six times. In contrast, the normal distribution is used for continuous outcomes. Probabilities from the normal distribution must be described in terms of areas under the curve. Recall that areas under a curve are usually found using calculus (Section 1.4). The normal distribution is so popular that there are many tables and software available, and calculus is not necessary. One such table is given as Table A.1 in the appendix.

With so many possible means and standard deviations, how can any table take all of the many normal distributions into account? The answer is that we really need only one normal curve, with a mean of 0 and a standard deviation of 1. This is referred to as the *standard normal* distribution. All normal distributions can be transformed into a standard normal by adding or subtracting (to get a mean of 0) and multiplying or dividing (to get a standard deviation of 1). More formally, if X is normal with mean μ and standard deviation σ, then

$$Z = \frac{x - \mu}{\sigma}$$

will behave as a standard normal.

[3] Johann Friedrich Gauss (1777–1855) German. One of the most influential mathematicians ever. He also made many contributions to physics.

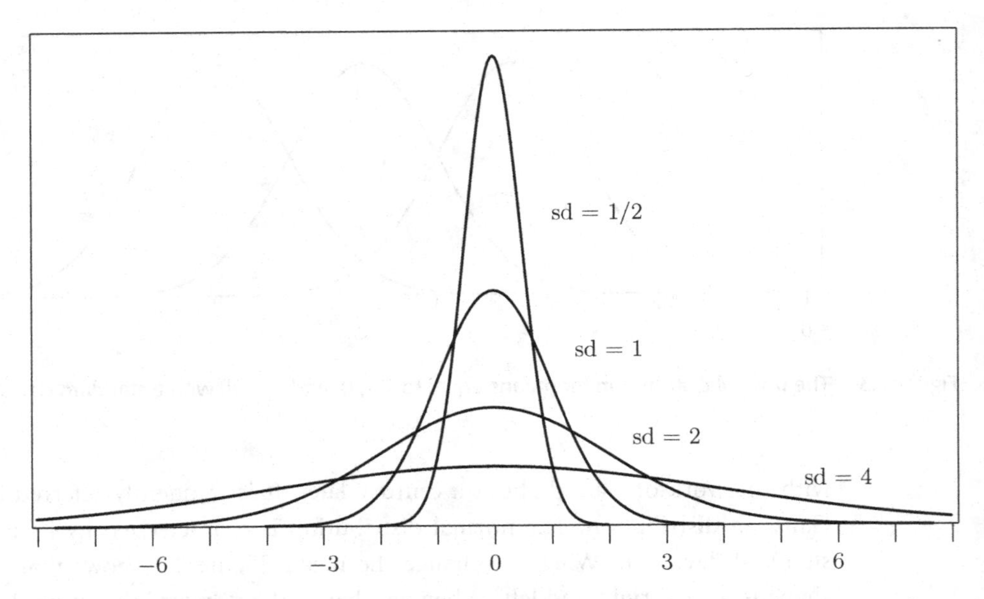

Figure 2.4 The normal distribution with mean 0 and different values of the standard deviation, as given.

Let us work out a few examples using Table A.1 in the appendix. We first notice in Figure A.1 that this table provides the area under the standard normal curve up to x for all values of x greater than 0.

That is, this table provides the shaded area

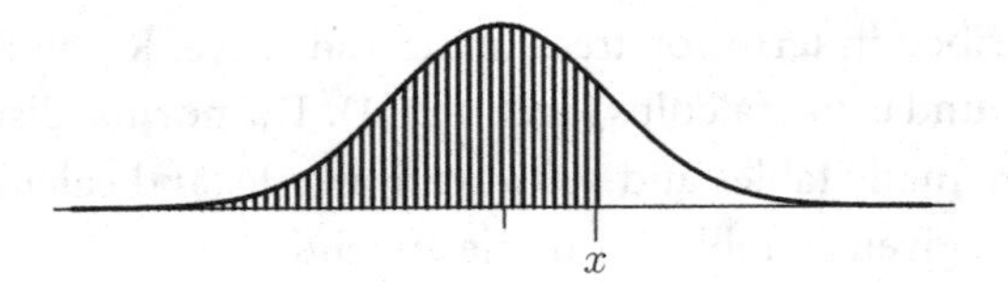

for all values of $x > 0$. Equivalently, the table in the appendix provides values of the function plotted on the right half of Figure 1.3, but this depiction of a shaded area is more intuitive.

So, for example, we have

$$\Pr[Z \leq 0.62] = .73237,$$

after looking up $x = .62$ directly from the table.

To find $\Pr[Z \geq 0.92]$, we note that the shaded area in

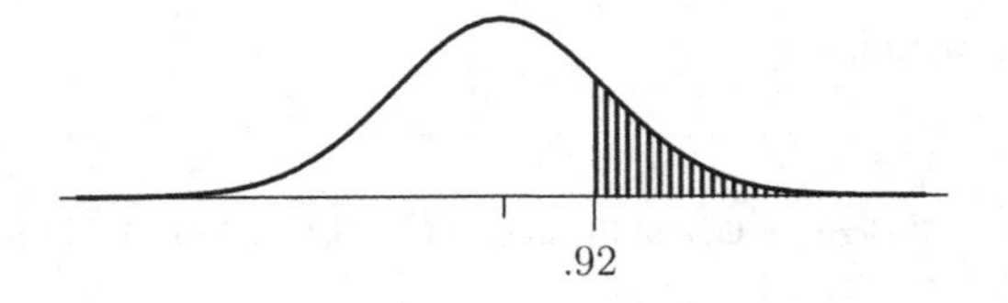

is 1 minus the shaded area in

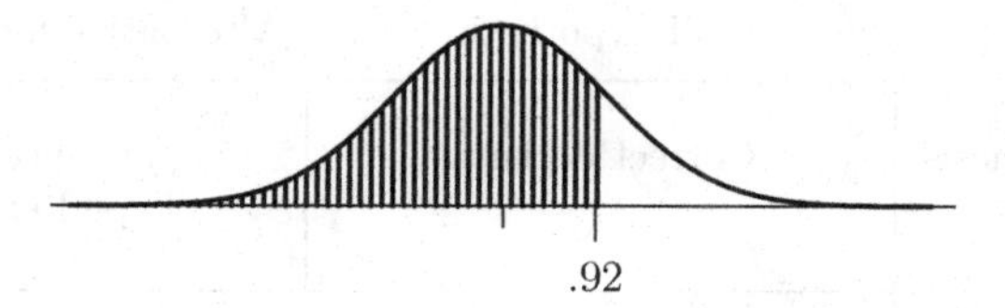

so that

$$\Pr[Z \geq 0.92] = 1 - \Pr[Z \leq 0.92] = 1 - .82121 = .17879.$$

Areas for negative values of x can be found by symmetry and using the fact that the total area under the curve is equal to 1.

As an example of this, in order to find $\Pr[Z \leq -1.31]$, we note that

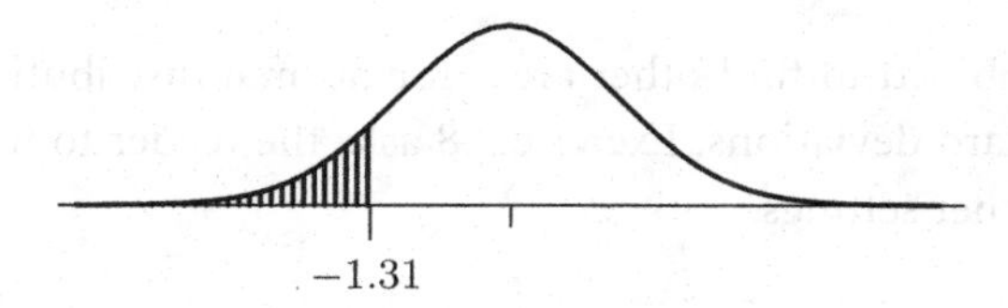

has the same area as

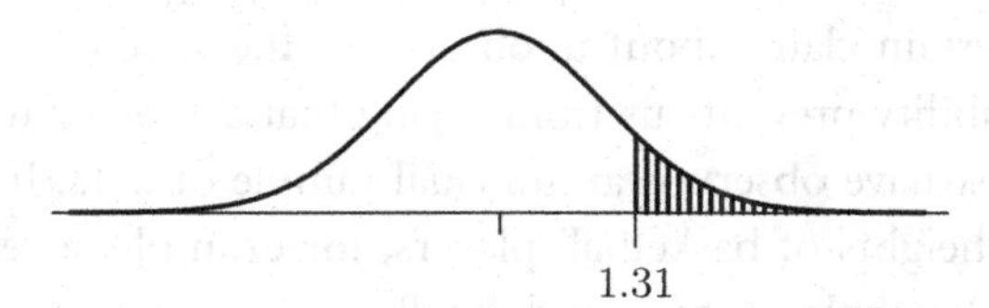

which is 1 minus the shaded area in

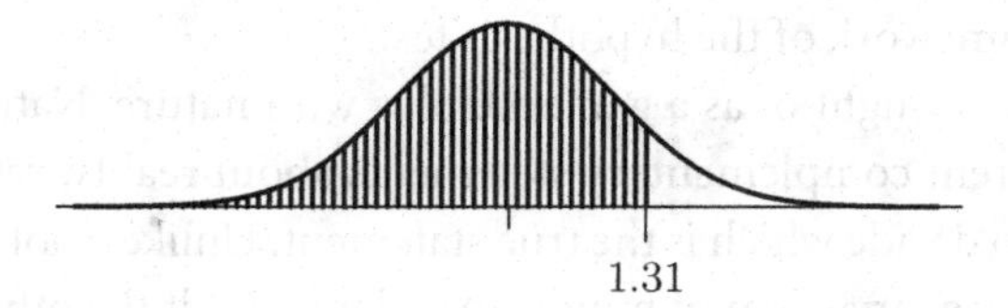

In this case we have

$$\Pr[Z \leq -1.31] = \Pr[Z \geq 1.31]$$

by flipping the figure over.

We also have

$$\Pr[Z \geq 1.31] = 1 - \Pr[Z \leq 1.31]$$

going from the shaded to the unshaded area.

		Your decision:	
		Null hypothesis	Alternative hypothesis
Nature decides:	Null hypothesis	Correct decision	Significance level Type I error
	Alternative hypothesis	Type II error	Power

Figure 2.5 A schematic of hypothesis tests. The significance level is the probability of incorrectly rejecting the null hypothesis. Power is the probability of correctly rejecting the null hypothesis.

Finally, we look up the value for $Z = 1.31$ in the table, giving us

$$\Pr[Z \leq -1.31] = 1 - .90490 = .09510.$$

These rules can be combined to find other areas for normal distributions with different means and standard deviations. Exercise 2.8 asks the reader to find other normal probabilities for other settings.

2.4 Hypothesis Tests

One of the important roles of statistics is to provide convincing evidence of the validity (or falsity) of a certain claim about unobservable the state of nature. Of course, the statistical variability prevents us from saying that a statement is 100% true, because we might just have observed an unusual sample of data. If we were only able to measure the heights of basketball players, for example, a reasonable conclusion would be that all people are over six feet tall.

Even if we can safely assume that our data is representative of the population, we still need to qualify our language with a certain measure of doubt about our conclusions. This is the framework of the hypothesis test.

A hypothesis test can be thought of as a game we play with nature. Nature picks from a choice of two different complementary statements about reality, referred to as hypotheses. Our job is to decide which is the true statement. Unlike a poker game, where we might have to pay a large sum of money in order to see if the other player is bluffing, in hypothesis testing we will never know if we made the correct decision. The objective is to pick the correct decision with high probability, but, unfortunately, we will never know with certainty which is correct. Figure 2.5 is a convenient way to illustrate all of the possible outcomes.

More specifically, a hypothesis test begins with a *null hypothesis* and a corresponding *alternative hypothesis*. The null hypothesis is typically a statement about the status quo, the way things are today. Examples might include stating that a new way of doing things is no better or worse that the way we have been doing them all along. The new "Drug A" is the same as the the standard treatment. "Brand X" detergent will get your clothes as clean as "Brand Y." These are all examples of typical null hypotheses.

The alternative hypothesis is sometimes the opposite of the null hypothesis, so we might say that Drug A is better, or Brand X detergent makes clothes cleaner. In both of these examples we are expressing a *one-sided alternative hypothesis* – one in which a specified direction is of importance. Drug A is either better or not, so maybe we should rewrite the corresponding null hypothesis as "Drug A is at least as good as Drug B" and the alternative hypothesis as "Drug A is better."

There are also *two-sided alternative hypothesis tests* that are of interest in settings where we are interested in whether or not a change has occurred and have no particular stake in the direction of the change. Suppose, for example, a new manufacturing process has been developed for manufacturing truck tires, and we want to determine whether the new method affects their lighter or darker color. Because nobody really cares what color the tires are (within reason), the null hypothesis of no color change is tested against the two-sided alternative of any change, with no clear preference for the direction of the change, lighter or darker.

The alternative hypothesis is more often expressed in terms of a quantitative difference from the null. So, for example, valid alternative hypotheses might be that Drug A will result in patients having 20% fewer colds this winter and that Brand X will make your clothes 30% brighter as measured in terms of reflected light. The two-sided truck tire example might be expressed as a difference of at least 10% lighter or darker. The reason for quantifying the difference between the two hypotheses is to specify the actual magnitude of a difference that is meaningful to us. If the difference is too small to be experienced, then it is probably not worth our while to convince others which of the two hypotheses is more likely to be valid.

The next step is to identify a statistical measure of the difference between these two hypotheses. After washing several piles of clothes, we measure the light reflectivity under two different detergents and then compare the two averages using the t-test, described in Section 2.5. Similarly, we might ask two groups of patients to take either Drug A or a placebo and then report back in the spring on the number of colds they experienced. We might look at the difference in the two rates.

How large should these differences be? Under the null hypothesis of no difference, the differences should be rather small. Of course, the size of the difference would depend on such factors as the sample sizes involved, the precision of our light meter, and the memories of our patients. Even after taking all of these factors into account, there will still be observed differences, and we will need to quantify the magnitude of these.

The magnitude of the difference is expressed as the probability that such a difference could have occurred by chance alone under the null hypothesis. This probability is called the *p-value*. The p-value is a measure of how unusual the observed outcome would be if all the conditions of the null hypothesis were valid. The p-value is also known as the *significance level*, or *statistical significance*.

> Statistical significance is the probability that such an outcome could have occurred by chance alone, under the null hypothesis.

What often happens in practice is that the author of an experiment will just report the p-value and leave it up to the reader to figure out what the null and alternative hypotheses are. Some of the journals that publish scientific studies are now asking authors to spell these hypotheses out. Similarly, every time we hear the expression "p-value," we should always be ready to ask about the null hypothesis, if it is not immediately obvious from the context.

Let us return to the interpretation of a p-value. If a really unusually small p-value is observed, this means that something occurred that would have a small probability of happening under the null hypothesis. At that point we will usually conclude that the null hypothesis is not valid and use the p-value as evidence for the alternative. More formally, we are said to *reject the null hypothesis* in favor of the alternative. Intuitively, if something very rare has just occurred, then we are moved to say that something must be wrong in our thinking. In this case, a small p-value suggests that perhaps the null hypothesis is not the correct explanation for the observed data.

Notice that the p-value is not the probability that the null hypothesis is true. This is a common misconception. The p-value is a measure of how tolerant we may be of unusual outcomes. This tolerance will vary depending on the circumstances. Another popular misconception is that observed values of p smaller than .05 are the only times we would reject the null hypothesis.

Although .05 is certainly a popular value, observing an outcome that occurs only 1 in 20 times need not cause us to reject an assumption that is held up to close scrutiny. Consider a situation where we are studying a newly developed but largely unstudied technology or drug that may show great promise. We may not be able to devote a lot of resources to testing it on a large sample size. In this situation we might use a more generous criterion to reject the null hypothesis that the new method is not any better. If we use a p-value of .10, for example, then we are giving the new idea a generous benefit of the doubt. Failing to reject the null hypothesis in this setting may result in a potentially great idea being discarded too early in its development.

At the other extreme, if we have a huge amount of data available to us, then we will need to have very strong evidence before we start making judgments and generalizations. Consider research based on the Surveillance Epidemiology and End Results (SEER) database. This program began in 1973 and is presently a complete census of all cases of cancer occurring in eighteen states and metropolitan areas across the United States. With such a huge sample size, we are able to test even the most subtly different pair of hypotheses with a very high probability of choosing the correct one.

Unfortunately, such close hypotheses may not be meaningful. Obtaining an extreme level of significance may not translate into a clinically recognizable advantage. An increase in lifespan measured in hours is not useful, regardless of how statistically significant the results may appear.

This leads us to the other problem of hypothesis testing seen in Figure 2.5, namely failing to reject the null hypothesis when we are supposed to. We need the ability to detect a difference when one actually exists. Just as with the uncertainty measured by the p-value (the probability of incorrectly rejecting the null hypothesis), the *power* is the probability of correctly rejecting the null hypothesis when the alternative is true. Again, refer to Figure 2.5 to clarify these different errors.

Power is the probability of correctly rejecting the null hypothesis when the alternative is true.

Power is a more difficult quantity to measure because it depends on the specific alternative hypothesis under consideration. Intuitively, if the null and alternative hypothesis are "further" apart in some sense, then less information is needed to tell the difference. In the abstract, it is easier to tell the difference between black and white than between two closely tinted shades of gray.

Let us take a more concrete example to illustrate this point. Suppose, in this example, we have a new method for predicting tomorrow's weather. The best methods available today are accurate 60% of the time. It will take us a very long time to prove the benefits of the new method if it is only accurate 62% of the time. This 2% improvement will be difficult to see unless we apply our new method for quite a while. That is, the power, or the probability of detecting the improvement, will be very low in this problem unless we are willing to invest a lot of time and energy into studying it.

Of course, some may argue that improving the accuracy from 60% to 62% is hardly worthwhile. Even if we had enough historical data and could claim an extreme statistical significance level (i.e., a very small p-value), there may be little to be gained if many people use the old forecasting method and would be reluctant to change over. This is another example of clinical versus statistical significance: The perceived improvement is too small to be appreciated despite the claims of statistical significance.

We can increase the power in this example by considering an alternative hypothesis in which we claim that the new forecast is accurate 80% of the time. There is a tradeoff with this approach. Although the difference between the old method with 60% accuracy and the new method with 80% accuracy is a greater improvement, we are also making a much larger claim that the new method must achieve. In words, we have greater power for testing hypotheses that are "further" apart, but at the same time, the method being tested has a much larger hurdle to jump over.

Let us end this section with a discussion of multiple comparisons. In the IMF/TB example described in Section 1.6, we pointed out that a large number of diseases might have been compared across the IMF loan and nonloan nations. What effect might these multiple comparisons have on the final results presented?

Suppose every disease compared would be declared statistically significant at the .05 level. This means that under the null hypothesis (there is no difference between the loan and nonloan nations), there is a 5% chance of rejecting that null hypothesis. If we did this for two different diseases, would there still be a 5% chance of rejecting the null hypothesis for either of these diseases? The answer is no. Two actions have occurred, each with probability .05 of occurring. The chance that at least one occurred will be greater than 5%. It is not clear exactly what that probability would be, but it is going to be larger than .05. As an extreme example, if hundreds of diseases were compared, then there is virtual certainty that a difference would be found in at least one disease at the .05 significance level.

What is the appropriate significance level to cite in this case? The answer to this question is not easy, because it is not clear whether the different diseases occur independently or not. A large number of TB cases might be associated with a high rate of other lung diseases, for example.

One way to correct for the multiple comparisons is to divide the necessary significance level by the number of comparisons being made. This is called the *Bonferroni*[4] *correction* to the significance level. In words, if two disease comparisons are made, then we must attain a statistical significance of .025 on either of these in order to claim a .05 significance level.

In the examples discussed in this book, we do not need to be concerned with the Bonferroni correction to significance tests. The examples we examine are exploratory and used to illustrate the statistical methods involved. In serious scientific examination, however, we need to be aware of such discovery biases and correct for them.

2.5 The Student t-Test

The Student t-test is the most commonly used method for statistically comparing the means of two different normal populations. The method assumes that there are two populations with normally distributed attributes. Observations are independently sampled from each of these populations. We want to compare the means of the populations by looking at the differences of the two sample averages.

> The Student t-test is used to draw statistical inference on the means of two populations.

[4] Carlo Emilio Bonferroni (1892–1960), Italian mathematician.

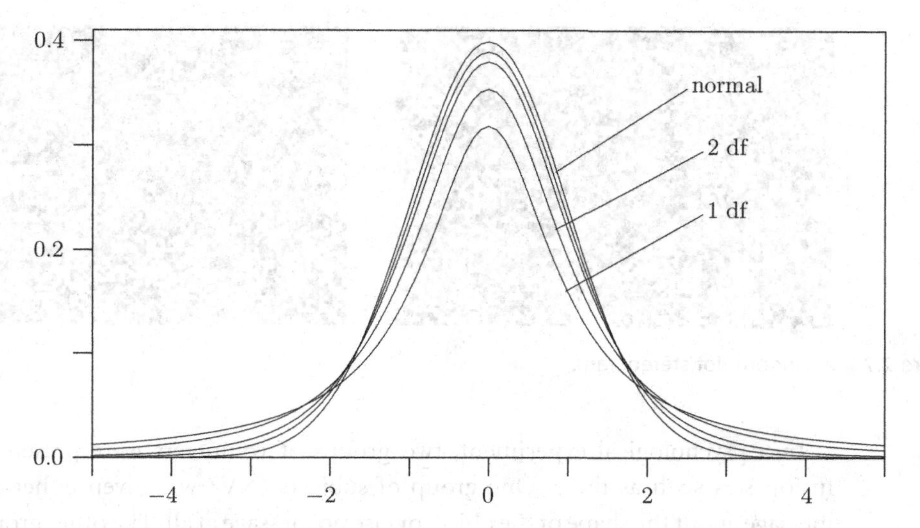

Figure 2.6 Student t distributions with 1, 2, 5, and 10 df and the normal distribution.

If the sample averages are very different, then we can reasonably conclude that the population means are different as well. The null hypothesis is that the two populations have equal means, and the alternative hypothesis is that the means are different.

The difference in the sample averages needs to be standardized by an estimate of the standard error. We usually assume that the standard deviations are the same in both of the underlying populations, but there are adjustments that SAS will make if this is not the case.

The *Student t distribution* is used to describe the behavior of the standardized difference of two sample means. The process of standardization means that the difference of the two averages is divided by an estimate of its standard deviation. In the case where the population standard deviations are the same, Figure 2.6 shows the distribution of the test statistic. These distributions are indexed by the degrees of freedom (df), which is 2 less than the number of observations in the two combined samples. As we can easily see, the larger the sample size, the more the Student t distribution looks like a normal. The concept of degrees of freedom is discussed again in Section 2.7.

Let us work out an example. Consider an example from a experiment on visual perception. The pair of boxes in Figure 2.7 appear to be sets of random dots. This is called a random dot stereogram. On closer examination, the stereograms appear to be identical. If you hold the figure close to your nose and allow your eyes to slowly come in and out of focus, another pattern appears. This requires some time and patience. If you do this carefully and correctly, an embedded figure will appear to float above the background.

Figure 2.7 A random dot stereogram.

In a psychological experiment, two groups of volunteers were presented with fusion sets such as these. One group of subjects (NV) was given either a verbal message about the shape of the object or else no message at all. The other group (VV) was given this same verbal information and also shown a drawing of the embedded figure. The fusion times (in minutes) for these two groups are presented in Table 2.1.

The average fusion times of the groups of subjects were 8.56 minutes for the verbal-only group and 5.55 minutes for the verbal and visual subjects. The standard deviations are 8 minutes and 4.1 minutes, respectively, in the two groups of subjects.

Table 2.1. Fusion times for two groups of subjects.

NV: Verbal message only									
47.2	22.0	20.4	19.7	17.4	14.7	13.4	13.0	12.3	12.2
10.3	9.7	9.7	9.5	9.1	8.9	8.9	8.4	8.1	7.9
7.8	6.9	6.3	6.1	5.6	4.7	4.7	4.3	4.2	3.9
3.4	3.1	3.1	2.7	2.4	2.3	2.3	2.1	2.1	2.0
1.9	1.7	1.7							
Average = 8.56 Standard deviation = 8.09									

VV: Verbal and visual messages									
19.7	16.2	15.9	15.4	9.7	8.9	8.6	8.6	7.4	6.3
6.1	6.0	6.0	5.9	4.9	4.6	3.8	3.6	3.5	3.3
3.3	2.9	2.8	2.7	2.4	2.3	2.0	1.8	1.7	1.7
1.6	1.4	1.2	1.1	1.0					
Average = 5.55 Standard deviation = 4.80									

Source: Frisby and Clatworthy (1975).
Online at http://lib.stat.cmu.edu/DASL/Stories/FusionTime.html.

These standard deviations are almost as large as the averages themselves, indicating that there is considerable variability in the subjects' fusion times. Let us look at the data values in Table 2.1. Most subjects resolved the fusion figure in a few minutes, but many must have struggled for more than 10 minutes.

Let us recall some of the basic principles of statistics that are outlined in Section 1.1 before we go any further. Specifically, the observed data in Table 2.1 is a sample of empirical experiences based on a number of volunteers. These observations are sampled from an almost infinitely large population that we will never be able to observe completely. The object of statistics is to use the observed, sampled data to make inferences about properties of this unobservable and almost infinitely large population.

Does a difference of three minutes in the observed averages suggest that there is a difference in the underlying population mean times? Could we have observed such a large difference in average fusion times if it did not matter whether subjects were given the additional visual information? Is the observed difference of three minutes between the two group averages a measure of the effect of the visual prompting, or could this difference be attributed to chance alone? On the basis of this sampled data, what can we say about the populations? The statistical question making inference on the population means can be examined using `proc ttest` in SAS. The program is given in Table 2.2.

In this program we read the fusion times and group indicator. The grouping values are alphabetical characters rather than numbers, so a `$` is needed in the `input` statement. The data is included here, but you can also read it from a separate file using the `infile` statement. Always follow a `data` step with a `proc print` and examine it closely so you can be sure that the data was read correctly. Reading the data incorrectly is a common source of error. Both `proc print` and `proc means` include a `by group` statement. This produces separate data listings and means for the two groups of subjects.

Before we proceed with the statistical examination of any data, it is always useful to plot the data to see if there are any things we can quickly learn. A useful graphical display for these data is the *boxplot.* The `proc boxplot` procedure in SAS produces the small side-by-side boxplots given in Figure 2.8 for each of the two groups of subjects. The medians are depicted by horizontal lines inside each box. The *median* is the value that divides the sample in half: half of the observed data are above this value and half are below. Statistical methods for comparing medians are given in Section 7.1.

The plus signs in the boxplots indicate the locations of the sample averages. The tops and bottoms of the small boxes locate the upper and lower *quartiles* of these data. The upper quartile is the point where 25% of the data is above and 75% below, with a similar definition for the lower quartile. The box extends from the lower quartile to the upper quartile and contains the location of the central half of the

Table 2.2. SAS program to compute the t-test comparing averages in the fusion experiment.

```
title1 'Fusion times in a psychological experiment';
data fusion;
   input time group $;
   if group='NV' then ngroup = 0; /* create a numerical group # */
   if group='VV' then ngroup = 1;
   jgroup = ngroup + rannor(0)/10;   /* jitter the group number */
   datalines;
  47.2     NV
  22.0     NV
   ......
   1.7     NV
   1.7     NV
  19.7     VV
  16.2     VV
   ......
   1.1     VV
   1.0     VV
run;

proc print;           /* Always print everything after a data step */
   by group;
run;

title2 'Simple summary statistics';
proc means;
   by group;
run;

title2 'Boxplot of the two groups';
proc boxplot;
   plot time * group;
run;

title2 'Compare the averages of the two groups';
proc ttest;
  var time;
  class group;
run;
```

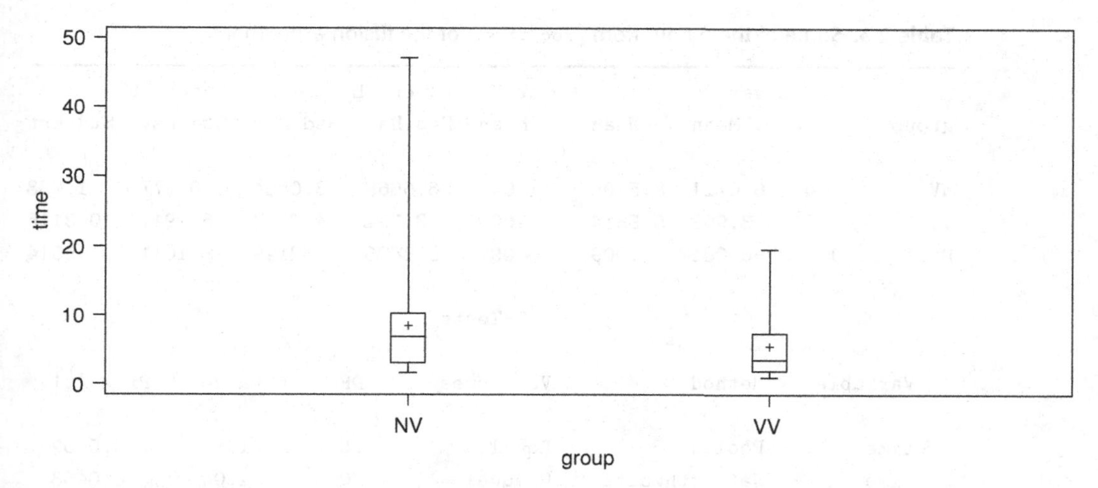

Figure 2.8 Boxplots for the fusion experiment.

observed data. The *whiskers* are the lines that extend above and below the quartile boxes to include the most extreme observations.

The boxplot allows us to perform a quick comparison of the data in these two groups. The means, medians, and quartiles all look very similar. The most notable feature is the extremes that extend above the boxes. These correspond to individuals who took a very long time to fuse their stereograms. The most extreme times occur in the NV group with no visual information about the image they were looking for.

In Figure 2.9 we scatter-plot the fusion times by group membership. The left half of this figure is the raw data. The group membership is binary valued, and this results in two vertical stripes. A bit more information can be seen when the group membership is *jittered*, or perturbed by a small amount of random noise. This noise

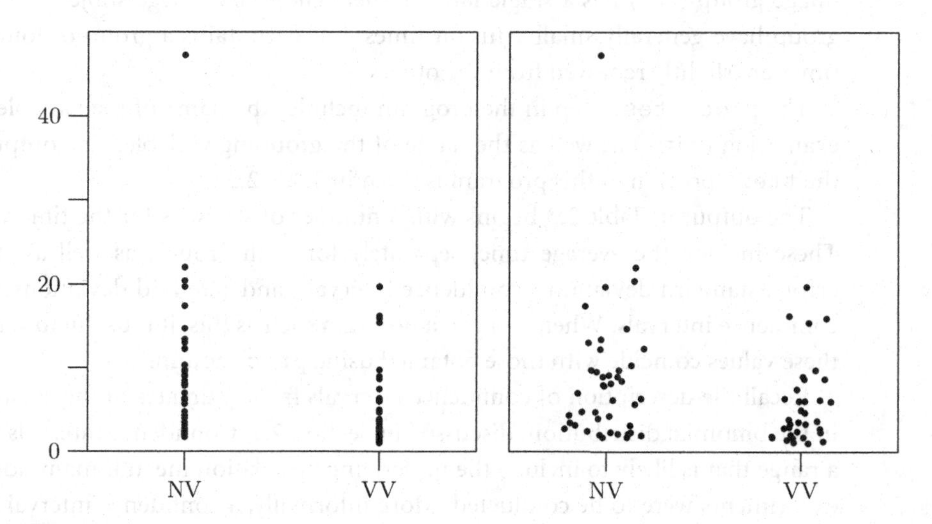

Figure 2.9 Fusion times by group and jittered group.

Table 2.3. Some of the output from `proc ttest` for the fusion experiment.

group	N	Lower CL Mean	Mean	Upper CL Mean	Lower CL Std Dev	Std Dev	Upper CL Std Dev	Std Err
NV	43	6.0721	8.5605	11.049	6.6668	8.0854	10.277	1.233
VV	35	3.902	5.5514	7.2009	3.884	4.8017	6.2912	0.8116
Diff (1-2)		-0.081	3.009	6.099	5.8826	6.8149	8.1011	1.5514

T-Tests

Variable	Method	Variances	DF	t Value	Pr > |t|
time	Pooled	Equal	76	1.94	0.0562
time	Satterthwaite	Unequal	70	2.04	0.0453

Equality of Variances

Variable	Method	Num DF	Den DF	F Value	Pr > F
time	Folded F	42	34	2.84	0.0023

is just enough to break up the pattern of the groups so we can see some of the patterns in the data.

The SAS program in Table 2.2 shows you how to add a small amount of normally distributed noise. This allows us to more easily count the number of individual observations and identify patterns. In the jittered plot we can see that the no-visual-image group (NV) has a single large outlier. The visual-image subjects in the VV group have generally smaller fusion times, but it contains a group of four whose times are slightly removed from the others.

The `proc ttest` step in the program includes the name of the variable we are examining (`time`) as well as the name of the grouping variable. The output from the `ttest` portion of this program is given in Table 2.3.

The output in Table 2.3 begins with a number of statistics for the time variable. These include the average time, separately for both groups, as well as standard errors, standard deviations, confidence intervals, and standard deviations of these confidence intervals. When you run a program such as this, it is useful to verify that these values coincide with those obtained using `proc means`.

Recall the description of confidence intervals from estimates of the p parameter in the binomial distribution, discussed in Section 2.1. Confidence intervals provide a range that is likely to include the underlying population mean if many additional experiments were to be conducted. More informally, a confidence interval is likely to contain the true underlying and unobservable population mean.

In the paragraph of the output, under the heading `T-Tests` we are given the Student statistics comparing the averages of the two groups of subjects in the fusion experiment. The `Pooled` method assumes that the variances are the same in the two populations. This method yields a p-value of .0562, providing a moderate amount of evidence that the two population means are not equal. Based on the discussion in Section 2.4, there is no way we will ever know this for certain. Instead, the p-value for this t-test is the probability of observing such a large difference in the sample averages if we assume that

- The two populations are sampled from underlying normal distributions
- The two populations have the same means and variances
- The subjects' times are independent

The alternative hypothesis is that the two groups of subjects have different means. The p-value tells us that the chances are .0562 of observing such a large difference in the two sample averages when all of these assumptions hold.

There are also t-tests that can be used when the variances are not equal. There are several ways of performing this test. The Satterthwaite method (also called the Welch-Satterthwaite method) used by SAS adjusts the degrees of freedom to account for unequal variances. This method gives a p-value of .0453, or just slightly smaller than the p-value obtained when we assumed that the population variances are equal.

These p-values are fairly close and both provide about the same moderate amount of evidence that the null hypothesis should be rejected. In conclusion, there is some evidence that the populations have different means on the basis of the observed data. It appears that visual information shortens the fusion time it takes people to resolve a random dot stereogram.

A p-value of .05 is not an automatic threshold for us to reject the null hypothesis, especially when these two methods yield p-values that are close in value. A change in the basic assumptions gave rise to a relatively small change in the resultant p-value. This should not result in an abrupt change in our actions.

The output of `proc ttest` given here ends with a statistical test of equality of variances. The null hypothesis is that both populations have the same variance. This test has a p-value of .0023, indicating that there is considerable evidence that the population variances are not equal.

Are the fusion times normally distributed? Some subjects took a very long time to resolve the figure. This provides evidence that the underlying distribution of fusion times in the general population may have a nonnormal distribution. Another approach to comparing these two groups of subjects is considered in Exercise 7.6, which reduces the effects of nonnormally distributed data and the influence of a few unusually large observations. Other aspects of this experiment are discussed in Exercise 2.5.

So, who was "Student"? His real name was William Sealy Gosset (1876–1937), and he worked as a quality engineer for the Guinness Brewery in Ireland in the early 1900s. His development of the t-test was considered a trade secret by his employer,

Table 2.4. Incidence of tumors in mice exposed to Avadex.

	Exposed	Control	Totals
Mice with tumors	4	5	9
No tumors	12	74	86
Totals	16	79	95

Source: Innes *et al.* (1969).

and he was not allowed to publicize his work. In order to publish his result and at the same time hide his identity, Gosset chose to publish his t-test in 1908 under the pen name "Student." Eventually he was found out, but the pen name remains. To this day, the well-known t-test is attributed to Student, rather than to the true name of its discoverer.

2.6 The Chi-Squared Test and 2 × 2 Tables

One of the most common ways of describing the relationship between two different attributes measured on each individual is to summarize these as frequency counts in a 2×2 table. An example is given in Table 2.4. This table summarizes an experiment in which ninety-five mice were either exposed to a fungicide (Avadex) or kept in unexposed, control conditions. After a period of time, all mice were sacrificed and examined for tumors in their lungs.

This table displays the discrete numbers of exposed and unexposed mice, as well as those with and without lung tumors. The totals in the margins of this table also provide the numbers of exposed (16) and unexposed (79) mice, as well as the overall numbers of mice with tumors (9) and those without tumors (86). These are sometimes referred to as *marginal counts* because they ignore the effects of the other variable in the table.

Such 2×2 tables are popular in the scientific literature because these tables provide a concise summary of the data and allow us to examine the relationship between two attributes measured on each individual. In the present case, the attributes are exposure status (exposed or control) and tumor status (yes/no). Both of these are binary valued. If one of the attributes is continuous valued, then it is common practice to convert this into a binary valued variable such as above or below the median value. In other words, even continuous-valued measures can still be displayed in a 2×2 table such as this.

The null hypothesis that is usually tested in a 2×2 table is that of *independence* of rows and columns. The expression of independence, by itself, is not intuitive until we translate this the present context. In the case of the data in Table 2.4, the two binary-valued measures are exposure (columns) and tumors (rows). Saying that columns and rows are independent is the same as saying that the rate of tumor formation is the same, regardless of whether the mouse was exposed to the fungicide. It is equally valid to say that tumor formation is independent of exposure status.

We then might think that the alternative hypothesis is that of *dependence*, but this is a poor choice of words. The data in Table 2.4 cannot be used to prove that exposure causes cancer any more than it can prove the light-hearted conclusion that tumors cause exposure. Causality is a much more difficult concept than can be demonstrated in such a simple data summary. Instead, the alternative hypothesis is that exposure and tumor formation are said to be associated or correlated. Noting this association is the best that a statistician can do. It remains to the scientific community how to interpret this association and whether or not it is meaningful.

One simple measure of association is the *cross-product ratio* or *odds ratio*, calculated as

$$\frac{4 \times 74}{5 \times 12} = 4.93$$

for the data in Table 2.4.

A value near 1 is indicative of independence. A value of the odds ratio greater than 1, as in this case, shows a positive association. That is, exposure to the fungicide is associated with higher rates of tumor formation.

There are many methods for assigning a p-value to these claims of association between the rows and columns of a 2 × 2 table. One of the oldest and most widely used is the *chi-squared test* (chi is pronounced *kī*, rhyming with "sky").

Use the chi-squared test to examine frequencies in a 2 × 2 table.

We calculate the chi-squared test by first finding the expected values of the counts under the null hypothesis of independence. The expected counts are found from the formula

$$\text{expected count} = \frac{(\text{row sum}) \times (\text{column sum})}{(\text{sample size})}. \tag{2.4}$$

As an example, the number of exposed mice with tumors is 4, and the expected number is

$$\frac{9 \times 16}{95} = 1.516.$$

The chi-squared statistic calculates the sum

$$\chi^2 = \sum \frac{(\text{observed} - \text{expected})^2}{\text{expected}}$$

over the four counts in the 2 × 2 table.

Specifically, for the data in Table 2.4 the value of this statistic is 5.408. The final step of obtaining a p-value is to look up this value in a table of chi-squared statistics. Just as with the t statistic, these are indexed by the degrees of freedom. A 2 × 2

Table 2.5. The SAS program to calculate measures of association in the fungicide data of Table 2.4.

```
data;
   input count tumor expos @@;
   datalines;
         4 0 0   5 0 1
        12 1 0  74 1 1
run;

proc print;
run;

proc freq;
   table tumor * expos  /  exact;
   exact or;
   weight count;
run;
```

table has 1 df. A small set of values of the chi-squared distribution are given in the appendix, Section A.2. From this table we can see that an observed value of 5.408 is just above the tabulated value 5.024, corresponding to a p-value of .025. (The correct p-value, obtained later using SAS, is .020.) This p-value provides a good rationale for rejecting the null hypothesis of independence of exposure and tumor growth and concluding, rather, that these two attributes are somehow related to each other.

Although the chi-squared statistic is easy enough to calculate by hand, this is best left to a computer. A small SAS program is given in Table 2.5 that uses `proc freq` to examine the frequencies in this 2×2 table. A portion of the output from this program appears in Table 2.6.

Yes, there is a lot of output from this program, but remember that 2×2 tables have been around for a very long time, and there are a tremendous number of ways to examine these four numbers. Let us concentrate on the most important parts of this output.

We note that the first line of the `Statistics` section of the output lists the chi-squared statistic, its value of 5.4083 with 1 df, and the p-value of .020. There are several other statistics listed, and these all have roughly the same p-value as well.

The printed `WARNING` is not as dire as it first appears. The validity of the chi-squared test is based on the assumption that all of the expected counts are large. (The expected counts were described in (2.4).) The approximation of the tabled p-value improves with larger expected counts. There is no absolute rule where the approximation suddenly becomes valid. The "larger than 5 rule" was suggested by

Table 2.6. A portion of the SAS output from the program in Table 2.5.

```
                 Statistics for Table of tumor by expos

       Statistic                        DF       Value      Prob
       ------------------------------------------------------
       Chi-Square                        1      5.4083    0.0200
       Likelihood Ratio Chi-Square       1      4.2674    0.0389
       Continuity Adj. Chi-Square        1      3.4503    0.0632
       Mantel-Haenszel Chi-Square        1      5.3514    0.0207
       Phi Coefficient                          0.2386
       Contingency Coefficient                  0.2321
       Cramer's V                               0.2386

        WARNING: 25% of the cells have expected counts less
                 than 5. Chi-Square may not be a valid test.

                          Fisher's Exact Test
                 ----------------------------------
                 Cell (1,1) Frequency (F)         4
                 Left-sided Pr <= F          0.9938
                 Right-sided Pr >= F         0.0411

                 Table Probability (P)       0.0349
                 Two-sided Pr <= P           0.0411

       Estimates of the Relative Risk (Row1/Row2)

    Type of Study              Value       95% Confidence Limits
    -------------------------------------------------------------
    Case-Control (Odds Ratio)  4.9333       1.1579       21.0182
    Cohort (Col1 Risk)         3.1852       1.2957        7.8299
    Cohort (Col2 Risk)         0.6456       0.3577        1.1653

                      Odds Ratio (Case-Control Study)
                  -----------------------------------
                  Odds Ratio                   4.9333

                  Asymptotic Conf Limits
                  95% Lower Conf Limit         1.1579
                  95% Upper Conf Limit        21.0182

                  Exact Conf Limits
                  95% Lower Conf Limit         0.8341
                  95% Upper Conf Limit        26.1606
```

Table 2.7. The underlying margins of Table 2.4 are the basis for exact tests.

	Exposed	Control	Totals
Mice with tumors	x		9
No tumors			86
Totals	16	79	95

W. Cochran[5] in the 1950s and remains with us to this day. SAS prints this warning to alert you of a potential problem.

One approach to this problem is to use a *continuity-adjusted chi-squared*, also known as the *Yates corrected chi-squared.* The continuity-adjusted chi-squared uses the formula suggested by F. Yates[6] in 1934,

$$\chi^2 = \sum \frac{(|\text{ observed} - \text{expected }| - .5)^2}{\text{expected}},$$

and then looks this value up in the chi-squared table.

The continuity-adjusted chi-squared is given in Table 2.6. Its value is 3.4503 with 1 df, and it has a p-value of .0632. This p-value is somewhat larger than that of the unadjusted chi-squared.

Another common approach that avoids any approximation to account for small sample sizes is the *exact test.* To understand how the exact test works, consider the empty shell in Table 2.7 obtained by deleting the data of the fungicide experiment. We keep the same marginal counts of exposed/control and tumor/healthy animals as before but omit the actual data on the inside of the table.

Let us denote the number of exposed mice with tumors by the symbol x. In this table we see that the value in this cell could assume any of the discrete values $0, 1, \ldots, 9$ consistent with the fixed marginal totals in this table. The observed value of x in the data is 4. More generally, if we assigned an arbitrary value to x in Table 2.7, then we could fill in all of the remaining cells of this 2×2 table. Also notice that it does not matter to which one of the four cells in the table we choose to assign a value; the other three entries would be similarly determined. The property that one cell determines all others is discussed in Section 2.7, where the concept of degrees of freedom is explained.

Without using an approximation or assuming very large sample sizes, exact tests are based on listing all ten of these possible outcomes and assigning a probability to each. Although this method is beyond the scope of the present book, note that if we use the `exact` option in `proc freq`, then SAS calculates both the approximate and exact significance levels.

[5] William Gemmell Cochran (1909–1980), statistician in Britain and the United States.
[6] Frank Yates (1902–1994), British statistician.

Table 2.6 shows that the observed value of $x = 4$ has probability .0349 in the paragraph following the heading `Fisher's Exact Test`. Notice that we are not interested in the probability of this outcome but, rather, the probability of this or a more extreme outcome. The concept of a p-value is the probability of the observed difference or larger, not the probability of the observed outcome. To repeat this concept, Exercise 2.6 points out that the probability of being dealt any specified hand of five cards may indeed be very small, but it is not necessarily a winning hand.

The exact test will enumerate the probability of the observed outcome along with every other outcome that is more extreme. In the case of the fungicide data output, the p-value is the probability of the observed value of 4 or a more extreme value of x. A value of $x = 4$ or greater has probability .9938, and a value of $x = 4$ or less has probability .0411. Notice that these two probabilities do not add up to 1. Exercise 2.7 goes over this in more details. We recognize .0411 to be the tail area of this distribution and that this is our exact significance level for these data. The SAS output of Table 2.6 includes both an asymptotic and an exact confidence interval for the odds ratio. These are obtained by either assuming that the counts are very large or else enumerating all possible outcomes consistent with the marginal totals of Table 2.7. Again, see Exercise 2.7 for details.

Although the name "exact" appears to bestow a greater level of precision and transparency, there is no real virtue in relying on these methods in every situation. In fact, it is generally recognized that exact tests often suffer from reduced power and may fail to detect the alternative hypothesis when it is valid.

In conclusion, the exact and asymptotic approximations to the p-value are reasonably close in this example (.0411 and .0200, respectively). The asymptotic 95% confidence interval (1.1579, 21.0182) for the odds ratio does not include 1. The 95% exact confidence interval (0.8341, 26.1606) for the odds ratio contains 1 because these require .025 in both "tails," but the exact significance level (.0411) is not quite extreme enough to exclude this value.

The chi-squared test and exact test will agree in large samples. With small samples or when these tests are discrepant, use the exact test.

With large sample sizes, the exact and chi-squared tests will come to roughly the same conclusions, as in this example. The conclusions of these two tests will be in better agreement as the sample size increases. If there is a large discrepancy in a small sample, then we should rely on the exact test.

2.7 What Are Degrees of Freedom?

We have seen this curious expression in two settings now: in the use of the t-test and when using the chi-squared test. What exactly are degrees of freedom, anyway?

More specifically, let's look at two situations where these words come up. The expression

$$\sum_{i}^{N} (x_i - \overline{x})^2$$

(where $\overline{x}$ is the average of the x_is), is associated with $N - 1$ degrees of freedom.

Similarly, in a 2×2 table of counts, we always say the chi-squared statistic has one degree of freedom.

The general rule is:

> Degrees of freedom are the number of data points to which you can assign any value.

Let's see how to apply this rule. When we look at the expression $\sum(x_i - \overline{x})^2$, there are N terms in the sum. Each term is a squared difference between an observation x_i and the average $\overline{x}$ of all the xs. Let us look at these differences and write them down. We have

$$d_1 = x_1 - \overline{x}$$

$$d_2 = x_2 - \overline{x}$$

$$\vdots$$

$$d_N = d_N - \overline{x}.$$

There are N differences d_i, but notice that these must always sum to 0. Adding up all of the values on the right-hand sides gives a sum of the xs minus N times their average. The d_i must sum to 0 no matter what values the x's are.

So how many differences d_i can we freely choose to be any values we want, and still have them add up to 0? The answer is all of them, except for the last one. The last one is determined by all of the others so that they all sum to 0. Notice also that it does not matter which d_i we call the "last." We can freely choose, $N - 1$ values and the one remaining value is determined by all of the others.

Now let us examine the use of degrees of freedom when discussing the chi-squared test. As an example, let us return to the data given in Table 2.4. The chi-squared statistic measures the association of rows and columns. In the present example, the association of interest is between developing lung cancer and exposure to the fungicide. The test is independent of the numbers of mice allocated to exposure or not and the numbers of mice that eventually develop tumors or not. The significance level of the test should only reflect the "inside" counts of this table and not these marginal totals.

Let us rewrite this table giving all of the margins, but without the values on the inside. This appeared earlier as Table 2.7. In this table we see that there are four missing numbers, but notice that any one of these determines the other three. If we knew the value of x (the number of exposed mice with tumors), for example, we could fill in the whole table using our knowledge of the marginal totals. That is, one value determines all of the others. There is one degree of freedom in this table.

If we look closely at Table 2.7, we can also see that the count labeled as x can only take on the values 0, 1, ..., 9, so that there are exactly 10 possible outcomes. The *Fisher exact test* exploits this property and constructs a hypothesis test of independence by enumerating all 10 of these outcomes. The details are beyond the present discussion, but the statistical significance of the exact test is provided in the SAS output of `proc freq`. These are described for this example in Section 2.6.

2.8 SAS, in a Nutshell

Among the most frustrating experiences since the invention of computers is human interactions with them. We are expected to remember passwords, endure long menus of telephone options just to get a simple answer, be deluged by spam, read error messages and help files that have no bearing on reality, and be patient when everything we have been working on for the past week has just vanished into thin air. Perhaps worst of all is the immediate feedback we receive when our intentions are misunderstood. There is no sense that a computer gave a moment's consideration to our request, however patiently we asked.

Having said all this, let us try to introduce SAS. First, you need to have SAS installed on your computer. You should also have a kind, understanding, patient friend nearby who is willing to drop everything and show you how to invoke the editor, submit a SAS job, retrieve the output, and finally print it out. If there is an error, you should learn to check the log file. The SAS log file can be surprisingly informative: not only does it point out your error, but it usually provides a list of possible options you might try to fix the problem. Sometimes SAS will detect an error, take a good guess at your intentions, fix it, and then keep going. Miracles do happen.

The easiest way to learn a computer skill is to find a program that works and then copy and modify it. The programs in this book are geared toward using this method of learning. After a while, you will want to consider additional options. When you reach this point, SAS offers an extensive Help File. Learn to use this valuable resource.

There are also two important reference books you might consider having nearby. Probably the best reference is Cody and Smith (2006). This book contains many useful SAS programs along with many of the options for commonly used statistical procedures. Delwiche and Slaughter published the *Little SAS Book*, which is full of all kinds of indispensable bits of information that will help you get started. It can't be recommended strongly enough.

To begin, your data might look like the listing in Table 2.8. This data on low-birth-weight babies will be examined at length in Chapter 3. Every line in the data represents information on a single baby, and each of the seven columns represents a type of information, called a variable. The seven variables in these data are (from

Table 2.8. A few lines of the low-birth-weight data. Columns are observation number; head circumference; length; gestational age; birth weight; mother's age; and an indicator for toxemia.

1	27	41	29	1360	37	0
2	29	40	31	1490	34	0
3	30	38	33	1490	32	0
4	28	38	31	1180	37	0
5	29	38	30	1200	29	1
6	23	32	25	680	19	0
7	22	33	27	620	20	1
.	.	.	.	.	.	.
.	.	.	.	.	.	.
.	.	.	.	.	.	.
99	28	41	33	1320	36	1
100	26	38	28	1080	36	0

Source: Pagano and Gauvreau (2000).

left to right) observation number; head circumference; length at birth; gestational age; birth weight; mother's age; and an indication of toxemia.

Your basic SAS program begins with a `data` step that reads the data into SAS and is followed by one or more procedures, identified with the keyword `proc`. The `procs` do things with the data. An example of the `data` step from Table 3.1 includes the code in Table 2.9.

The SAS code in Table 2.9 begins with a `title` that will appear on the top of every page of the output. When your desk is covered in paper, you will appreciate having a heading that explains what this material refers to. The `infile` statement identifies a file containing the data. Your `infile` statement may need to include information

Table 2.9. A short SAS program.

```
title1 'Data on low birth weight infants';
data regn;
    infile 'birthwt.dat';
    input headcirc  length  gestage  birthwt  momage  toxemia;
        label
            headcirc = 'head circumference'
            gestage  = 'gestational age'
            birthwt  = 'birth weight'
            momage   = 'mother''s age'
            toxemia  = 'indication of toxemia';
run;

proc print; /* Always print out everything after the data step */
run;
```

about the computer drive and directory. This information will be specific to your computer and different from the examples in this book. Again, your helpful friend may be needed to get you started with this.

The `input` statement lists all of the variables in the order these are listed in your data. Every statement ends in a semicolon (";"). Omitting semicolons will probably be your most common source of errors. After your `data` step, you should always print out all of the data using `proc print;`. This step will reveal a major source of problems. The rest of your program will not work correctly if you don't begin with the correct data.

In addition to titles, you should also get in the habit of putting comments into every program you write. Comments go anywhere and are an important aspect of writing good computer code. Comments begin with a * and end with a semicolon, as in

```
* Write anything useful in this comment ;
```

or in the form bracketed with delimiters as in:

```
/* This is another form of a SAS comment */
```

You should use almost as many lines of comments as actual SAS code. There are several important reasons for this. In the short term, you will never remember what this program does or why it was written when you look at it again, only a few weeks after it was written. Second, in larger projects, programs are always part of a team effort and are shared by several individuals. If you can't remember what the program is supposed to do, then your co-workers will be even more confused without comments.

You should avoid using variable names such as `x` that provide no useful information about their role. In addition to comments, there is also a `label` statement that allows you to provide a brief description of a variable in case the name alone does not provide an adequate explanation of its meaning. Finally, SAS statements can begin anywhere on the line, but if you indent lines, as in the example in Table 2.9, it is easier to see what parts of the code belong to which steps.

Small datasets can be read with the actual data listed as part of the `data` step following a `datalines;` statement. It is also possible to read Excel files directly into your `data` step. You can read and process dates and text in SAS, work with tab-delimited data, and export your results in Postscript or hypertext for use on a web page. All of these topics are beyond the present discussion but are covered in Delwiche and Slaughter's *Little SAS Book*.

2.9 Survey of the Rest of the Book

Having reviewed all of the mathematical and statistical prerequisites, let us step back a moment and see what we are going to do with them and where we are going.

We begin with a dataset measuring attributes on several individuals. The low-birth-weight infant data of Section 2.8 is a good example. All of the attributes or columns of this data are referred to as *variables.* Often one of these variables is of greatest importance to us, and we sometimes refer to it as the *outcome variable.* (Other authors will refer to this as the response variable or dependent variable.) The outcome variable is more important than any other data measured on each individual. We often refer to this variable by the symbol y. The object of this book is to show how we might explain the different values of the outcome variable y in terms of other information. Other variables measured on every individual are usually denoted by x and sometimes called *independent variables* to distinguish them from the outcome y. We sometimes call y the *dependent variable* because its value will be explained using x. In the following chapter we show how to explain the infant weight values y based on the length x of the infants. The concept of dependent variable is entirely a construct of our mathematical modeling framework and does not mean to imply a cause-and-effect relationship.

We begin with a detailed discussion of the situation where y follows a normal distribution, in part because this is the most commonly encountered situation. Much research has gone into this setting, and many diagnostics and graphical displays are available to facilitate the corresponding statistical analysis. Once we understand how to model the outcome y as a normally distributed quantity, we can generalize to other settings where the outcome y might be binary valued, for example, or represent discrete counts.

Let us look back at the chi-squared test and t-test as examples. For the t-test, the outcome y has a continuous, normal distribution, and the explanatory or group membership variable is binary valued. In the chi-squared test in a 2×2 table, we might think of the row category explaining the column category or vice versa, and the dependent outcome variable y is binary valued. The explanatory variable x is binary valued in both of these examples. In the examples of subsequent chapters, the explanatory variable can also be continuous. We also demonstrate in those chapters how to combine the effects of multiple explanatory variables. The January temperatures in various cities (outcome) can be explained in terms of the latitude, as well as the altitude above sea level. We will need to combine the effects of latitude and altitude in explaining differences in temperature. One effect may be more important than the other, and we will need to assess the relative effects of other explanatory measures.

2.10 Exercises

2.1 How could we use the data in Figure 1.4 to argue that the economy is improving? Use the same data and discuss how this shows that the economy is in decline. Also, are the axes in these graphs correct?

2.2 I pass a certain intersection very often and have learned that I will have to stop for the traffic light 80% of the time. If I pass through this intersection eight times, what is the probability that I will have to stop for the traffic light six or more times?

2.3 In a day-care center there are eight preschool children. Suppose that the probability is 1/4 that one has a cold on given day.

a. Use the binomial distribution to estimate how many children you expect will have a cold on a given day. What is the standard deviation of this number?

b. What is the probability that all eight children have a cold today? What is the probability that three or more have a cold today?

c. Is this an appropriate use of the binomial distribution? Why or why not?

2.4 a. In a test of a hypothesis, does the power increase or decrease when the difference between the null and alternative hypotheses increases? Why?

b. Similarly, what kinds of alternative hypotheses have the greatest power? Should we consider these? Why?

c. When the sample size increases, if the null hypothesis and the significance level remain the same, what kinds of alternative hypotheses can we test using the same level of power?

2.5 a. What is the population in the fusion experiment described in Section 2.5? Is it possible to consider examining every subject in the population?

b. Each of the subjects was given either verbal-only or verbal and visual information. Should we be interested in what their outcomes might have been if they were randomized to the other group? If each subject was tested twice, once with verbal-only and once with verbal and visual information, would it matter which condition was given first? What additional biases would this type of experiment introduce? In a *crossover experiment*, all subjects would experience both of the two different types of settings, but in a random order. That is, some would experience verbal-only first and then the verbal and visual information, whereas the others would receive these in the reverse order.

2.6 a. In the middle of a poker game, one of the players declares that he holds a "kangaroo flush." His cards are 3♢, 6♡, 7♣, 9♢, and J♠. Of course there is nothing remarkable about this hand, but the player claims that the probability of holding these exact five cards is extremely small. What is the probability of being dealt a kangaroo flush? On the basis of this extremely small probability, the player claims that his cards must beat every other possible poker hand. What do you say about this argument?

b. Explain why the exact significance level of Table 2.4 is not the probability of observing this table. Instead, the significance level is the probability of observing this table or any other more extreme table.

c. List all of the tables that are more extreme and show that the odds ratios of these tables are larger than those of the observed table.

2.7 Why do the two tail probabilities add up to more than 1 in the exact test given in Table 2.6?

2.8 Use Table A.1 in the appendix to find these probabilities for the normal distribution.

a. Find $\Pr[-2.18 < Z < .38]$ for a standard normal Z.

b. Find $\Pr[1.16 < Y < 2.72]$ for a normal Y with mean 1.35 and a standard deviation of 2.2.

Hint: $(Y - 1.35)/2.2$ will behave as a standard normal, so we have

$$\Pr[1.16 < Y < 2.72] = \Pr\left[\frac{1.16 - 1.35}{2.2} < \frac{Y - 1.35}{2.2} < \frac{2.72 - 1.35}{2.2}\right]$$
$$= \Pr[-0.09 < Z < 0.62],$$

where Z behaves as a standard normal.

2.9 In a clinical trial of chronic granulomatous disease (CGD, a hereditary immune disorder) 128 patients were randomized to either a placebo or to gamma interferon and then followed for about 1 year. Among the 63 treated patients, 14 experienced at least one infection for a total of 20 observed infections. In the placebo group, 30 patients experienced at least one infection and 56 total infections were recorded.

a. Express the numbers of treated or placebo and infection-free or not patients as a 2×2 table. Use the chi-squared test to see if gamma interferon was effective.

b. Would this be an appropriate way to compare the number of infections in the placebo and treated group?

c. Could we use the binomial distribution to compare the total number of infections? Here is how we might proceed: In total, $20 + 56 = N$ infections were recorded. Of the 20 infections in the treated group, these occurred in $\widehat{p} = 63/128$ fraction of the sample. How can we use the binomial model to obtain a p-value for these data? Comment on the validity of this approach.

2.10 What is the hidden geometric shape in Figure 2.7?

2.10.1 Maintaining Balance

It is difficult to maintain your balance when you are concentrating on something else. In an experiment involving aging, 9 elderly volunteers (6 men, 3 women) and 8 young male volunteers tried to keep their balance while reacting to a randomly timed noise. They stood, barefoot, on a specially designed platform that measured their motion. Each time they heard the noise they were supposed to press a hand-held button, all the while trying not to move. The data is given in Table 2.10.

Use a t-test to compare forward/backward motion distances in the elderly and young volunteers. Does age appear to make a difference in the responses? Use a t-test to compare these groups. Is there evidence that the observed values are not normally distributed? Are there unusual observed values that influence the t-test? Should these be omitted, or should they be included in your examination of the data? Can you make an argument for both of these actions?

Table 2.10. Measures of motion in a balance experiment.

	Motion		
Subject number	Forward and backward	Side to side	Age group
1	19	14	elderly
2	30	41	elderly
3	20	18	elderly
4	19	11	elderly
5	29	16	elderly
6	25	24	elderly
7	21	18	elderly
8	24	21	elderly
9	50	37	elderly
1	25	17	young
2	21	10	young
3	17	16	young
4	15	22	young
5	14	12	young
6	14	14	young
7	22	12	young
8	17	18	young

Source: Teasdale, Bard, LaRue, and Fleury (1993) and online at http://lib.stat.cmu.edu/DASL/Stories/MaintainingBalance.html.

Repeat your examination using the side/side distances. Is your conclusion any different from the forward/backward motion?

How might we combine these separate measures of motion into a single number? Try it. You will need to define a new variable in the `data;` step of your program. Print it out to make sure it is correct. Is it useful in comparing the two groups of volunteers?

2.10.2 Reading Scores

Two groups of children participated in an experiment to see if their reading scores could be improved. One class of twenty-one children was presented with eight weeks of directed reading activities, and another control class did not receive this additional training. The scores from a standardized reading test are given in Table 2.11.

Did the additional directed reading activities improve the reading scores? Use a t-test and boxplot to support your conclusions. Do the test scores appear to be normally distributed within each of the two groups of children? Are the variances comparable? Is there any other information that you would find useful in your analysis of these data?

Table 2.11. Reading scores for third-grade children.

Additional directed activities									
24	43	58	71	43	49	61	44	67	49
53	56	59	52	62	54	57	33	46	43
57									
No additional activities									
42	43	55	26	62	37	33	41	19	54
20	85	46	10	17	60	53	42	37	42
55	28	48							

Source: http://lib.stat.cmu.edu/DASL/Stories/DRPScores.html.

2.10.3 A Helium-Filled Football

If we filled a football with helium, would a kicker be able to punt it farther? In an attempt to answer this important sports-related question, two identical footballs were presented to an amateur player who alternately kicked each as far as he could. He was unaware that one football was filled with helium, the other with regular air from a pump. The kicking took place outdoors, on a windless day. The trial number and distances (in yards) kicked are given in Table 2.12.

Why did the trials alternate between the two footballs? What biases would this remove from the experiment? The kicker did not know what the experiment was about. What biases would it introduce if he was told what was going on? A test subject who is unaware of the treatment is called *blind.*

Table 2.12. Distances two different footballs were kicked.

Trial	Air	Helium	Trial	Air	Helium	Trial	Air	Helium
1	25	25	2	23	16	3	18	25
4	16	14	5	35	23	6	15	29
7	26	25	8	24	26	9	24	22
10	28	26	11	25	12	12	19	28
13	27	28	14	25	31	15	34	22
16	26	29	17	20	23	18	22	26
19	33	35	20	29	24	21	31	31
22	27	34	23	22	39	24	29	32
25	28	14	26	29	28	27	22	30
28	31	27	29	25	33	30	20	11
31	27	26	32	26	32	33	28	30
34	32	29	35	28	30	36	25	29
37	31	29	38	28	30	39	28	26

Source: http://lib.stat.cmu.edu/DASL/Stories/Heliumfootball.html.

Those evaluating the subject might provide unintentional or subtle messages about the experiment. An experiment in which those doing the evaluation are also blinded is called *double blind.* What biases might be avoided if those measuring the distance of the football kicks were also blinded as to the purpose of the experiment?

Plot the distances kicked by the trial number. Is there evidence that the kicker improved as the experiment continued? Can you explain why this might be the case?

Look at a boxplot of the kicking distances for each of the two footballs. Is there evidence of extremely long or short kicks? Some might argue that kicks of less than 15 or 20 yards are flubbed and should be neglected. Or maybe not.

What does the t-test tell us? Is there evidence of a difference between the two footballs? What other information would you find helpful in deciding if a helium-filled football provides an advantage in terms of kicking distance? Should a professional player be used, for example?

3

Introduction to Linear Regression

In this book we develop mathematical models for explaining the variability of measurements made on an outcome of interest. The aim is to try to explain the different values of this outcome in response to other information available to us. Random variation in the values of the response makes this difficult, and at best we will only be able to make a statement about the typical or average value of the response under a given set of circumstances. Let us make this clear with an example in which we try to explain the different birth weights of a group of 100 low-birth-weight babies using only information about their length.

3.1 Low-Birth-Weight Infants

One of the health problems associated with low-birth-weight infants is just that: their low weight is associated with a myriad of health problems. A "low birth weight" is any value lower than 1,500 grams. Figure 3.1 plots the length and birth weight of 100 low-birth-weight infants born in one of two Boston-area hospitals.

In this figure we see a rough relationship between birth weight and length. In general, larger birth weight is associated with greater length. Despite a small number of notable exceptions in this plot, we can see that most of the infants follow a general pattern. The large "cloud" of observations along the right half of this figure defines the general pattern of the data. The values of length were rounded to the nearest centimeter, and this explains the vertical "stripes" that appear in Figure 3.1.

The aim of this chapter and the following is to fit the given straight line to data of this type and assess its adequacy in explaining the response. Of course a straight line is not going to explain the differences in all of the birth-weight values, but for a given value of length, we can make a statement about the average birth weight that would be expected at that length. Similarly, we are not making a prediction about the birth weight beyond suggesting where the average might be. Prediction is not a good word to use with this activity because of its association with fortune tellers and crystal balls. We are also not trying to prove a cause-and-effect relationship. It would be

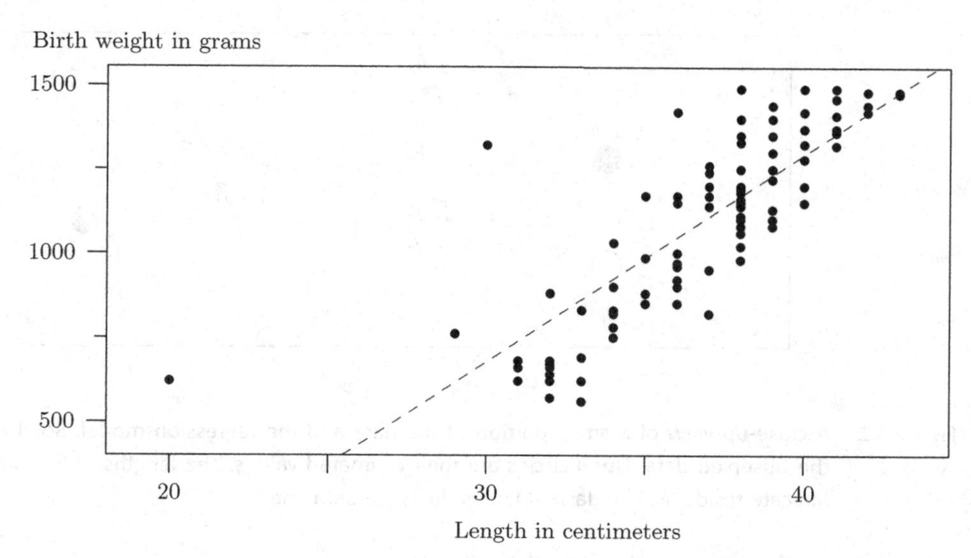

Figure 3.1 **Birth weight and length of 100 low-birth-weight infants along with the fitted least squares regression line.**

foolish to try to "prove" that greater length causes greater birth weight, or vice versa. Statistics alone cannot prove cause-and-effect relationships. In the present example, both length and birth weight are the result of other factors, and the cause-and-effect relationship is beyond the scope of this book. On the other hand, an infant's length can easily be estimated using readily available imaging technologies before birth, so it is a reasonable exercise to provide a good estimate of the ultimate birth weight.

The following section describes how the fitted line in this figure is determined, and in Section 3.3 we show how to find this in SAS.

3.2 The Least Squares Regression Line

A line is determined by its slope and intercept. In this section we show how these two parameters are estimated. Along the way, we also need to explain how the best-fitting line is going to be defined. All of the numerical calculations involved will be done by the computer, so there is no need to dig out the pocket calculator. Even so, it is important for the user of these methods to understand the steps involved in fitting these mathematical models.

Our data consists of ordered pairs of coordinates: $(x_1, y_1), (x_2, y_2), \ldots, (x_n, y_n)$. In terms of the low-birth-weight infants, the xs are the lengths and the ys are the birth weights. The aim of this section is to explain how to obtain a regression line model

$$y = \alpha + \beta x$$

for the data.

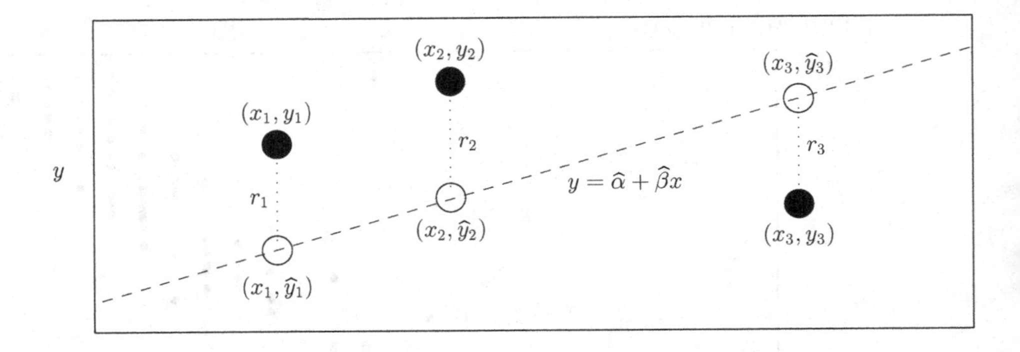

Figure 3.2 A close-up view of a small portion of the data and the regression model. Solid circles are the observed data. Open circles are their estimated values. The lengths of the dotted lines indicate residuals. The dashed line is the regression line.

This equation is a mathematical model for the data. A quick look at Figure 3.1 reminds us that there is no reason for this line to pass through any of the data points. A model is a simplified version of reality. The line provides an intuitive summary of the relationship of weight and length for typical infants but is not indicative of any one of them.

A more accurate description of what is going on is to write a separate equation for each (x_i, y_i) pair. There is only one underlying line for the whole dataset, but we also need to take into account the fact that the individual data points do not lie exactly on the line. Some observations will be above the line and others will be below. As a compromise, let us write

$$y_i = \alpha + \beta x_i + r_i,$$

where r_i is the difference between the observed value y_i and where it is expected to be if it appeared exactly on the line.

We call these r_i the *residuals* because they represent what is left over after fitting the line. In other words, there is one line with slope β and intercept α. At any given length x_i of the ith infant, the observed weight y_i will be close the estimated value on the line $\alpha + \beta x_i$. The residual is the difference between the observed value and where it would be expected if it appeared exactly on the line. The choice of "best fitting" line is determined by these residuals. In Section 4.4 we also see that the residuals are useful in identifying any inadequacies of the model.

To determine the most appropriate line, we need to estimate both the intercept α and the slope β for this line and define a criterion by which we are to obtain these estimates. The process of estimation is motivated by the depiction of the data given in Figure 3.2. In this figure we imagine the regression line passing three data points, depicted by solid circles. The regression line is shown as a dotted line. This is an extreme close-up view of a very small part of the full data. There are many other data points, but they are outside the range of this figure.

For each of the three observations in Figure 3.2, we can see where these observations would be if the line represented a perfect fit to the data. These perfectly fitted, or *estimated*, data points appear as open circles along the dashed line. Note that the estimates are obtained as changes in the y values only. The estimated value is not identified as the closest point to the observed data on the regression line. The implications of this convention are that the x values are assumed to be known to a high degree of precision and all of the statistical variability takes place along the vertical y axis. In the case of the low-birth-weight infants, for example, we assume that the length is known with some degree of precision on the basis of a CT scan, and the infant's weight is the only variable we wish to explain.

In linear regression we know x and are estimating the mean of y for that value of x.

The coordinate pairs of the estimated observation on the regression line are denoted by $(x_i, \widehat{y}_i)$, where the carets ($\widehat{\ }$) on the $\widehat{y}$s are indicative of an estimated value. (We pronounce $\widehat{y}$ as "y hat.") Similarly, the estimated intercept and slope are denoted by $\widehat{\alpha}$ and $\widehat{\beta}$, respectively.

Equally important in Figure 3.2 are the *residuals* or differences between the observed and estimated values. Mathematically, we define

residual = observed − expected

or how far the observed data is from where we would expect it to be in a perfectly fitting model.

The lengths of the three residuals are indicated by dotted lines in Figure 3.2. Values of r_1 and r_2 are positive numbers because the observed data is larger than what the model expects; r_3 is negative. In this and subsequent chapters we see that the residuals play an important role in determining the adequacy of the models we build for data, and help in identifying unusual observations in the data. Briefly, the residuals represent the shortcomings of a mathematical model in its representation of the observed data.

Let us look more closely at the residuals for our straight-line model. If we knew the values of the slope β and intercept α of the regression line, then the perfectly fitted observation corresponding to the observed pair (x_i, y_i) would be

$$\widehat{y}_i = \alpha + \beta x_i$$

and the residual r_i is exactly zero because of the perfect fit.

That is, $\widehat{y}_i$ is the value of y on the line at the value x_i. The values of $\widehat{y}_i$ appear as the open circles in Figure 3.2. We can write our definition of the ith residual as the observed y_i minus its expected value

$$r_i = y_i - \widehat{y}_i$$

or as

$$r_i = y_i - (\alpha + \beta x_i). \tag{3.1}$$

This last representation of the residual will allow us to estimate the parameters α and β of the regression line. Ideally we would like all of our residuals to be "small" in some sense. The principle of least squares provides the appropriate guidance on how to achieve this.

Estimation using least squares minimizes the sum of squared residuals.

Using the guidance of least squares, the aim is to estimate α and β by minimizing

$$\sum_i (\text{residual}_i)^2.$$

Of course, we can't see α and β in this last expression, but if we look back at (3.1) we can write this as

$$\sum_i (y_i - \alpha - \beta x_i)^2. \tag{3.2}$$

The objective, then, is to find the values of α and β that minimize this quantity. We should immediately recognize this minimization as a problem from calculus. A quick overview of the principles of calculus appears in Section 1.4. We do not actually go through all the details, but the reader should recognize the steps that need to be taken to solve the problem.

Specifically, we need to differentiate (3.2) with respect to α and set this equation to zero. We also need to differentiate (3.2) with respect to β and set this second equation equal to zero. These steps result in two equations in two unknowns: α and β.

These two equations are

$$\sum_i \text{residual}_i = 0 \tag{3.3}$$

and

$$\sum_i x_i \text{ residual}_i = 0. \tag{3.4}$$

As written, we can't see the α and β, but they are in there. Exercise 3.1 asks you to rewrite these two equations to make this clear.

There is no reason for us to actually solve these two equations: the computer does this for us. The computing is covered in the following section, but it is important to see what the computer is actually doing in order to obtain the estimates $\widehat{\alpha}$ and $\widehat{\beta}$. Before that, let us describe the implications of these two equations.

Equation (3.3) asserts that the residuals sum to zero or, more importantly, have an average value of exactly zero. Intuitively, this is a nice property. If the residuals represent the differences between the observed data and their expected values along the regression line, then we would want the line to represent the average values and not be either too high, on average, or too low. Equation (3.3) assures us that the regression line is centered about the data. If $\bar{x}$ and $\bar{y}$ are the averages of the xs and ys, respectively, then the point of averages $(\bar{x}, \bar{y})$ is a point on the regression line.

The second equation (3.4) states that the residuals are uncorrelated with the explanatory x values. We discuss correlation later in Section 4.1, but for the moment the implication is that the regression line contains all of the linear information that can be extracted from the explanatory variables. The least squares regression line obtains all of the linear information available in the x values, and there is nothing left but the residual noise. A plot of the explanatory values (or fitted values) against the residuals of our model should show only random white noise with no apparent pattern or trend.

3.3 Regression in SAS

Before we go any further, let's get SAS to fit a regression line. The data appears in a file, and printing it gives output similar to Table 2.8. Each line represents the data on one infant. The columns represent the items or variables measured on each baby. There are 100 infants represented here, so we only include a few of the first and last of these.

A short SAS program that reads the data, plots the (x, y) values, and finds the least squares slope and intercept is given in Table 3.1. The `data` step reads the data. The `infile` tells SAS where to find the data. You will need to change this line for the specific directory on the computer that you are using. The `input` statement gives names to the columns in the data. The use of these additional columns of data in more complex statistical models is discussed in Chapter 5. A more elaborate `data` step for this data is given in Table 2.9.

Get in the habit of using a `proc print` following a `data` step to make sure that SAS reads your data correctly. The `data` step is a common source of errors, and printing out all of your data is a quick way to check your program. The `gplot` procedure produces a nice scatter plot of the data. This is another useful way to check the validity of your data.

The `reg` procedure does the actual fitting of the regression model. The `model` statement specifies the dependent y variable (birth weight, in this case) on the left side of the equals sign, and the x variable (length, in this example) is listed on

Table 3.1. SAS program to read the low-birth-weight data and perform a linear regression.

```
title1 'Data on low birth weight infants';
data regn;
   infile 'birthwt.dat';    /* you will need to change this */
   input headcirc  length  gestage  birthwt  momage  toxemia;
run;

proc print; /* Always print out everything after the data step */
run;

proc gplot;
   plot birthwt * length;
run;

proc reg;
   model birthwt = length / p r i;
   output residual=res predicted=fitted;
run;
proc print; /* print residuals and regression diagnostics */
run;
proc gplot;
   plot res*fitted; /* Plot residuals and fitted values */
run;
quit;
```

the right. There is no need to tell SAS to include an intercept, because this is the default.

There is a lot of output from this program, but right now we want to concentrate on the portion that appears in Table 3.2. These are the least squares estimates of the intercept ($\widehat{\alpha} = -1171.25$) and slope ($\widehat{\beta} = 61.65$). Exercise 3.3 asks you to interpret these values.

Both of these estimated parameters are associated with a standard error. The ratio of the parameter estimate divided by its standard error is listed under the

Table 3.2. Parameter estimates from the program in Table 3.1.

Parameter Estimates

Variable	DF	Parameter Estimate	Standard Error	t Value	Pr > |t|
Intercept	1	-1171.25305	163.46909	-7.16	<.0001
length	1	61.65408	4.41915	13.95	<.0001

label `t Value`. This statistic is used to test the null hypothesis that the underlying parameter being estimated has a population value of zero. (Use a pocket calculator to verify the values in this column.)

The rightmost column provides a p-value to test the statistical significance of this hypothesis. In Table 3.2 the two p-values provide very strong evidence that both the population slope and the intercept are nonzero. Notice the statistical inference taking place in this statement: The estimated sample slope ($\widehat{\beta}$) and intercept ($\widehat{\alpha}$) are far enough from zero to lead us to conclude that the population slope (β) and intercept (α) are also nonzero.

Why is this statement about statistical significance so important? A test of the slope is the primary reason for performing a linear regression in the first place. Our aim is to see if the x variable (length) has any value in explaining the outcome or dependent y variable, birth weight. If we concluded that the regression slope was 0, then we could learn little about birth weight from knowing the baby's length. One of the most important tasks in proposing a statistical model is to demonstrate its value as an estimator of y. The demonstration of a statistically significant slope is one of the strongest pieces of evidence that a data analyst can provide for the usefulness of a regression model. A test of significance of the intercept is usually not of interest to us, but see Exercise 3.3 for more details on the intercept in the present example.

The program also demonstrates how you can capture the fitted values $\widehat{y}_i$ and the residuals r_i. The most important diagnostic available to us is a plot of the residuals following a model fitting. This plot can disclose a variety of problems with a mathematical model of real data. These will be discussed in Section 4.4. The program produces a plot using `proc gplot` of the residuals against the fitted values.

3.4 Statistics in the News: Future Health Care Costs

The expansion of costs of U.S. federal health care programs as a percentage of the total economy is of concern, and details of this can be seen in Figure 3.3. The average age of the population is increasing in many industrialized nations. Older people consume more health care per person than the rest of the population.

The top line in this figure anticipates a huge rise in federal spending on health care programs and is cause for concern. Then again, the bottom line in this figure indicates a trend that is only slightly increasing. Many of the assumptions made here may not be valid in the future. A lot has changed, and we should anticipate even more changes in future health care costs as well.

All of the estimates in this figure are based on assumptions that may or may not continue to be valid even in the near future. Technology can rapidly change, and new medical discoveries may become commonplace. Congress could pass a law tomorrow, for example, creating a new system of universal private health care. This might happen, of course, but the idea illustrates that a lot could quickly change. The predictions in this figure about events seventy-five years in the future could prove

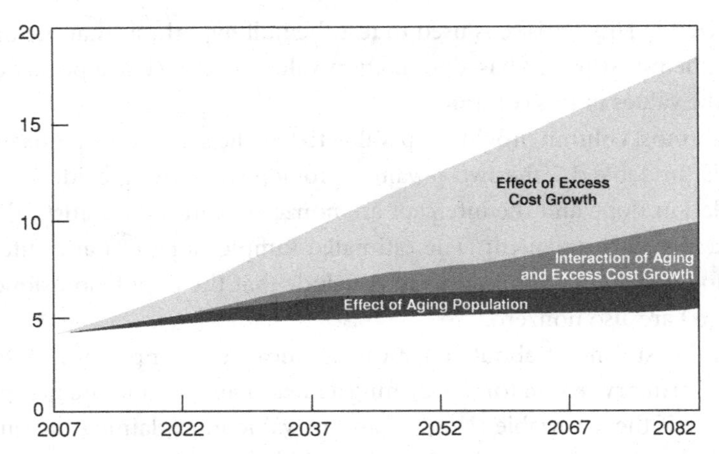

Figure 3.3 **Future health care cost estimates as a percentage of gross domestic product.** ***Source:*** **Congressional Budget Office.**

to be wildly inaccurate. Look at the wide range of possibilities between the three estimates.

Extrapolate at your peril.

There is a danger of *extrapolating* beyond the data. The ability to fit regression lines does not give us license to describe events beyond the available data. There is no certainty that the conditions that generated the data will continue to hold. Linear regression can be abused in the wrong hands. Extrapolations, especially predictions about future events, should be made sparingly and need to be identified as such.

3.5 Exercises

3.1 Rewrite the two equations in (3.3) and (3.4) to convince yourself that these really are two equations in two unknowns α and β. You will need to refer back to (3.1) to answer this question. If you are feeling very brave, try to solve these two equations for $\widehat{\alpha}$ and $\widehat{\beta}$.

3.2 Reread Section 2.7 and guess how many degrees of freedom are associated with the sum of squared residuals given at (3.2).

3.3 a. The estimated slope in Table 3.2 is 61.65. Interpret this number. Specifically, what can you say about the average weights of two infants who differ by 1 cm in length?

b. The estimated intercept in Table 3.2 is a large negative number. Is that cause for concern? How do we interpret the intercept in this model?

3.4 Use SAS to estimate the regression model explaining infant weight from gestational age. Provide a simple interpretation for the value of the slope in the fitted equation.

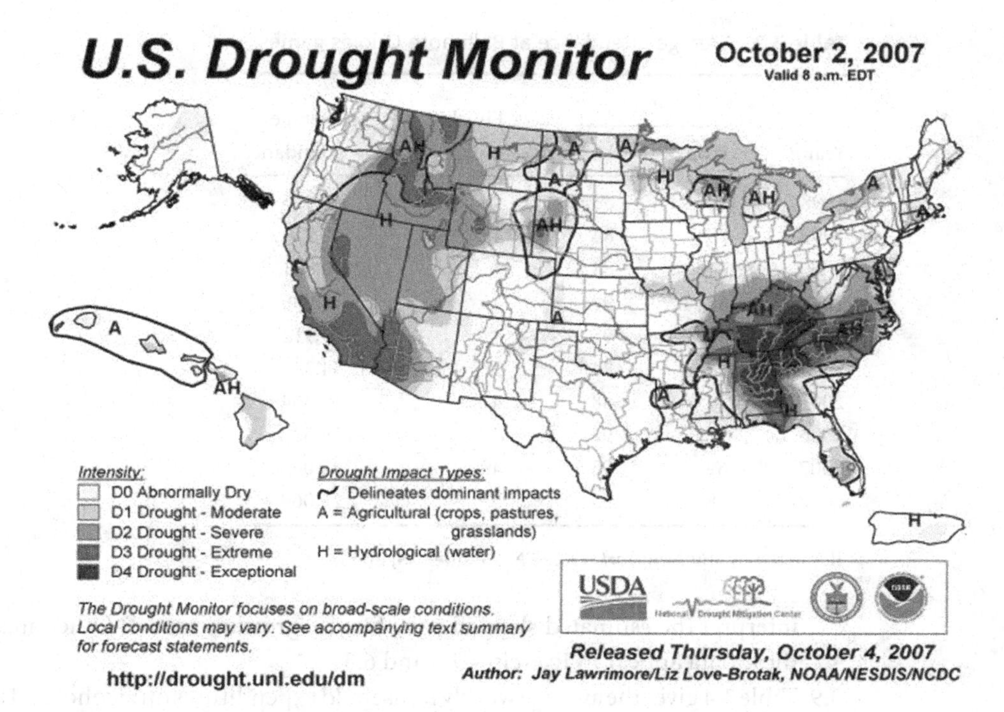

Figure 3.4 Map of drought conditions in the United States.

3.5 There is often some imprecision about the gestational age, but length can be measured fairly accurately. Use SAS to model gestational age from length. Why might this exercise be useful?

3.6 The map in Figure 3.4 shows drought conditions in the United States in the fall of 2007.[1] The lack of rainfall was most acute in the Southeast. Is this a map of the observed data, the expected mean values, or the residuals from the expected values? Which one of these three would be the best way to describe the weather conditions?

3.7 Examine the three weather maps in Figure 1.1. Identify which of these represents the raw data, which is the expected, and which of these is the residual. Which of these is most useful to you? For example, is it better to know that Florida was warm, or that Florida was expected to be warm, or that Florida was much colder than anticipated?

3.8 The Baltimore Orioles have not had a winning season in the decade since 1997, and their fans have not been kind to them. The average attendance per home game is given in Table 3.3 for the years 1998 through 2008.[2] Perform a linear regression modeling average attendance on the year. You might subtract 1997 from every year so that 1997 becomes year zero, or the baseline year. How do you

[1] Available online at http://www.ncdc.noaa.gov/img/climate/monitoring/drought/nadm/nadm-200709.jpg.
[2] Available online at http://www.nytimes.com/2008/11/28/sports/baseball/28orioles.html.

Table 3.3. Average attendance at Baltimore Orioles games.

Year	Games Won	Games Lost	Finishing rank	Average attendance
1998	79	83	4	45,496
1999	78	84	4	42,914
2000	74	88	4	40,681
2001	63	98	4	38,686
2002	67	95	4	33,112
2004	78	84	3	34,344
2005	74	88	4	32,404
2006	70	92	4	26,582
2007	69	93	4	27,060
2008	68	93	5	25,000

Reported by the *New York Times*, November 28, 2008.

interpret the estimated slope in your fitted regression model? Other analyses of these data appear in Exercises 5.4 and 6.3.

3.9 Table 3.4 gives the average weekly household expenditures on alcohol and tobacco (measured in pounds sterling) for each of the regions of Great Britain as reported by official 1981 government statistics.[3]

Plot the data and fit a model explaining values of one expenditure from the other. Why would you think that one of these variables should provide a good explanation for the values of the other?

From these data, can you conclude that households that consume more tobacco are also those that consume more alcohol? The people who smoke may or may not be the same people who drink alcohol, for example. Such macro data as these tells us only about aggregate behavior and cannot always be used to explain data at the individual level.

3.5.1 Statistics in the News: Savings for Medicare

Rather than assign a fixed dollar amount for medical equipment and supplies, Medicare will open the prices for some of these items to competitive bidding. This changes the way in which Medicare reimburses suppliers for medical supplies. Some of these items (diabetic test strips and nutritional supplies) are consumed, and others (hospital beds and wound therapy pumps) are leased.

Naturally, not everybody is pleased with this change. The news article[4] that accompanied the data in Table 3.5 also included a description of the intense lobbying effort mounted against these changes by certain medical equipment suppliers.

[3] Available online at http://lib.stat.cmu.edu/DASL/Datafiles/AlcoholandTobacco.html.
[4] Available online at http://www.nytimes.com/2008/06/25/business/25leonhardt.html.

Table 3.4. Average weekly household expenditures (in £) on alcohol and tobacco in Great Britain.

Region	Alcohol	Tobacco
North	6.47	4.03
Yorkshire	6.13	3.76
Northeast	6.19	3.77
East Midlands	4.89	3.34
West Midlands	5.63	3.47
East Anglia	4.52	2.92
Southeast	5.89	3.20
Southwest	4.79	2.71
Wales	5.27	3.53
Scotland	6.08	4.51
Northern Ireland	4.02	4.56

Perform a linear regression, explaining the new price y using the current price x. Notice that the largest percent savings are generally associated with the least expensive items. Why do you think this might be the case? Which changes do you think might produce greater savings: a large percentage change in an item that is consumed in large amounts (such as the test strips) or a similar change in an expensive, specialized wheelchair that only a few patients will need? Try to use linear regression to explain the percentage savings using the current price. Does this regression line have a useful interpretation?

3.5.2 Arsenic in Drinking Water

Arsenic is a potent poison, and ingesting or inhaling even small amounts can be fatal. It has been linked to a variety of different cancers as well. Long after death, arsenic

Table 3.5. Changes in the way Medicare pays for certain medical supplies.

Type of equipment	Current price	New price	Percent savings
Diabetic test strip, per 50	$36	$20	43%
CPAP respiratory device, per month	105	67	36
Enteral nutritional pump supplies, per day	12	9	30
Folding wheeled walker	112	78	30
Oxygen concentrator, per month	199	141	29
Hospital bed, per month	140	99	29
Standard power wheelchair	4024	3033	25
Wound therapy pump, per month	1716	1389	19
Power wheelchair with tilt system	8741	7530	14

Source: Centers for Medicare and Medicaid Services.

Table 3.6. Arsenic levels in well water and toenails of twenty-one New Hampshire residents.

Age in years	Sex (1 = M, 2 = F)	Drinking use	Cooking use	Arsenic in water (ppm)	Arsenic in toenails (ppm)
44	2	5	5	0.00087	0.119
45	2	4	5	0.00021	0.118
44	1	5	5	0	0.099
66	2	3	5	0.00115	0.118
37	1	2	5	0	0.277
45	2	5	5	0	0.358
47	1	5	5	0.00013	0.080
38	2	4	5	0.00069	0.158
41	2	3	2	0.00039	0.310
49	2	4	5	0	0.105
72	2	5	5	0	0.073
45	2	1	5	0.046	0.832
53	1	5	5	0.0194	0.517
86	2	5	5	0.137	2.252
8	2	5	5	0.0214	0.851
32	2	5	5	0.0175	0.269
44	1	5	5	0.0764	0.433
63	2	5	5	0	0.141
42	1	5	5	0.0165	0.275
62	1	5	5	0.00012	0.135
36	1	5	5	0.0041	0.175

Source: Statlib.

is detectable in the hair of the victim, so cases of poisoning can be discovered years after the fact. In some places, arsenic is present in the ground water, slowly affecting those who drink from these sources. In the United States, municipal water sources are regularly tested, but private wells are not.

The data in Table 3.6 was part of an epidemiology study of drinking water in New Hampshire.[5] Researchers from Dartmouth interviewed each of twenty-one residents who relied on private wells for much of their water for drinking or cooking. Each reported how much they relied on their private wells. (Household drinking and cooking use levels were coded as follows: 1, up to 1/4; 2, 1/4; 3, 1/2; 4, 3/5; and 5, over 3/4.) A sample of a toenail was taken from each resident and assayed for its arsenic content.

The arsenic levels in the water and toenails are measured in parts per million (ppm). A quick look at these values in Table 3.6 shows that the toenail arsenic levels

[5] Statlib is available online at http://lib.stat.cmu.edu/.

are all much higher than the water levels. This is consistent with the concentration of arsenic in the hair, long after ingestion.

Ideally, we might also want to know how long each resident had lived at that address and relied on the well water. In Chapter 5 we see how to take into account the additional effects such as age, sex, and level of household well water use.

For the present, use SAS to fit a linear regression using well arsenic level to explain the toenail levels. Verify that the fitted model is

$$\text{Toenail level} = 0.15504 + 12.98558 \times \text{Well water level.}$$

Are you concerned that the intercept is not zero? That is to say, with no exposure, there should also be no arsenic in the toenail. Can you offer another explanation for the nonzero estimated intercept in this model?

We can fit a regression model in SAS with a zero intercept. The code to do this uses the `noint` option as follows:

```
proc reg;
   model artoe = arwater / noint;
run;
```

Run this program and verify that the fitted model is

$$\text{Toenail level} = 14.86808 \times \text{Well water level.}$$

This model is interpreted as meaning that toenail levels are *proportional to* well-water levels of arsenic. Does this model offer a better interpretation than the linear regression model with an intercept?

Why is the slope in the zero-intercept model (14.868) larger than the slope in the model with an estimated intercept (12.986)? It may help to plot the two fitted models in order to answer this question.

3.5.3 Statistics in the News: Dermatologists' Fees

Dermatologists treat disorders of the skin, but also perform cosmetic surgery. The article associated with the data in Table 3.7[6] points out that there is a great divide between these two different roles. Some doctors will specialize in one or the other of these. Those who practice both cosmetic and medical surgery may have separate waiting rooms, appointment procedures, and treatment rooms for their patients, much as the airlines will segregate their first-class passengers from those paying to fly coach.

Medical procedures include the removal of moles and warts but also examination of cancerous and precancerous lesions. These are medically necessary procedures and are covered by Medicare and private insurance. Similarly, the reimbursement rates for these procedures are regulated by the amounts that insurance will cover. Cosmetic

[6] Available online at http://www.nytimes.com/2008/07/28/us/28beauty.html.

Table 3.7. Dermatologists' fees for medical and cosmetic procedures.

Medical procedure	National average Medicare reimbursement	Estimated time spent by doctor
Abscess treatment	$96	15 to 20 minutes
New patient visit	62 to 91	5 to 30 minutes
Visit with skin cancer exam	60 to 90	5 to 20 minutes
Wart removal	89	up to 5 minutes
Mole biopsy	88	1 to 7 minutes
Psoriasis photo-therapy	75	20 seconds
Destruction of pre-cancerous lesion	67	30 seconds to 5 minutes
Cosmetic procedure	National average physician fee	
Laser skin resurfacing	$2,418	30 to 40 minutes
Fat injection	1,546	20 minutes
Chemical peel	718	5 to 10 minutes
Restylane injection	576	5 to 6 minutes
Laser vein treatment	462	5 minutes
Laser hair removal	387	2 to 5 minutes
Botox injection	380	1 to 10 minutes

Source: Inga Eitzey Practice Group, American Society for Aesthetic Plastic Surgery, Dr. Mark Knautz and Dr. Kenneth Mark.

procedures are elective and are paid for out-of-pocket by the patient. Similarly, there is little oversight on how fees for cosmetic procedures are set. The data in Table 3.7 makes it very clear that these different classes of procedures represent very different fees for the doctors.

There is no need to resort to statistics to make the case that these different types of procedures have a different fee schedule. Instead, let us see how the fee schedule is determined, separately for medical and cosmetic procedures. Table 3.7 includes a rough estimate of the amount of time the doctor will spend in performing each of several types of procedures. Is there evidence that the fees charged are related to the time involved? Can we use linear regression to estimate the charge for a procedure based on the amount of time it takes to perform? There will be a separate regression line for medical and cosmetic procedures. Statisticians at insurance companies regularly use statistical methods such as these in order to determine reimbursement rates.

What assumptions do we need to make in order for this exercise to make sense? Do the various procedures (both medical and cosmetic) require additional equipment or drugs? This additional information would be useful in assigning a fee to a procedure. In this exercise we will need to assume that all procedures have roughly the same

Table 3.8. Breast cancer mortality rates in different countries.

Mortality rate	Mean annual temperature	Mortality rate	Mean annual temperature
102.5	51.3	104.5	49.9
100.4	50.0	95.9	49.2
87.0	48.5	95.0	47.8
88.6	47.3	89.2	45.1
78.9	46.3	84.6	42.1
81.7	44.2	72.2	43.5
65.1	42.3	68.1	40.2
67.3	31.8	52.5	34.0

Source: http://lib.stat.cmu.edu/DASL/Stories/Breastcancer.html.

overhead costs to the doctors. Where the time is given as a range, we might replace these with the midpoint, or perhaps use the longest estimate of time as a worst-possible case.

What other information would you like to see before being able to estimate the fees charged? Table 3.7 does not include the relative frequencies of these various procedures. Should a commonly performed procedure, for example, be associated with a lower cost than one rarely performed, all other things being equal?

3.5.4 Breast Cancer Survival and Climate

It is well known that some diseases have an environmental component. In a study of mortality rates in breast cancer, Table 3.8 provides the data for mean annual temperature in regions of Great Britain, Norway, and Sweden. Higher mortality rates translate into shorter survival times.

Fit a linear regression, estimating mortality rates from mean annual temperature. What is the equation of the fitted line? Look at a scatter plot of mortality and temperature. Notice how two observations represent much colder climates than the remainder of the data. Do these two observations follow the general trend in the data? Is it reasonable to use your regression model to estimate mortality rates in the range of temperatures for which there is no data? Why do you think that women in colder climates have better survival rates? What additional data would help you in answering this question?

Is this an observational study or a randomized experiment? Reread Section 1.6 and compare these two different types of data. What are the similarities and differences between the IMF data and this breast cancer data in the way that the data is collected and conclusions are drawn? Are we comfortable drawing conclusions from this study? What reservations did we have with drawing conclusions from the IMF data? Do you have the same reservations with this data?

Table 3.9. Rates per 100,000 persons of the leading causes of death for all ages in the United States, 1950–2004.

Year	All cause mortality	Heart disease	Cancer	Stroke	Respiratory diseases	Unintentional injury
1950	1,446.0	586.8	193.9	180.7		78.0
1960	1,339.2	559.0	193.9	177.9		62.3
1970	1,222.6	492.7	198.6	147.7		60.1
1980	1,039.1	412.1	207.9	96.2	28.3	46.4
1985	988.1	375.0	211.3	76.4	34.5	38.5
1990	938.7	321.8	216.0	65.3	37.2	36.3
1995	909.8	293.4	209.9	63.1	40.1	34.4
1996	894.1	285.7	206.7	62.5	40.6	34.5
1997	878.1	277.7	203.4	61.1	41.1	34.2
1998	870.6	271.3	200.7	59.3	41.8	34.5
1998*	870.6	267.4	202.1	62.8	43.8	35.6
1999	875.6	266.5	200.8	61.6	45.4	35.3
2000	869.0	257.6	199.6	60.9	44.2	34.9
2001	854.5	247.8	196.0	57.9	43.7	35.7
2002	845.3	240.8	193.5	56.2	43.5	36.9
2003	832.7	232.3	190.1	53.5	43.3	37.3
2004	800.8	217.0	185.8	50.0	41.1	37.7

* Adjusted because of a change in definitions.
Source: National Center for Health Statistics, *Health, United States, 2007.*

3.5.5 Vital Rates

Government agencies go to great effort to collect vital information on the well-being of the population. This data is made freely available to the public at no cost. One such table, selected from a large volume[7] is given in Table 3.9 and presents the rates of the five leading causes of mortality in the United States from 1950 to 2004. In the year 1998 a definition was changed, and the data for that year is presented both with and without the adjustment.

Much can be learned by studying tables such as these. Use linear regression methods to show that some rates such as heart disease and stroke have decreased over the years given in this table, but other rates such as those of cancer or respiratory diseases are flat or perhaps increasing.

Can you explain this finding? Despite the high level of funding for research, are we losing the "war on cancer" as some have claimed? Can you offer a different explanation? Perhaps the large drop in deaths due to heart disease is to blame for the lack of a decline in cancer rates. People who would have died of heart disease before 1970 are now living long enough to develop cancer.

[7] The document for 2007 is available online at http://www.cdc.gov/nchs/data/hus/hus07.pdf.

4

Assessing the Regression

How do we know if our linear regression is any good? We can take the results from Table 3.2 and test the null hypothesis that the regression slope is zero. That is, could this apparent regression have happened by chance alone, if x and y were really unrelated? What tangible benefit can we claim for performing a linear regression? The analysis of variance described in this chapter allows us to actually quantify the information gained when we examine a linear regression model. Even more importantly, is a straight line an appropriate summary for these data? Maybe there is a better explanation that describes a curved relationship between x and y. Finally, if there are remarkable exceptions to the linear pattern, how can we identify these observations? This chapter and the following use plots of the residual values to identify a large number of problems that can arise in fitting mathematical models to real data.

4.1 Correlation

The correlation coefficient is a single-number summary expressing the utility of a linear regression. The correlation coefficient is a dimensionless number between -1 and $+1$. The slope and the correlation have the same positive or negative sign. This single number is used to convey the strength of a linear relationship, so values closer to -1 or $+1$ indicate greater fidelity to a straight-line relationship.

The correlation measures the strength of a linear relationship.

The correlation is standardized in the sense that its value does not depend on the means or standard deviations of the x or y values. If we add or subtract the same values from the data (and thereby change the means), the correlation remains the same. If we multiply all the xs (or the ys) by some positive value, the correlation

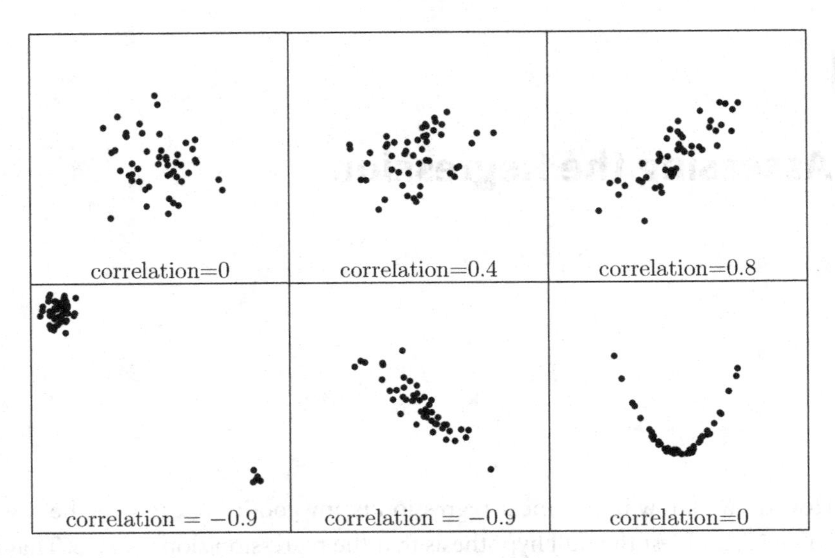

Figure 4.1 Simulated datasets illustrating different correlations.

remains the same. If we multiply either the *x*s or the *y*s by a negative number, the sign of the correlation will reverse.

As with any oversimplification of a complex situation, the correlation coefficient has its benefits, but also its shortcomings. A variety of values of the correlation are illustrated in Figure 4.1. Each of these separate graphs consists of 50 simulated (computer-generated) pairs of observations. A correlation of 0 in the upper left of Figure 4.1 shows no indication of a linear relationship between the plotted variables. A correlation of 0.4 does not indicate much strength, either. A correlation of either 0.8 or −0.9 indicates a rather strong linear trend. Notice that the sign of the correlation is the same as that of the slope.

It is possible to have a high correlation with little or no linear trend. The correlation of −0.9 in the lower-left example is more the result of the small number of unusual individual observations than an indication of a true trend in the data. The big separated group in the upper-left corner is more representative of the population and exhibits no trend at all.

Similarly, a zero correlation does not indicate that these measures are unrelated. In the lower-right example of Figure 4.1, we see that the two variables have a very strong relationship but that it is not a *linear* relationship. The correlation coefficient is useful only in measuring the strength of a linear relationship.

The lessons we learn by looking at the plotted data in Figure 4.1 is that the correlation coefficient conveys an indication of a trend, but we still need to look at the scatter plot in order to understand the true nature of our data. Just as we say that a picture is worth a thousand words, we could say that a single number cannot possibly describe every situation we are likely to encounter. Despite these shortcomings,

Table 4.1. The correlations between U.S. and other foreign stock markets.

Country	Correlation with the S&P 500
Germany	0.89
France	0.88
Spain	0.85
MSCI EAFE	0.85
Britain	0.81
Italy	0.75
Mexico	0.74
Brazil	0.68
South Korea	0.67
Singapore	0.66
Hong Hong	0.55
China	0.53
India	0.43
Russia	0.35
Japan	0.29

Source: Standard & Poor's.

the correlation coefficient remains one of the most important summaries of the relationship between measurements on two variables.

The correlation coefficient is often expressed as its square and referred to as R^2 or *r-squared.* This definition is useful when we generalize linear regression to multivariate models in Chapter 5, where we consider models in which there are several explanatory variables. Just as with the correlation, the value of R^2 remains unchanged if we subject either of the two variables to a linear transformation. That is, we can add or subtract, multiply or divide (by a nonzero value) either the x or y variables, and the resulting values will have the same value of R^2.

4.2 Statistics in the News: Correlations of the Global Economy

In an article about investing,[1] Table 4.1 presents the correlations between returns in several foreign stock markets with that of the United States. The Standard and Poor's 500 (S&P 500) is a weighted average of prices of the stocks of the 500 largest U.S. companies and is a surrogate for almost all of the U.S. stock market. The correlation of each country's data with the S&P 500 is taken over the previous five years. The MSCI EAFE Index, a weighted average of several countries' data, is also given here.

[1] Available online at http://www.nytimes.com/2007/06/03/business/yourmoney/03fund.html.

Some countries, notably Germany, France, and Spain, have stock markets that closely follow that of the United States. The article suggests that such investments would not provide any diversity and it would not be worth the additional risks of sending money overseas. Stock markets in India, Russia, and Japan, for examples, have much lower correlation with those in the United States and would provide greater diversification.

Notice how a large amount of data has been reduced to a single number: the correlation. As we saw in Figure 4.1, the correlation can be useful in some settings but may oversimplify more complex relationships. Domestic problems, such as a flood, may affect one country's economy but not others. Global changes in oil prices, for example, can affect many nations. The correlations in this table reflect all of these events, but do not offer an explanation or provide critical details that might be helpful.

The article that accompanies this data concludes that investments in Japanese stocks would provide a good counterbalance to those in Europe and the United States. An investment in Japan would not necessarily provide better returns, but instead might be less volatile. One market zigs while the other zags, so to speak. A small variability is reassuring when it comes to one's savings. Table 4.1 suggests a way in which investors could reduce the variance of their investment returns by diversifying across countries, but it does not explain how to increase the mean. (Which do you feel is more important: the mean rate of return, or the volatility experienced along the way?) The correlation is standardized, so it doesn't directly measure either of these.

Finally, notice that there are no negative correlations in this data. It would be useful to know if there were stock markets that moved in opposite directions, one rising while the others fell. This would provide a useful way to hedge one's bets.

4.3 Analysis of Variance

Just as a statement from an accountant details how money was earned and spent, the analysis of variance (frequently abbreviated as ANOVA) is the statistician's table to explain, partition, and allocate variability in the data. To continue this analogy, variability is the currency of statistics. If all data always fell perfectly on a straight line, there would be no need for us to study statistics. Similarly, the ANOVA details the departure from a straight-line relationship.

What is the variability that we are going to examine? Let us look back at Figure 3.2 to see where the variability occurs. Notice that the residuals are defined in terms of the vertical differences so that all of the variability occurs along the y axis. All of the variability occurs within the dependent variable that we want to explain.

The variability of these values is measured by

$$\text{Total sum of squares} = \sum (y_i - \bar{y})^2 \tag{4.1}$$

Table 4.2. The analysis of variance produced by the SAS program in Table 3.1.

```
                         Analysis of Variance

                                        Sum of           Mean
Source                      DF         Squares         Square    F Value

Model                        1         4800035        4800035     194.65
Error                       98         2416708          24660
Corrected Total             99         7216743

Root MSE             157.03593    R-Square     0.6651
Dependent Mean      1098.85000    Adj R-Sq     0.6617
Coeff Var             14.29093
```

This expression, divided by $n - 1$, is denoted by s^2. We use s^2 to estimate the variance of y in the absence of any knowledge of an explanatory variable x. The expression for s^2 was given in (1.1). The analysis of variance allows us to quantify the benefit of knowing x and using it as an explanatory variable in a linear regression. This benefit is expressed as a reduction in the variability of the y values.

In the analysis of variance, (4.1) is called the *total sum of squares.* In Section 2.7 we saw that this expression is associated with $n - 1$ degrees of freedom. This quantity is listed by SAS as `Corrected Total` in Table 4.2 under the `Source` column. There are 100 observations in the data, so this value is listed with 99 df. The total sum of squares, as with the accounting analogy, is the total amount of variability we have to work with. Ultimately we want to show how much of this variability is reduced by knowing x and how much is lost to random variability that we cannot otherwise explain.

The *error sum of squares* is just that: the sum of squared residuals, defined at (3.2), that we want to minimize. The computer finds the values of the slope and intercept that minimize this quantity. The error sum of squares is the value at its minimum. For the example, this value is listed as `Error` in Table 4.2 under the `Source` column.

$$\text{Error sum of squares} = \sum (\text{residual}_i)^2$$

There are 100 residuals in this example, but these are subject to two linear restrictions given at (3.3) and (3.4). Specifically, the residuals sum to 0 and are uncorrelated with the explanatory x values. These two restrictions result in a loss of 2 df, so Table 4.2 lists the error sum of squares with $100 - 2 = 98$ df.

Some books and computer programs will also call this quantity the *residual sum of squares.* Still other books and computer programs will call this the *unexplained variability* or the *unexplained sum of squares* because it represents the noise that is left over after fitting the linear regression model.

The residuals represent departures from the model, and the model is fitted in a way that makes the error sum of squares as small as possible. Intuitively, the residuals represent the part of the data that cannot be explained by the model; hence the name.

If the total sum of squares measures the whole amount of variability present in the data and the residual sums of squares is the unexplained portion of this, then the difference must be the part that is explained by the model. This difference is called the *model sum of squares* in the SAS output of Table 4.2. Expressed another way:

Total sum of squares = Model SS + Error SS

In other words, the total amount of variability in the values (the y_i) that we want to explain can be decomposed into the sum of the amount explained by the model (knowing the xs), and the remainder is random noise or error. We can verify that this relationship in the ANOVA is indeed the case with the numbers in the example of Table 4.2.

Just as the sums of squares add up in this table, so do the degrees of freedom. The degrees of freedom for the model sum of squares are equal to 1 in this example. When we build more complex models involving additional explanatory variables in Chapter 5, the model df will equal the number of explanatory variables in those models. For the time being, our model has only one x variable.

The R^2 is an important measure that reflects how much of the total variability is explained by the model. Specifically, we define the R^2 as

$$R^2 = \frac{\text{Model sum of squares}}{\text{Total sum of squares}} .$$

We should look back at the SAS output in Table 4.2 and use a calculator to verify that this is indeed the case. When R^2 is written in this fashion, we see that it also has the popular interpretation

R^2 is the percent of total sum of squares explained by the model.

The values in the `Mean Square` column of Table 4.2 are obtained by dividing the sums of squares by their degrees of freedom. Again, a quick calculation should convince you of this.

The last entry for the ANOVA in Table 4.2 is the `F value`, which is calculated as

$$F = \frac{\text{MS(model)}}{\text{MS(error)}} .$$

The F statistic (sometimes called the *F ratio*) provides a statistical test of the contribution of the model in explaining the total variability of y. If we think of the model sum of squares as the explained variation and the error sum of squares as the unexplained part, we want this ratio to be large. Another way to think about F is the signal-to-noise ratio. Ideally, we want a strong signal in the numerator relative to the noise component in the denominator. There are tables of the F statistic, but SAS will usually provide a p-value, so there is no real need to refer to them.

The p-value of the F statistic provides a significance test that the slope of the regression model is zero. We have already seen such a test in the computer output in Table 3.2. When there is only one explanatory variable, we have $t^2 = F$. In this particular example, we have $t = 13.95$ for the slope in Table 3.2 and $F = 194.6$ in Table 4.2. We can verify that

$$13.95^2 = 194.6,$$

so here is another check on the relationships that exist in the analysis of variance. In Chapter 5, when we talk about more than one x variable in the model, F tests whether *all* of the slopes are zero.

Below the ANOVA in Table 4.2 are a series of other useful statistics. These include the squared correlation coefficient ($R^2 = 0.6651$). The adjusted R^2 is described in Section 5.6 when we discuss multiple linear regression.

Perhaps the most important number of all in this table is denoted by `Root MSE` or root mean squared error. In this table we can verify that

$$\texttt{Root MSE} = \sqrt{24660} = 157.04$$

is indeed the square root of the mean square for error in the analysis of variance.

This value represents the estimated standard deviation of the residuals. Recall that residuals represent the differences between the observed and expected values for our regression line. The root mean squared error represents the standard deviation or magnitude of this difference. This number tells us how far the observed data are from the fitted line. Of course there will be outliers and exceptions to the rule, but if we assume that observations are normally distributed about the regression line, we now have an estimate of the standard deviation of that normal distribution. This brings us to the assumptions we make about the linear regression model, which are described in the following section.

4.4 Model Assumptions and Residual Plots

The computer can always calculate whatever you ask it to, but cannot be expected to judge the validity or appropriateness of the methods used. The p-value for the F statistic in the analysis of variance represents a calculation by a machine that does not know anything about how your data was obtained. In order for the model to accurately explain the data and for your p-value to represent a meaningful test of the null hypothesis, we need to make some assumptions about the data.

Many diagnostics about the regression model can be derived using plots of the residuals of the fitted model. The residuals can easily be obtained and examined, but the crucial concept is that these are sampled from a larger, unobservable population.

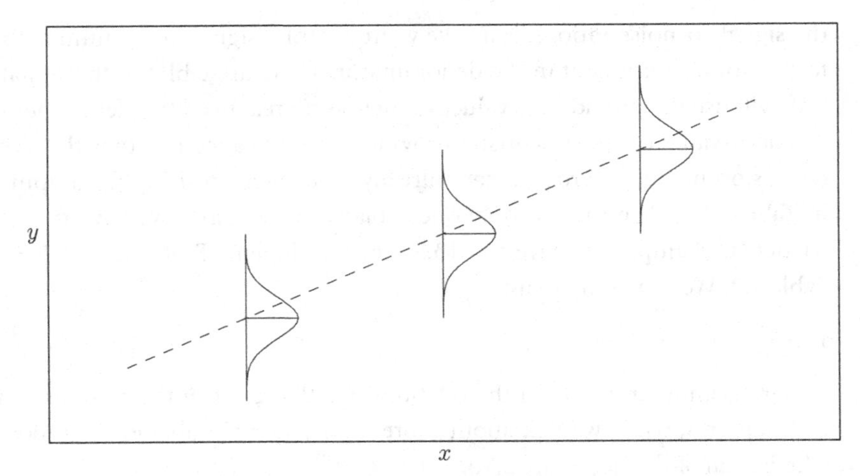

Figure 4.2 The idealized regression model is a series of normal distributions centered along the regression line.

In Section 1.1 we made this distinction between sampled data and the larger population. As with all statistical inference, a sample (in this case, of residuals) is used to infer properties of a much larger population. This population is referred to as the *error distribution*. The residuals are an observed sample of errors.

The model assumptions are expressed in terms of the error distribution. These are

1. Errors are independent
2. Errors have constant variance
3. Errors have mean zero
4. Errors follow a normal distribution

Think of the regression model as a series of normal distributions centered along the regression line. Figure 4.2 will help you to visualize this. At any given value of x, there is a y value sampled from the normal distribution whose mean is equal to $\alpha + \beta x$. The standard deviation of this regression line is estimated by the root mean squared error, described in the previous section.

All of the assumptions we need to make about the model are concerned with the errors. We cannot observe the errors, and we only have a sample of residuals from that population. The most important message, then, is that we must take the residuals very seriously. We cannot abrogate our responsibility and ask for a statistical test of these assumptions to let us off the hook. One of the most important tools available to us is to

Plot and examine the residuals for your model.

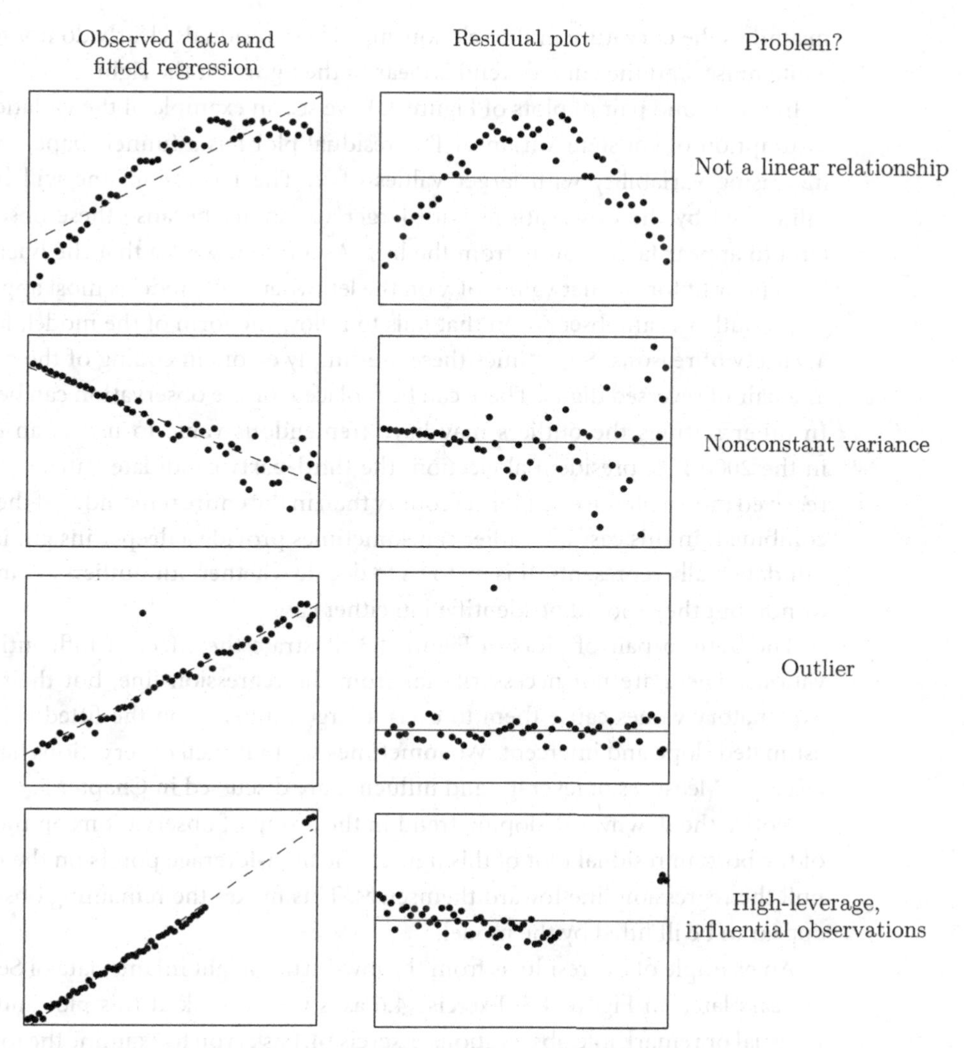

Figure 4.3 Simulated datasets illustrating different problems that residual plots may uncover.

This one simple technique is, by far, the most powerful and yet simplest way to diagnose many of the problems that may exist in a regression model. The true difficulty will be for the user of these methods to verify that the assumptions are met. The computer cannot do this for us. We need to examine these plots and try to infer whether the model is appropriate or not. The residual values are typically plotted on the vertical axis, and the horizontal axis might be either the explanatory value x or the estimated value $\widehat{y}$.

Figure 4.3 presents a set of four problems in data analysis that might arise when we perform a linear regression. In most cases the residual plot will magnify the problem and make it more easily apparent and diagnosed. At the top of this figure we see that the relationship between x and y is not a straight line. The residual plot magnifies the curvature in the relationship. These residuals clearly do not represent white noise, and the curved trend is clear in the figure on the right.

In the second pair of plots of Figure 4.3, we see an example of the violation of the assumption of constant variance. The residual plot has a funnel shape, indicating increasing variability with larger values of x. The regression line will be overly influenced by the observations with larger variability because these observations tend to appear farther away from the line. As a result, we see that the linear model has a poor fit for smaller values of x on the left where the model is most appropriate.

An outlier is an observation that fails to follow the form of the model, for any of a variety of reasons. Sometimes these are simply errors in coding of the data, such as a pair of reversed digits. These can be replaced, or the observation can be deleted. In other settings the outliers may have tremendous value to us. As an example, in the 2000 U.S. presidential election, the third-party candidate Patrick Buchanan received more votes in one Florida county than in the entire remainder of the country combined. In this case an outlier can sometimes provide a deeper insight into what our data really represents. It is up to us to decide whether our outliers are important or not, but they should be identified in either case.

The bottom pair of plots in Figure 4.3 illustrate the effect of influential observations. These are not necessarily far from the regression line, but their unusual explanatory values cause them to exert a large influence on the fitted value of the estimated slope and intercept. We sometimes say that such observations have a high leverage. Measures of leverage and influence are discussed in Chapter 5.

Notice the downward-sloping trend in the group of observations on the left side of the bottom residual plot of this figure. The high-leverage points on the right side pull the regression line toward themselves. This makes the remaining observations appear to be ill fitted by the model.

An example of the residuals from the low-birth-weight infants data of Section 3.1 appears later, in Figure 4.5. Exercise 4.6 asks you to look at this plot and identify unusual or remarkable observations. Exercise 4.1 asks you to examine the four model assumptions described in this section for a dataset appearing in the news.

4.5 Exercises

4.1 Figure 4.4 is a graph of U.S. airline profits since 1978 plotted by year. Suppose we were to produce a linear regression on profit using the year as the explanatory variable. Look at the four important assumptions in Section 4.4. Which of these model assumptions are violated when we perform this linear regression?

4.2 What is the largest correlation that can be achieved with exactly three pairs of observations? Draw a scatter plot to show how this can be achieved. Similarly, can a correlation of exactly 0 be achieved with three pairs of observations? What might this scatter plot look like?

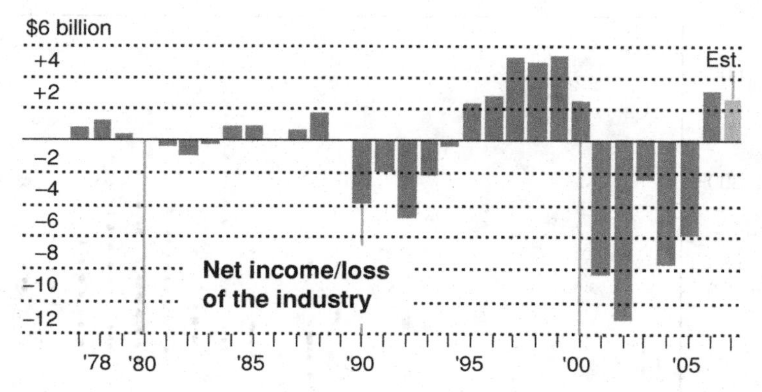

Figure 4.4 Airline profits since 1978. *Source:* The *New York Times*, April 17, 2008, page C10.

4.3 Suppose I found the correlation between x and y. If I add 5 to all of the x values, what is the new correlation between x and y? If I multiply all the y values by 3, what is the new correlation? If I multiply all the values of x by -2, what is the new correlation between x and y?

4.4 I prepared an analysis of variance for homework, but my dog ate it. All that is left is given in Table 4.3. Can you fill in the parts that are missing?

4.5 Look back at the arsenic data examined in Exercise 3.5.2. Examine the residuals for this fitted regression and compare your plot to those in Figure 4.3. Identify the individual with the highest arsenic exposure. Is this observation influential in the regression model? What happens to the fitted regression coefficients when this one individual is deleted and the model is refitted?

4.6 a. Look at the low-birth-weight data on infants from Chapter 3. The residuals from the regression in Figure 3.1 are given in Figure 4.5. What do you learn by looking at this figure? Can you identify outliers or highly influential observations? The variability of the residuals seems to decrease with the fitted value. Why does this appear to be the case? Remember what it means for an infant to have a low birth weight.

b. Fit some other regression models to this data. Draw some graphs of observed values and the residuals from your regression. Comment on what you see. See

Table 4.3. Part of the output for Exercise 4.4.

Source	df	Sum of Squares	Mean Square	F value
Model	1			4.0
Error			8.0	
Total	21			

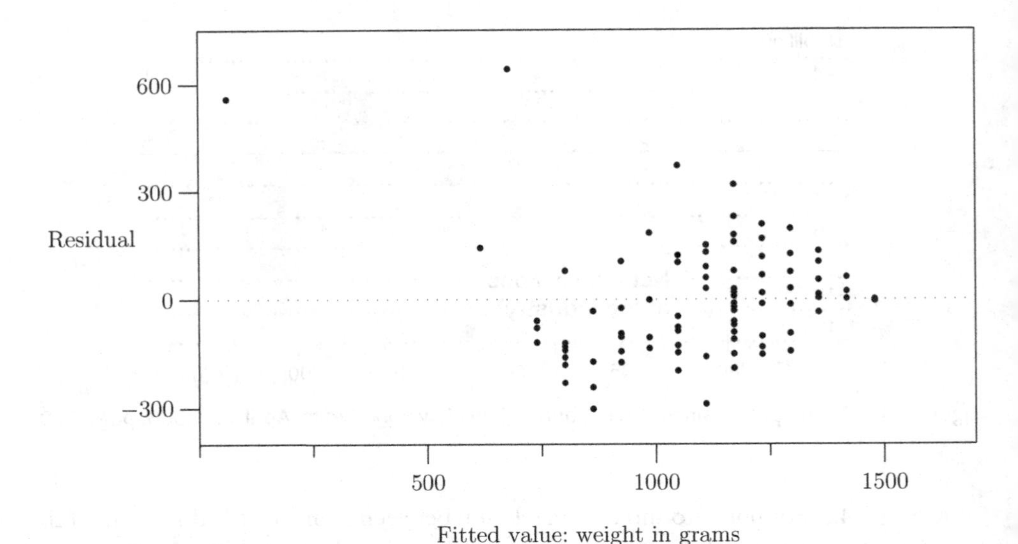

Figure 4.5 Residuals for low-birth-weight babies.

if you can find outliers and or influential observations. Identify the equation of your linear regression. Cite statistical measures of significance levels.

Why did you choose the explanatory x and response y variables that you did? Is linear regression appropriate for this pair of values in the dataset? Are there other variables that you would like to know about that are not given here? What additional knowledge do you have about infants that you can use to provide a better understanding of the examination of this data?

4.5.1 Statistics in the News: Food Imports

Following reports of tainted pet food, seafood, toothpaste, and pharmaceutical additives from China, the data in Table 4.4 appeared,[2] demonstrating that food shipments are refused by U.S. customs officials from other countries as well. Common sense indicates that the number of shipments refused should be related to the total number of shipments. The numbers of shipments are not provided, but instead the table gives the total value of all food imports for each of the countries listed.

Plot the value of the total food imports (as the explanatory variable x) against the number of shipments refused y. What do you see? Does the slope go in the direction you expected it to? Can you provide an explanation for this?

Notice the very large influence in this graph of the total food imports from Mexico. The total value of these imports is about as great as that of all of the other listed countries' imports combined. Why do you think this may be the case?

Relatively few shipments from Mexico are refused relative to their total import value. What do you think is the reason for this? Look at the most frequent reasons

[2] Available online at http://www.nytimes.com/2007/07/12/business/12imports.html.

Table 4.4. Food import shipments refused at the border by the FDA. Those countries with the largest number of refusals are listed.

Country	Number of shipments refused	Frequency of most common refusal	Total value food imports
India	1,763	256	$1.2B
Mexico	1,480	385	9.8
China	1,368	287	3.8
Dominican Rep	828	789	0.3
Denmark	543	85	0.4
Vietnam	553	118	1.1
Japan	508	143	0.5
Italy	482	138	2.9
Indonesia	460	122	1.5

given for food refused from Japan, Denmark, and Italy to see if this may be the case. These countries also export relatively small amounts of food to the United States.

Fit the linear regression with all of the data and then again excluding Mexico. Is the fitted model different? Comment on the change in correlation and the statistical significance in the $F-$ratio.

The total import value data covers the calendar year 2006 but does not exactly coincide with the time period for the food shipment refusal data. What additional data would you need to see if imports from China were being given greater scrutiny following news reports? What additional information would you need in order to tell if food imports from all source countries were being examined more closely following the news?

4.5.2 Statistics in the News: Women Managers

It is not news that large numbers of women are entering the workforce, but there are often complaints about the "glass ceiling" that prevents their promotion to the ranks of management. The data in Table 4.5 compares the promotion rates in ten different countries. For each country we have the percentages of women employed as managers in the years 1985 and 2005. The newspaper article[3] points out that although Japan has passed several antidiscrimination laws, the laws are rarely enforced, and there is a cultural reluctance to initiate lawsuits. There has also been little change in South Korea, but the other Asian nations of Singapore and Malaysia have made large advances in promoting women to management positions.

Use linear regression to explain the 2005 rates in terms of the 1985 rates. Plot the raw data. Is there evidence that the variance is not constant? Explain why this might be the case. Examine the fitted regression coefficients and explain these values in terms of the original data.

[3] Available online at http://www.nytimes.com/2007/08/06/world/asia/06equal.html.

Table 4.5. Percentage of management jobs held by women in 1985 and 2005.

	Percent of female managers	
Country	in 1985	in 2005
Philippines	21.9	57.8
United States	35.6	42.5
Germany	25.8	37.3
Australia	17.6	37.3
Britain	32.9	34.5
Norway	22.0	30.5
Singapore	12.0	25.9
Malaysia	8.7	23.2
Japan	6.6	10.1
South Korea	3.7	7.8

Source: New York Times, August 6, 2007.

Suppose we wanted to examine the percentage change in these rates. Construct a new variable that is defined as the 2005 rate divided by the 1985 rate. Perform a linear regression to explain this new variable from the 1985 rate. Notice that the slope is negative. Does this mean that those countries with the lowest 1985 rates tended to have the greatest percentage increase in women managers? Can you provide a different interpretation of this regression slope?

4.5.3 Statistics Is More Than Just Numbers

Francis J. Anscombe[4] was the founder of the Statistics Department at Yale University. He created the four datasets given in Table 4.6. These are the most amazing datasets ever! If you examine only the statistics from the computer output, you might be led to think that these four were the same data.

In this exercise, pick any two of these four datasets and see how similar the computed numbers appear when you regress y on x. Run SAS programs you are familiar with, such as `means`, `univariate`, and `reg`. Which summary statistical measures are the same for the pair of datasets you choose? If you are unsure, try looking at a third dataset. In what ways are the datasets different? You might begin, for example, by noting, that the first three datasets all have identical values for their x variable.

When you are done, look at the scatter plot of x and y values for the datasets you examined. Note how very different these are. Describe each dataset in a sentence or two. Notice how all of the summary statistics fail to tell us what the data actually is.

[4] Francis John Anscombe (1918–2001). British statistician.

Table 4.6. The four datasets from Anscombe (1973), listed as (*x*, *y*) pairs.

First dataset							
10	8.04	8	6.95	13	7.58	9	8.81
11	8.33	14	9.96	6	7.24	4	4.26
12	10.84	7	4.82	5	5.68		
Second dataset							
10	9.14	8	8.14	13	8.74	9	8.77
11	9.26	14	8.10	6	6.13	4	3.10
12	9.13	7	7.26	5	4.74		
Third dataset							
10	7.46	8	6.77	13	12.74	9	7.11
11	7.81	14	8.84	6	6.08	4	5.39
12	8.15	7	6.42	5	5.73		
Fourth dataset							
8	6.58	8	5.76	8	7.71	8	8.84
8	8.47	8	7.04	8	5.25	8	5.56
8	7.91	8	6.89	19	12.50		

Which description is more meaningful: the graph or the summary statistics? Which would you rather have?

The conclusion of this exercise is an important lesson:

> Statistics is much more than formulas and numbers.

It is possible to summarize data in any number of ways and still miss the point. You might think that the mean and standard deviation contain just about all you need to know about your data, and if you do, you could be way off the mark. A correlation could represent a wide variety of different situations. We saw this in the examples of Figure 4.1. You might reread the example appearing in Section 1.6 to see how the statistical methods can be carefully applied and still yield absurd conclusions.

5

Multiple Linear Regression

We often have several possible explanatory variables that may be of use in helping us model the outcome variable. Some of these have more explanatory value than others, some may be redundant, and others may be totally useless.

Multivariate models bring a new set of challenges and tools for modeling data. The reward for our efforts is that we are often able to summarize a large amount of data in a succinct fashion.

5.1 Introductory Example: Maximum January Temperatures

The dataset listed in Table 5.1 provides the maximum January temperature for many U.S. cities. Also given are latitude (degrees north from the equator); longitude (degrees East/West); and altitude above sea level in feet. The start of a SAS program is given in Table 5.2.

The regression model fitted by the SAS program in Table 5.2 is

$$\text{maxt} = \alpha + \beta_1\text{lat} + \beta_2\text{long} + \beta_3\text{alt} + \text{error}. \tag{5.1}$$

The model specifies that the maximum January temperature is linearly related to each of latitude, longitude, and altitude, separately. The SAS program estimates the intercept α and each of the regression slopes β_1, β_2, and β_3. We interpret this model to mean that the maximum January temperature is the sum of the individual effects of latitude, longitude, and altitude. There is an intercept (α) and three regression slopes that need to be estimated. In such a model we sometimes say that temperature is *corrected* for the separate effects of these three explanatory variables.

In the `model` statement of `proc reg`,

```
model maxt = lat long alt;
```

from the program in Table 5.2, we put the dependent variable that we wish to explain on the left of the "=" sign and provide a list of the explanatory variables on the right. The SAS programming is then no more difficult than what we saw in Chapter 3. The

Table 5.1. Maximum January temperature (T, in degrees Fahrenheit), latitude, longitude, altitude in feet above sea level, and the name for the some of the largest U.S. cities. Data from Mosteller and Tukey (1977, pp. 73–4), with a corrections.

T	Lat	Long	Alt	Name	T	Lat	Long	Alt	Name
61	30	88	5	Mobile AL	59	32	86	160	Montgomery AL
30	58	134	50	Juneau AK	64	33	112	1,090	Phoenix AZ
51	34	92	286	Little Rock AR	65	34	118	340	Los Angeles CA
55	37	122	65	San Francisco	42	39	104	5,280	Denver CO
37	41	72	40	New Haven CT	41	39	75	135	Wilmington DE
44	38	77	25	Washington DC	67	30	81	20	Jacksonville FL
74	24	81	5	Key West FL	76	25	80	10	Miami FL
52	33	84	1,050	Atlanta GA	79	21	157	21	Honolulu HI
36	43	116	2,704	Boise ID	33	41	87	595	Chicago IL
37	39	86	710	Indianapolis IN	29	41	93	805	Des Moines IA
27	42	90	620	Dubuque IA	42	37	97	1,290	Wichita KS
44	38	85	450	Louisville KY	64	29	90	5	New Orleans LA
32	43	70	25	Portland ME	44	39	76	20	Baltimore MD
37	42	71	21	Boston MA	33	42	83	585	Detroit MI
23	46	84	650	Sault Ste Marie	22	44	93	815	Minneapolis MN
40	38	90	455	St Louis MO	29	46	112	4,155	Helena MT
32	41	95	1,040	Omaha NE	32	43	71	290	Concord NH
43	39	74	10	Atlantic City NJ	46	35	106	4,945	Albuquerque NM
31	42	73	20	Albany NY	40	40	73	55	New York NY
51	35	80	720	Charlotte NC	52	35	78	365	Raleigh NC
20	46	100	1,674	Bismark ND	41	39	84	550	Cincinnati OH
35	41	81	660	Cleveland OH	46	35	97	1,195	Oklahoma City
44	45	122	77	Portland OR	39	40	76	365	Harrisburg PA
40	39	75	100	Philadelphia PA	61	32	79	9	Charleston SC
34	44	103	3,230	Rapid City SD	49	36	86	450	Nashville, TN
50	35	101	3,685	Amarillo TX	61	29	94	5	Galveston TX
37	40	111	4,390	Salt Lake City	25	44	73	110	Burlington VT
50	36	76	10	Norfolk VA	44	47	122	10	Seattle WA
31	47	117	1,890	Spokane WA	26	43	89	860	Madison WI
28	43	87	635	Milwaukee WI	37	41	104	6,100	Cheyenne WY
81	18	66	35	San Juan PR					

output in Table 5.3 lists (among other things) estimates for the intercept (α) and each of the three regression coefficients (βs) along with their standard errors.

Northern cities are colder than most, as are cities at high altitudes. We should not be surprised to see the corresponding negative estimated slopes in Table 5.3 because these represent negative correlations.

Let us interpret the output in Table 5.3. The estimated regression coefficient for latitude (-1.95981) is negative. We can intuit that for every degree north of the

Table 5.2. Part of a SAS program for the January temperature data.

```
options linesize=78 center pagesize=60 number;

title1 'Max Jan Temp: Lat, Long, and Altitude for Major US Cities';
data cold;
   infile 'c:\hot.dat';  /* You will need to modify this line */
   input
      maxt  lat  long  alt  city $  18-35;
   longe=180-long;       /* reverse east and west */
   label     /* Get in the habit of labeling variables of complicated
                  data sets so you will remember what they are   */
     maxt = 'maximum January temperature'
     lat  = 'degrees latitude'
     long = 'degrees longitude'
     longe= 'longitude east'
     alt  = 'altitude above sea level - ft'
     city = 'city name' ;
run;

proc print;  /* Always print it all out */
run;

proc gplot;
   title2 'A map of the major U.S. cities';
   plot longe * lat;
run;

title2 'Explain max Jan temperature';
proc reg;
   model maxt = lat long alt; /* specify the y and x variables */
   output residual = resid;
run;

title2 'Bubble plot residuals by longitude';
proc gplot;
   bubble resid*longe = alt;  /* greater altitude: larger bubbles */
run;

quit;
```

Table 5.3. Part of the output from the SAS program in Table 5.2.

Analysis of Variance

Source	DF	Sum of Squares	Mean Square	F Value	Pr > F
Model	3	11170	3723.26033	129.41	<.0001
Error	57	1640	28.77002		
Corrected Total	60	12810			

Parameter Estimates

Variable	Label	Parameter Estimate	Standard Error	Value	Pr > |t|
Intercept	Intercept	100.94498	5.19332	19.44	<.0001
lat	degrees latitude	-1.95981	0.10481	-18.70	<.0001
long	degrees longitude	0.21003	0.04129	5.09	<.0001
alt	altitude	-0.00164	0.00051794	-3.17	0.0024

equator, the temperature drops by almost 2 degrees Fahrenheit. This estimate is more than 18 times its estimated standard error (0.10481), so latitude has a huge effect in explaining the different temperatures of the various cities. Similarly, altitude plays a large role in explaining the different temperatures. Cities at higher altitudes are colder; hence the negative estimated regression coefficient. For every 1,000 feet above sea level, the estimated temperature drops 1.64 degrees. The estimated intercept ($\widehat{\alpha}$) in this table and other analyses of these data are described in Exercise 5.7.2.

Estimates of the regression coefficients ($\alpha, \beta_1, \beta_2, \beta_3$) for the model in (5.1) are obtained by SAS using least squares. Specifically, these are obtained by making the sum of squared errors as small as possible. This approach for estimating regression parameters was covered in Section 3.2 for a model with a single explanatory variable. The same approach is followed here in multiple regression models, except that SAS will minimize an expression similar to (3.2) with respect to several regression slopes.

The output of `proc reg` in multiple regression includes the analysis of variance given in Table 5.3 and can be compared to the output given in Table 4.2. The largest difference we see is that the model sums of squares will have 1 df for every regression slope that appears in our model. As with simple linear regression, the sums of squares and df will add up just as in Exercise 4.4. The mean squares are again defined as sums of squares divided by their degrees of freedom. The F statistic provides a significance test of the null hypothesis that all of the regression slopes are zero in the population.

Here are some things to think about as we proceed. What about northern cities at high altitude? Is their January temperature the sum of its parts, or is there a synergy?

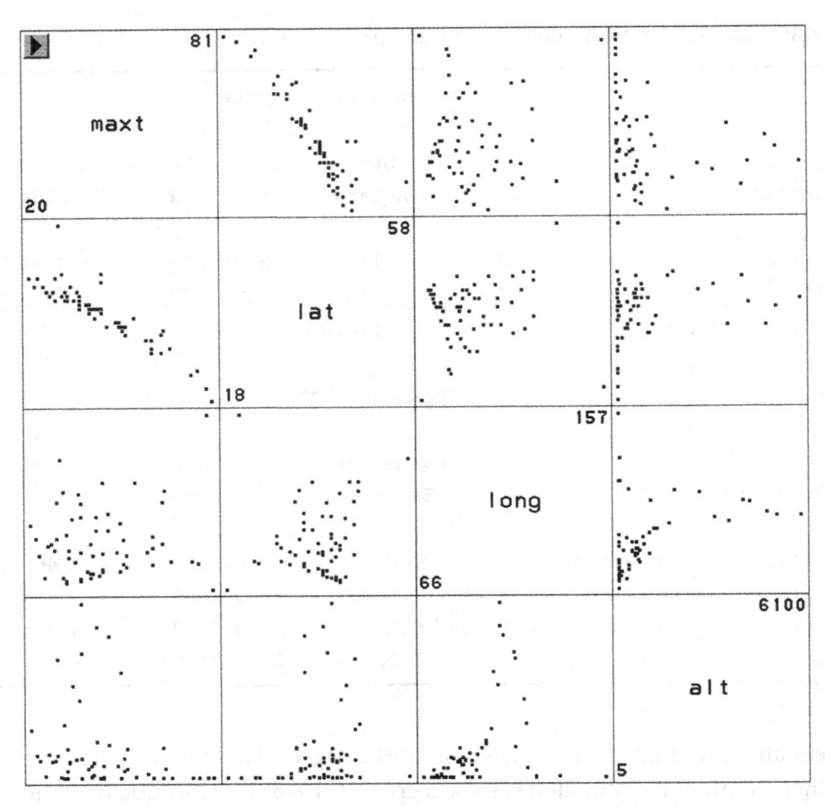

Figure 5.1 A matrix scatter plot of every January temperature variable plotted against every other using `proc insight`.

Synergy occurs when two factors combine to produce a greater effect than either one individually, working together like a well-practiced sports team. Think of it as a situation in which $1 + 1 = 3$. We address synergy in Section 6.3. The present chapter describes several measures of influence. Before we get to these topics, we look at a variety of graphical displays for multivariate data such as these.

5.2 Graphical Displays of Multivariate Data

Before we describe some of the methodology used with multivariate regression methods, let us examine some of the popular methods for graphically displaying such data. A moment's reflection will reveal that the display of multivariate data is a challenging task: it is very difficult to display several different kinds of information simultaneously on a two-dimensional piece of paper. A bit of creativity has been needed and used to create these displays. This section introduces a few of these methods.

The scatter plot is well known to the reader. The display in Figure 5.1 provides a "matrix" of scatter plots for every pair of variables in the linear regression model.

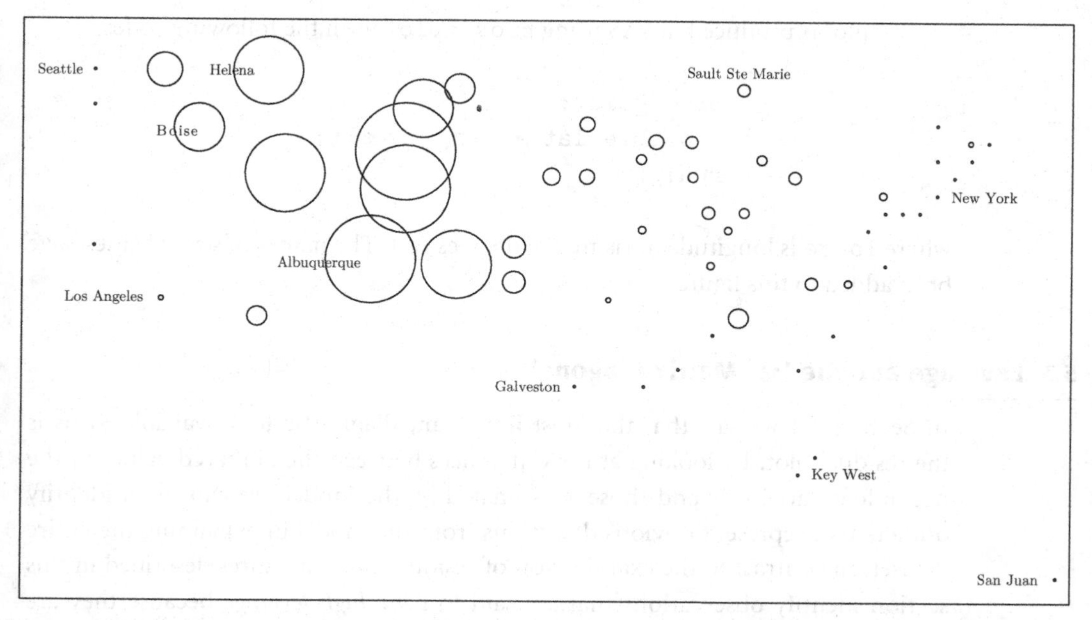

Figure 5.2 A bubble plot map of U.S. cities, omitting Juneau and Honolulu. Several key cities are identified. The bubble sizes are proportional to altitude.

The diagonal of this display provides the names of the variables and the range of their values. Each plot is provided twice as a pair of graphs that are transpositions of each other. Specifically, in the first row, the maximum temperature is the vertical axis and is plotted against all other variables. In the first column, the maximum temperature is again plotted against all other variables, but now along the horizontal axis. This figure is produced in `proc insight`, a largely interactive SAS procedure that also allows you to select and highlight individual observations across all of the plots.

When we look at Figure 5.1, we see that the only really "linear" relationship is between temperature and latitude, given in the two plots in the upper-left corner of this figure. These relationships are negatively correlated because more northerly cities are generally colder.

These plots also reveal that altitude is not well correlated with any of the other variables. The plots in the last row and column show plots of altitude against all other variables. Most of the U.S. cities are located at or near sea level, so the altitude values tend to be small. There are a few highly influential, high-altitude cities with values that are much larger than others.

The bubble plot of Figure 5.2 provides a three-dimensional map of the U.S. cities. Values of latitude and longitude locate the cities in a familiar manner. The sizes of the circles are related to their altitude. The resulting figure is called a `bubble plot` because of its overall appearance. In addition to the familiar map of the United States, we also see that the largest altitudes are in the West, medium altitudes occur in the Midwest, and coastal cities, as their name implies, are situated at sea level.

This plot is produced in SAS using `proc gplot` as in the following code:

```
proc gplot;
  bubble lat * longe = alt;
run;
```

where `longe` is longitude measured in degrees east. The names of several cities have been added to this figure.

5.3 Leverage and the Hat Matrix Diagonal

In Section 4.4 we saw that the most important diagnostic tool available to us is the residual plot. By looking at the differences between the observed values of the dependent variable y and those $\widehat{y}$ estimated by the model, we can often identify outliers that represent obvious deviations from the model in explaining the entire dataset. In contrast to the examination of residuals, the measures described in this section identify observations that are said to have *high leverage* because they are outliers in terms of their explanatory x variables.

For an example of leverage, let us look back at Figure 4.3. The bottom pair of plots in this figure exemplify a dataset in which a small number of points with unusual explanatory x values have a large leverage on the fitted model. If the problem is due to the y value, then we attribute this to outliers or observations that fail to follow the model. Outliers are usually identified by plotting the residuals. Leverage points, however, may be due to unusual values of the explanatory variables, and these may be more difficult to identify in multiple linear regression.

If we had only one explanatory variable, a simple plot of the data would reveal high-leverage observations because of their extreme values. Look back at the low-birth-weight infant data in Figure 3.1 that is repeated here as Figure 5.3. Notice how one very short infant appears at the far left of this figure. The data on this one infant has a large effect: it pulls the fitted regression line toward itself, resulting in a line that appears to overestimate the weights of the other smallest infants in the data. For this reason, we say that such an observation has a high amount of leverage because it is so far away from the other data values of the explanatory variable.

Why are high-leverage observations so difficult to identify? The problem with multivariate regression models is that a group of several explanatory variables may have collectively unusual values but may not be extreme in any one of them. For two weather-related examples, a chilly day (but not the coldest) along with a light drizzle (but not the heaviest rain) may result in an experience of the worst weather. As another example, the wind chill factor is a combined measure of cold and wind in which a particular temperature on a windy day feels equivalent to a much colder temperature without the wind. The weather feels extreme even though the temperature may not be unusually low.

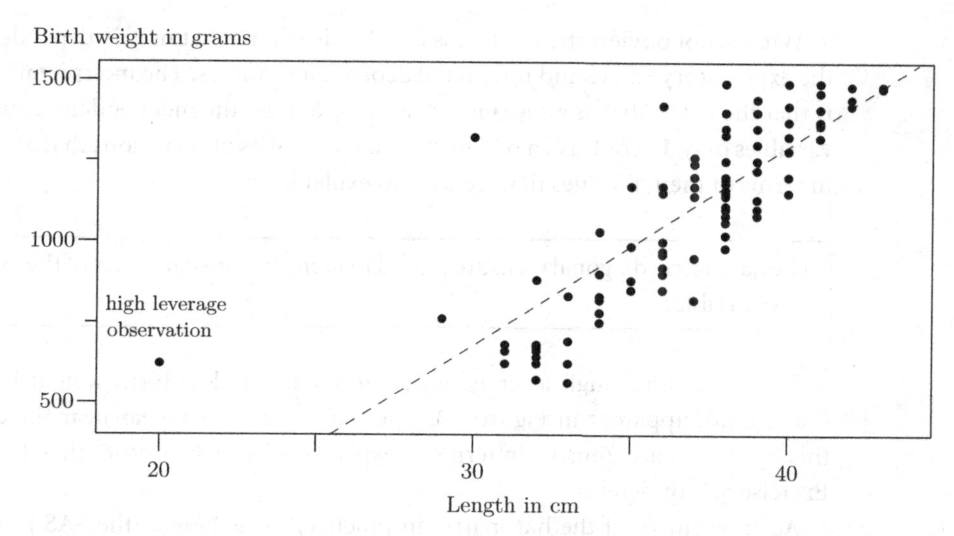

Figure 5.3 Birth weight and length of 100 low-birth-weight infants along with the fitted least squares regression line.

The *hat matrix diagonal* is a popular method for describing leverage in multivariate regression. The mathematical form of the hat matrix is more than we need here, but we can express it in a simple form that will make it easier to remember. The hat matrix has the property that

$$\text{Hat matrix} \times \text{Observed} = \text{Expected}.$$

That is, the hat matrix acts on the observed y values, collectively, and transforms these into the fitted or expected $\widehat{y}$ values. Written another way, we have

$$\text{Hat} \times Y = \widehat{Y}. \tag{5.2}$$

In this last expression we see that the hat matrix "puts the hat on Y"; hence the name. This transformation is smooth in the sense that each observed y value contributes to each and every fitted value, including its own. Ideally we want this process to be uniform, where all of the observations are used equally to help estimate all of the fitted values.

The diagonal of the hat matrix shows how much each individual observation contributes to its own fitted value. In the ideal situation, all observations would provide an equal amount to their own fitted values, along with some information about the others as well. Ideally this would all be about the same for each observation in the data.

Observations that contribute much more than others to their own fitted values are suspect and should be identified. In an extreme setting, an observation that provides all of the information about its own fitted value is not really following the model at all. For this to happen, the values of the explanatory variables of this observation will have to be very unusual.

What is not obvious from expression (5.2) is that the hat matrix depends only on the explanatory values and not on the dependent y values. The interpretation, then, is that the hat matrix is a measure of leverage among the independent, explanatory variables only. In contrast, a plot of residuals identifies observations that are unusual in terms of their Y values that we wish to explain.

The hat matrix diagonal measure is used to identify unusual values of the explanatory variables.

There are other high-leverage observations in the low-birth-weight baby data that are not apparent in Figure 5.3. These observations appear near the center of this figure and are unusual in terms of explanatory variables other than length. See Exercise 5.3 for details.

As an example of the hat matrix in practice, let us look at the SAS program in Table 5.2. At the end of this program, add the lines

```
proc reg data=cold;
   model maxt = lat long alt / p r influence ;
   output out=inf h=h p=p r=r;
run;
proc gplot data=inf;
   plot h * p;
run;
```

This program produces a large number of diagnostic measures with the `influence` option, and these are explained in the following section. This SAS code creates a new dataset called `inf` containing both the original data and a number of measures of influence. The hat influence is included in this dataset, denoted by the variable named `h`.

Figure 5.4 plots the hat matrix diagonal against the fitted values (called `p`) for this regression model. This plot has the familiar "U" shape that is common to most hat matrix plots. We can intuit that the extreme highest and lowest observed values of the explanatory variables are also furthest from the center of the data and will exert the greatest influence. Observations near the center of the data should have the least leverage. When there are many explanatory variables, it is difficult to determine which observations are near the center and which are somewhat closer to the "edge." This is where the hat matrix and regression diagnostics described in the following section become most useful.

In the present plot for the January temperature data, Juneau and Honolulu have the most extreme longitude and latitude values and also have the highest leverage. San Juan is far to the south of the continental United States and is also influential. Cheyenne is not the most extreme in terms of its fitted value, nor is it extreme in its

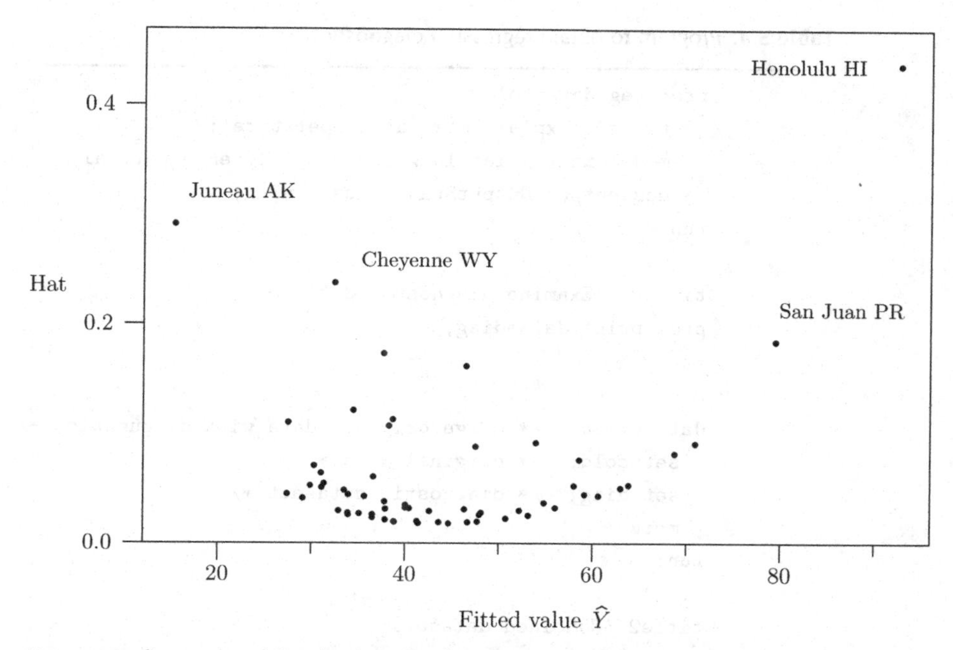

Figure 5.4 Hat matrix diagonal and fitted values for the January temperature data.

latitude. However, many U.S. cities are located at sea level, so the extreme altitude of Cheyenne has high leverage.

An informative graph in some situations is to plot the hat diagonals against the residuals of a model. The hat matrix identifies extremes in the explanatory variables, and extreme residuals locate poorly fitted observations in terms of their response variable. Combining these two diagnostics allows us to identify poorly fitting observations and their leverage at the same time. The plot of residual and hat matrix diagonals for the January temperature data is given later, in Figure 5.7.

5.4 Jackknife Diagnostics

These are a set of useful diagnostic measures that are used to describe how influential an observation is on the overall fit of the model. The *jackknife* is a simple idea: delete an observation, refit the model without that observation, and then see how much the fitted model changes without it. If an observation is deleted from the dataset and the new fit is very different from the original model based on the full dataset, then that observation is said to be *influential* in the fit.

> The jackknife measures how much the fitted model changes when one observation is deleted and the model is refitted.

Each individual observation is deleted in turn, and then a new model is fitted corresponding to each deleted observation. The omitted observation is then replaced

Table 5.4. Program to obtain regression diagnostics.

```
proc reg data=cold;
   title2 'Explain max Jan temperature';
   model maxt = lat long alt / p influence partial;
   ods output OutputStatistics = diag;
run;

title2  'Examine diagnostic data set';
proc print data=diag;
run;

data combo;   /* merge original data with diagnostics */
  set cold;   /* original data */
  set diag;   /* diagnostic data set */
  merge;
run;

title2 'Combined datasets';
proc print data=combo;
run;
```

before the next observation is deleted. Many different things can change, and a number of comparisons can be made between the model fitted with the full data and the model fitted from jackknifed data. The SAS program that produces these diagnostics is given in Table 5.4.

Put these program lines after the `data` step of the program in Table 5.2. The `/ p influence partial` options produce the fitted value, measures of influence, and partial residual plots that are described later, in Section 5.5. The program in Table 5.4 produces a new SAS dataset called `diag` that contains the diagnostic measures. This dataset is merged with the dataset containing the original data to produce a new dataset called `combo`. As with all programs that involve creating and modifying existing datasets, be sure to use `proc print` until you are certain that everything is working as you wanted it to.

Let's go over a list of the diagnostics that SAS produces. The first of these is the hat matrix diagonal that was covered in the previous section.

The `dffits` measures the change in the fitted value for each observation, both with and without that observation in the data. SAS will jackknife (delete) the ith observation, refit the model, and use these new fitted regression coefficients to estimate the value of the deleted observation. This jackknifed estimate is denoted by $\widehat{y}_{(i)}$ where the subscript in parentheses indicates that the ith observation has been omitted. That is, $\widehat{y}_{(i)}$ is the estimated value of y_i from the model that is fitted from data in which this observation has been deleted.

Finally, `dffits` is equal to the difference

$$\widehat{y}_i - \widehat{y}_{(i)}$$

where the fitted observation $\widehat{y}_i$ is estimated from the full dataset. This difference is standardized by the jackknifed hat matrix diagonal and mean square for residual in order to give the `dffits` a comparable variance for all observations.

A good strategy is to plot the `dffits` and look for any values with wide changes. Your visual inspection is probably the best way to judge problems with the data. A common suggestion is to be suspicious of any observation with a `dffits` with an absolute value greater than

$$\sqrt{p/n},$$

where p is the number of parameters in the model and n is the sample size. This is just a suggestion, and your own inspection should provide the best guidance.

There is also a diagnostic called *Cook's D* that combines all of the individual `dffits` for each observation into a single statistic. Cook's D measures how much all fitted values change when the ith observation is jackknifed.

In addition to the usual residual (observed minus expected), there is also a standardized student residual `RStudent`, which includes a measure of hat diagonal that takes into account the change in estimated regression coefficients when this observation is jackknifed. These residuals should be comparable to the usual residuals in most settings. As is the case with usual residuals, observations with values of `RStudent` greater than 2 in absolute value are worth noting.

Another useful jackknife diagnostic is the change in the estimated regression coefficients (including the intercept) when an observation is deleted and the model is refitted. These are collectively called `dfbeta`. There will be a `dfbeta` for every observation and every regression parameter in your model. When you run the program in Table 5.4, you will see the list of these variables and how SAS names them. The `dfbeta` changes in the estimated regression coefficients are standardized to make them comparable, but, as with the other diagnostics described in this section, your visual judgment is probably the best way to examine these.

Finally, the covariance ratio is a jackknife measure of the stability of the estimated fitted values $\widehat{Y}$. These are similar to the hat matrix diagonals discussed in the previous section and are referred to as `CovRatio` in SAS. Values of the covariance ratio should be close to 1 in value. These diagnostics are similar (but not identical) to the `dffits`, and SAS often refers to both of these as `CovRatio`, so you should be careful about which one you are using.

An influential observation usually also has high leverage, but a high-leverage point does not have to be influential. At the bottom of Figure 4.3 we see a set of high-leverage points, but deleting any one of these might not appreciably alter the fitted model. This is a subtle distinction, but in any case we should be prepared to

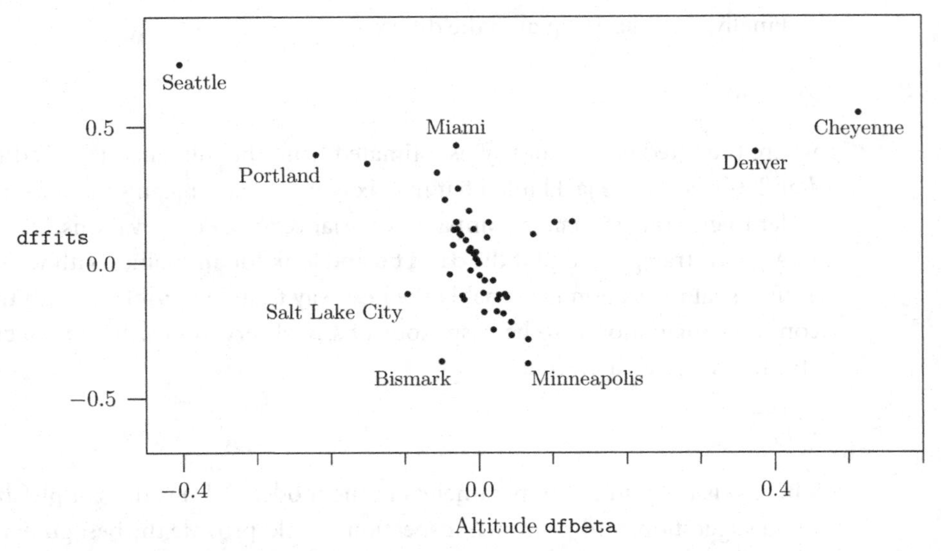

Figure 5.5 The `dffits` and altitude `dfbeta` for the January temperature data, excluding Juneau and Honolulu.

identify unusual observations and determine whether they are influential, have high leverage, or are outliers.

So, how do we make use of all of these different diagnostics? The short answer is that some trial and error is necessary. Not all of these diagnostics will help identify unusual observations in every setting. One useful strategy is to plot one against another and use that to identify influential observations in two directions at a time. An example of this is the plot of `dffits` and altitude `dfbeta` for the temperature data, given in Figure 5.5.

In this figure we exclude the cities Juneau and Honolulu, two very influential observations that have already been identified. Other unusual cities appear to have influence and are identified. These include Cheyenne and Denver, two cities with very high altitudes. Also appearing in this figure are Seattle and Portland, two cities that are far north but unusually warm (and rainy) due to Pacific currents.

5.5 Partial Regression Plots and Correlations

In multiple linear regression there are several explanatory variables, and these will usually be correlated with each other. This leads us to ask how to attribute the contribution of each one toward explaining the outcome variable. In the low-birth-weight infant data, for example, length is useful in explaining birth weight. But length and birth weight are also related to all of the other variables in the data. How can we separate the contributions made by each of these individual explanatory variables?

Table 5.5. SAS program to produce partial regression plots and correlations.

```
proc reg data=lowbw;
   model birthwt = headcirc  length  gestage  momage  toxemia
        / partial influence p r pcorr1 pcorr2;
   ods output OutputStatistics = diag;
run;
```

At this point, we do not have a tool to address this question. The analysis of variance, for example, provides an *F*-ratio testing the null hypothesis that all of the population regression coefficients are equal to zero. This is useful in making a statement about the utility of the whole model, but it does not examine individual contributions. We can make use of SAS output, as in Table 5.3 that tests for statistical significance of individual regression coefficients, but this also fails to take into account the multivariate relationships between the various explanatory variables.

One way to address the question of the individual contribution of each explanatory variable is through the use of partial correlations and partial regression plots. These are obtained using the `/ partial` option in `proc reg`. An example program is given in Table 5.5. The diagnostic dataset can be merged with the original data, as we saw in the program of Table 5.4. Always print out all new datasets and verify that these are what you expect.

Let us describe the partial regression plot. Consider the role that infant length plays in explaining the birth weight. In Figure 5.6 we plot birth weight by length. The correlation between these two variables is 0.82, indicating a strong linear relationship.

How much of this relationship depends on the other variables available to us? After all, length depends on head circumference, for example, as does birth weight. How much of the relation between length and birth weight remains after we take into

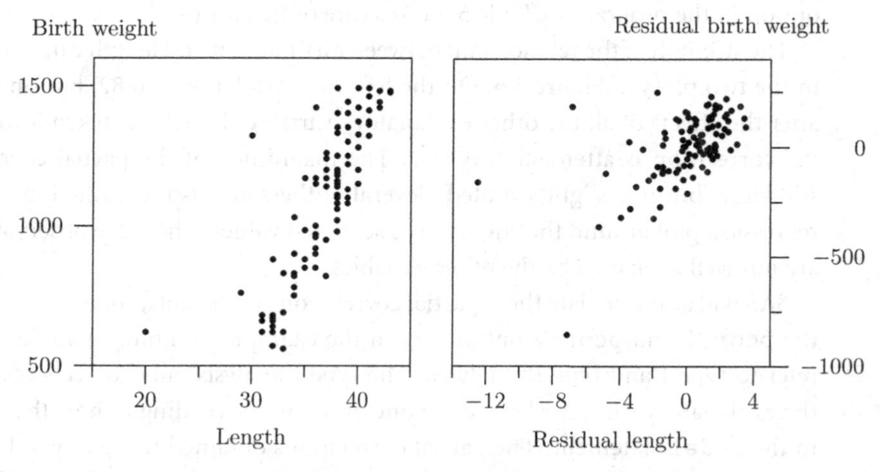

Figure 5.6 Scatter plot of birth weight by length and the partial regression plot after correcting for all of the other variables.

account the effects of head circumference as well as the other explanatory variables? To answer this question requires that we examine a *partial regression plot* such as the one given in Figure 5.6.

Specifically, the partial residual birth weight for length is the residual that remains after we fit the regression with all of the variables except for length. Similarly, the length residual is the residual that remains after we fit a linear regression with all of the other explanatory variables (not including birth weight).

That is, the partial regression plot in Figure 5.6 plots the residuals from the regression

```
proc reg;
   model birthweight = headcirc gestage momage toxemia;
run;
```

on the vertical axis. These are called the partial birth weight residuals because length is not included in the model.

The partial regression plot contains the partial length residuals from the regression

```
proc reg;
   model length = headcirc  gestage  momage  toxemia;
end;
```

along the horizontal axis. These residuals are from a regression of length on all the other explanatory variables. These explanatory variables do not include birth weight, which is the variable we want to explain.

The two variables plotted in the partial regression plot are corrected for the linear effects of all the other variables available in the regression model. This plot is a scatter diagram of the two sets of residuals from two regression models. We don't actually have to perform all the steps involved in creating this figure, because the `/ partial` option in the program in Table 5.5 takes care of this for us.

The strength of the relationship between birth weight and length can be compared in the two plots of Figure 5.6. On the left, the correlation is 0.82, but on the right, after the effects of all the other explanatory variables have been taken into account, the correlation is attenuated to 0.57. The magnitude of the partial correlation is still large, but it is slightly muted. Several outliers are also identified in the partial regression plot around the edges of the scattered values. These are observations that are not well explained by the other variables.

SAS will also calculate these partial correlation coefficients, squared, when we use the `pcorr1` and `pcorr2` options, as in the example program of Table 5.5. These refer to type I and type II analyses. The type I analysis only corrects residuals for the explanatory variables before the one of interest according to how they are listed in the `model` statement. The partial correlations obtained using a type I approach depend on the order in which they are listed in the `model` statement. The type II analysis is the method we described previously and treats every explanatory variable as though it were the last one added to the model. The type II approach is preferred in most circumstances.

5.6 Model-Building Strategies

So far in this chapter we have learned how to use SAS and fit regressions with several explanatory variables. Sections 5.3 and 5.4 describe how to identify outliers and influential observations. In this section we describe the model-building process. When faced with many possible explanatory variables, how do we find a simple model that explains the dependent variable well? Which explanatory variables need to be included in the model? Which of these are not useful or are redundant?

There are several approaches we can take to make this task easier. The three we describe are stepwise selection (sometimes called *forward selection*), backward selection, and all possible regressions. In *stepwise regression*, the program adds explanatory variables to the model, one at a time. This proceeds until no variable not already in the model can be added to make a significant improvement. In *backward selection*, the program begins with all the possible explanatory variables in the model and then eliminates those that do not make a contribution that crosses a specified threshold. In *all possible regressions*, as the name implies, the program fits all possible models and then presents several among the best of these.

Let us illustrate stepwise regression using the low-birth-weight data. Recall that we are building a model to be used to explain the different birth weights of the infants in this dataset. We continue the program in Table 2.9. The program lines

```
title2 'Forward stepwise selection';
proc reg;
   model birthwt =  headcirc length gestage momage toxemia
         / selection=f;
run;
```

request that SAS perform a forward selection procedure by including the `/ selection=f` option.

A portion of the output from this program is given in Table 5.6. This output summarizes the steps taken by `proc reg`. At the first step, the infant length variable was included in the model. At the next two steps, the head circumference and then the indication of toxemia were added. No further variables were found to make a statistical contribution, and the model building stopped at that point. This contribution is often set as a minimum statistical significance level to be achieved.

Each model in this stepwise regression output is provided with its corresponding value of R^2. Notice that these values increase as more terms are added to the model. The `Partial R-Square` is the change in R^2 comparing each model with the one at the previous step. These indicate successively smaller improvements as stepwise regression identifies the most useful explanatory variables for the model, but

Table 5.6. A portion of the stepwise regression output for the low-birth-weight baby data.

Summary of Forward Selection

Step	Variable Entered	Label	Number Vars In	Partial R-Square	Model R-Square
1	length		1	0.6651	0.6651
2	headcirc	head circumference	2	0.0962	0.7613
3	toxemia	indication of toxemia	3	0.0104	0.7717

Summary of Forward Selection

Step	C(p)	F Value	Pr > F
1	42.0945	194.65	<.0001
2	4.4209	39.10	<.0001
3	2.1258	4.38	0.0390

subsequently added variables make smaller contributions. There is also an F statistic for each new variable added to the model. These also indicate successively smaller incremental contributions with each stage of the model.

The stepwise model-building process ends at the point when length, head circumference, and toxemia are in the model. The omitted variables (gestational age and mother's age) are judged to have no additional explanatory value, given the other three variables already in the linear model.

Backward stepwise regression is similar to forward stepwise, except that it begins with all of the explanatory variables in the model and then removes, one at a time, those that make the least contribution. The SAS code for running a backward regression is

```
title2 'Backward stepwise regression method';
proc reg;
   model birthwt =  headcirc length gestage momage toxemia
         / selection=b;
run;
```

using the `/ selection=b` option. We will not include the output from this program.

Some fans of stepwise regression prefer the backward method over the forward selection because every explanatory variable gets a chance of being included in the final model chosen. Others might argue that backward regression is unnecessarily complicated right at the beginning. In this example of the low-birth-weight infants, both the forward and backward programs end at the same place, namely the model with same three explanatory variables: length, head circumference, and toxemia. In this example it doesn't matter which stepwise direction was used, because they both come to the same conclusion. This might not be the case in other examples. In further refinements of forward stepwise regression, some strategies may allow for the exclusion of a variable once it is included. Similarly, backward regression might later consider including a variable again after it has been removed.

Critics of stepwise methods will be quick to remind you that the level of statistical significance will be distorted because a number of significance tests have been performed without taking their multiplicity into account. A discussion of multiplicity of tests and their Bonferroni correction is given in Section 2.4. Even if we were willing to make this correction, it is not clear how many comparisons were made by the stepwise procedure.

It is possible that neither forward nor backward methods obtain the best model. We might also wonder how far the best is from second best and whether a much simpler model might do almost as well. This is the approach taken by the all-possible-regressions method. Before we explain the all-possible-regressions method, let us explain some criteria we might use to decide what we mean by "best."

First, remember that we use statistics to simplify things. We begin with a large amount of data and need to make a concise generalization about things. Along the way, we want to point out exceptions to the rule in terms of outliers. At the same time we aim to provide a brief statement that will quickly be grasped by our intended audience.

There is a penalty for building overly complicated models.

A model with many explanatory variables will confuse your audience. A model with almost as many estimated parameters as observations will fit the data well but does not simplify things. Complicated rules do not serve their intended purpose.

Fitting a model with a large number of explanatory variables can result in an unrealistically large R^2 statistic. Adding a large number of explanatory variables can inflate this statistic. In model building, it is not fair to compare two models with different numbers of explanatory variables, because the larger model will have an unfair advantage. It sees intuitive that a price should be paid for providing an unnecessarily complex model that was supposed to simplify things. At the extreme, if each observation is used to explain its own value, then the R^2 will equal 1; however, such a model is useless. See Exercise 5.1 for more information about such a strategy for model building.

The *adjusted* R^2 statistic takes the number of explanatory variables p into account. The definition is

$$\text{Adjusted } (R^2) = 1 - \frac{(N-1)(1-R^2)}{N-p}$$

where R^2 is the usual or unadjusted value, p is the number of parameters in the model, and N is the sample size.

If the sample size N is much larger than the number of explanatory variables, then the adjusted R^2 will not be very different from the usual R^2. SAS prints out both the R^2 and the adjusted R^2 in the output from `proc reg`. If these two statistics are very different in value than this is indicative of an overly fitted model with too many explanatory variables, relative to the sample size.

Another useful statistic in model building is C_p, defined as

$$C_p = \frac{\text{Error SS(p parameters)}}{s^2\text{(for the full model)}} - N + 2p,$$

where s^2 is the mean square for error of the full model and N and p are the sample size and number of explanatory variables, as before. This statistic is used to compare a "full" model including all of the explanatory variables to a smaller model with p parameters. Smaller values of C_p are preferred, because these represent both a small root mean square error of the model and fewer terms in the model.

In addition to stepwise regression, all possible regressions is another popular automated model-building strategy. In all possible regressions, SAS will fit every possible regression model by alternately including and excluding every combination of the explanatory variables listed in the `model` statement. To obtain the all-possible-regressions model in SAS, we write

```
title2 'Selecting the best of all possible regression models';
proc reg;
  model birthwt =  headcirc  length  gestage  momage  toxemia
        / selection=cp adjrsq r best=5;
run;
```

The `/ selection=cp adjrsq r` option instructs SAS to use the C_p criterion in ordering the best models and also to list the adjusted and unadjusted R^2 statistics. The `best=` option specifies the largest number of different models SAS will list after examining all possible choices of explanatory variables. A portion of the output from this program segment appears in Table 5.7.

In this table, we see the five best possible models, ordered by their C_p statistics, arranged from smallest (best) to largest. At the top of the list is the best of these, corresponding to the same model selected by the forward and backward regression models, namely the model with length, head circumference, and toxemia.

Notice that the corresponding values of R^2 are not similarly ordered in Table 5.7. There is no reason that ordering by one criterion corresponds to the same ordering by a different criterion. The adjusted R^2 values are ordered according to the C_p statistic in this example, but this will not always be the case. The adjusted R^2 statistics in this table do not differ markedly from the unadjusted R^2 values. This is because

Table 5.7. Some of the output for all possible regressions in the low-birth-weight infant data.

Number in Model	C(p)	R-Square	Adjusted R-Square	Variables in Model
3	2.1258	0.7717	0.7646	headcirc length toxemia
4	4.0198	0.7720	0.7624	headcirc length gestage toxemia
4	4.1208	0.7718	0.7621	headcirc length momage toxemia
2	4.4209	0.7613	0.7564	headcirc length
3	5.8098	0.7628	0.7554	headcirc length gestage

the sample size ($N = 100$) is much larger than the numbers of variables ($p = 2$, 3, or 4).

A closer examination of Table 5.7 reveals that there is a model with only two explanatory variables (length and head circumference) that has an R^2 and adjusted R^2 that are almost the same as any other three- or four-variable model listed in this table. All other things being equal, we should prefer a simpler explanation of the data. Of course, always be ready to examine the residuals for outliers and seek out influential observations. In terms of the information given in this table, this simpler model would make a good candidate for further examination.

Let us conclude this section with a brief discussion of the methods covered here. In each of the three methods (forward, backward, and all possible) described in this section for building a regression model, we are asking the computer to decide which variables to include in our model. This relieves us of some of the responsibility we have for our data. We often have some good knowledge of the variables involved and their relationships with each other and the dependent variable. Why was data on each of the different variables collected? Was there a reason for each variable's inclusion in the dataset, or did somebody suggest that we collect as much as we could in the hope that something might prove to be useful?

In the field of *data mining*, researchers start with huge databases and look for any and all useful patterns. With many possible choices for models, it is easy to find a well-fitting, statistically significant model. We also need to make sure that the model makes practical sense, or it will not provide any useful value.

> We are not finished with any regression until we interpret our final model.

We cannot simply say a model is the one that the computer suggested. Besides the diagnostics (outliers, residuals, influence) discussed earlier in this chapter, we also need to be able to defend the model in terms of the underlying science of the problem that gave rise to the data. Does it make sense? Do the explanatory variables in the model have some valid or intuitive reason for being there?

5.7 Exercises

5.1 Consider a model with just as many explanatory variables as observations. How many degrees of freedom would the residual sums of squares have? What would be the numerical value of the residual sums of squares in this setting? What would the value of the unadjusted R^2 be? Similarly, how can we make the R^2 large? Is this a useful strategy for building a model of our data?

5.2 Look at the arsenic exposure data in Exercise 3.5.2 and examine whether there are differences in sexes. Is the self-reported amount of well water used for drinking and cooking useful in explaining toenail arsenic levels? In Exercise 4.5 we identified an influential observation in these data with an extremely high exposure level. Do your conclusions change when this person is deleted from the regression model? Should this person's data be deleted in order to meet the assumptions of the statistical model? Do the jackknife diagnostics tell you anything else? Is it possible that this observation is the most important and informative of all?

5.3 Examine the low-birth-weight infant data using all of the explanatory variables available. Plot the hat matrix diagonal against the fitted value and notice two very influential observations. One of these influential observations had an extreme length and is identified in Figure 5.3. Locate one other observation with an extremely large influence. Notice that this infant is extreme neither in length nor in weight. Why is this observation influential?

5.4 Reexamine the attendance figures for the Baltimore Orioles in Exercise 3.8. In addition to the year number, does the finishing position of the team affect the average attendance? For most of the years in Table 3.3, the baseball team finished in fourth place, but there were a few years with different rankings. Are the finishing ranks in these years influential in explaining the average attendance?

In the "record" column of Table 3.3, the first number represents the number of games that the Orioles won that season. Is the number of games won a useful statistic in explaining the average attendance? Can you interpret the regression slope on the number of games won? Another analysis of this data appears in Exercise 6.3.

5.7.1 University Endowments

Universities need lots of money to operate. Not all of this is covered by tuition and grants. University endowments act as large savings accounts that can be used as needed for building new and refurbishing existing facilities, and to hire new faculty and staff. Most of the money comes either as contributions from alumni or as returns on investments. Some of these endowments have grown to huge sizes over

Table 5.8. The ten largest university endowments.

University	2007 endowment in $ billions	Percent change 2006–7	Per student in $ millions
Harvard	34.6	19.8	1.8
Yale	22.5	25.0	2.0
Stanford	17.2	21.9	1.2
Princeton	15.8	21.0	2.2
U. of Texas System	15.6	18.0	0.1
MIT	10.0	19.3	1.0
Columbia	7.1	20.4	0.3
U. of Michigan	7.1	25.4	0.1
U. Pennsylvania	6.6	24.9	0.3
Texas A & M System and Foundations	6.6	16.8	0.1

Source: NACUBO and TIAA-CREF.

the years. Data on the ten largest endowments (at the time of this writing) is given in Table 5.8.[1]

This table provides data on the ten largest total endowments along with the change over the previous year and the share of the endowment on a per-student basis. We can obtain an approximation to the number of students in the university using the ratio

$$\text{Number of students} = \frac{\text{Endowment}}{\text{Endowment per student}}.$$

Remember to multiply this ratio by 1,000 because the endowments are measured in billions of dollars but the per-student values are in millions.

The amount of a university endowment is principally due to return on investments and, to a smaller degree, to contributions from former students and their families. Similarly, the percent change over the previous year's endowment is also made up of these two factors. Build a linear model and see if you can explain the 2007 endowment value from the number of current students and the percent change over the previous year.

Which of these two explanatory variables offers greater value in explaining the size of the endowments? Similarly, should the university put more effort into raising money from former students or seeking greater investment returns?

5.7.2 Maximum January Temperatures

Use SAS to plot a map of the United States by drawing a scatter plot of the latitude and longitude values. Where are Miami, New York, Alaska, and Hawaii? Are they where they should be?

[1] Available online at http://www.nytimes.com/2008/01/25/education/25endowments.html.

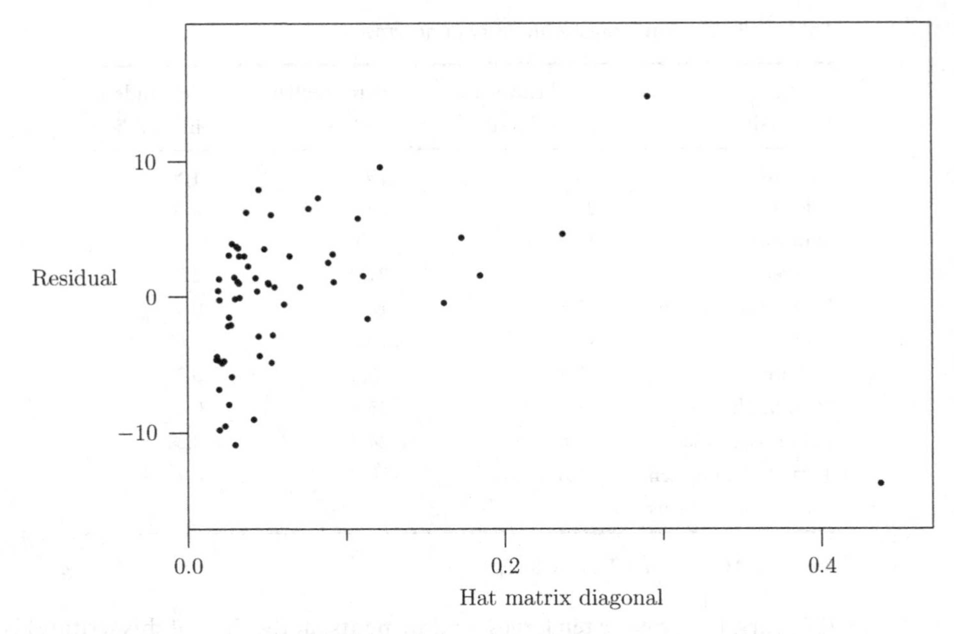

Figure 5.7 Hat matrix diagonal and residuals for the maximum January temperature data.

Fit a linear model explaining temperature from the other covariates. Plot your residuals and look for outliers. Explain these. Identify influential points using the diagnostics described in this chapter. Explain any influential observations that you find.

What role does the intercept play? Does its value have meaning? Hint: Look at a map to find the location with a zero latitude, longitude, and altitude. Learn why residents of Ghana claim to live near the center of the earth.

Try putting both longitude and longitude-squared in the same model. Try something wild that nobody else ever thought of. Does your R-squared or root-mean-squared-error improve your ability to explain the temperature values? What evidence can you provide that your model is any good?

There are some very large outliers in this data. Carefully identify these cities. Large positive and negative residuals occur in Alaska and Hawaii. These observations are also highly influential, as we see in Figure 5.7. Are you surprised by learning the identity of the outliers? Does your intuition help you or hinder you? Can you explain why these residuals are so extreme in their respective directions?

5.7.3 Statistics in the News: Heart Surgery Mortality

Table 5.9 presents a summary of survey data obtained from hospitals in the Philadelphia area in 2005. The newspaper article[2] concentrates on coronary bypass surgery and the costs of patient care. The article questions whether the mortality outcome is related to the cost of the procedure.

[2] Available online at http://www.nytimes.com/2007/06/14/health/14insure.html.

Table 5.9. Hospital costs and mortality following bypass surgery in a survey of hospitals in the Philadelphia area. Death rates are summarized as being greater (+), lower (−), or close (0) to expected.

	Average paid to hospital		Postsurgical		In-hospital deaths	
Hospital	By Medicare	By private insurance	length of stay (days)	Cases	Number	Rate
Lower Bucks	30	95	7.1	74	2	0
Hahnemann University	50	78	8.1	153	9	+
Albert Einstein	45	73	6.1	116	6	+
Graduate	40	70	5.2	43	2	+
Crozer-Chester	35	66	5.8	102	1	0
U of Pa Hospital	45	62	6.6	145	3	0
Temple University	42	58	7.1	114	4	0
Thomas Jefferson Univ.	43	50	7.6	173	3	0
Main Line Paoli	30	45	6.5	105	3	0
Penn Presbyterian	35	43	6.5	221	5	0
Mercy Fitzgerald	42	45	7.0	90	9	+
Brandywine	30	43	5.3	57	1	0
Pennsylvania	39	41	6.5	91	5	0
Abington Memorial	37	37	7.2	153	6	0
Main Line Bryn Mawr	30	36	6.3	86	4	0
Main Line Lankenau	30	35	5.4	299	2	−
Frankford	38	30	6.5	231	1	0
Doylestown	25	30	5.6	182	2	0
Chester County	29	24	5.8	91	1	0
Phoenixville	.	18	5.5	60	0	0

Source: Pennsylvania Health Care Cost Containment Council.

This table provides the following data variables:

- Average costs paid by Medicare
- Average costs paid by private insurance
- Average postsurgical length of hospital stay, in days
- Number of cases treated
- Number of in-hospital deaths

The number of deaths should always be expressed as a rate, or the ratio of the number of deaths to the number of cases. Otherwise, hospitals that treat many patients would also appear to have too many deaths.

Consider the average total cost per patient as your dependent variable. Total cost is the sum of the amounts paid by Medicare and private insurance. Is the average number of hospital days related to the average total costs paid by insurers? Suppose you use the average length of hospital stay as your dependent variable. Can this variable be explained well by the average costs paid?

Create a new variable that is the ratio of Medicare to private insurance costs for each hospital. Is this ratio related to either length of stay or mortality rate? Private insurance patients are more likely to be employed or have greater financial means. Hospitals with greater private insurance claims may also have healthier patients than hospitals with a larger percentage of Medicare reimbursements.

This table also includes a column indicating whether the mortality was higher or lower than expected. Do you agree with these measures? Do these summaries correspond to the residuals in your regression model?

Another examination of the mortality data in this figure is given in Section 10.6.1.

5.7.4 Characteristics of Cars, 1974

Let's go back to the days when leaded gasoline cost less than $1.00, before catalytic converters, back to the time of an earlier energy crisis, back when Nissan was called Datsun. But look: after all these years, Toyota still makes the Corolla.

The data in Table 5.10 lists eleven different characteristics of cars that were made in 1973–4. The data was originally published in a 1974 issue of *Motor Trend* magazine, and another statistical analysis appears in Henderson and Velleman (1981). Besides the make and model, these are the variables:

- mpg: Miles per U.S. gallon
- cyl: Number of cylinders
- disp: Displacement (in cubic inches)
- hp: Gross horsepower
- rar: Rear axle ratio
- wt: Weight (lb/1,000)
- qsec: 1/4 mile time
- V/S: Cylinders form a "V" (1) or are in a straight line (0)
- T: Transmission (0 = automatic, 1 = manual)
- G: Number of forward gears
- C: Number of carburetors

There is a lot that can be said about the data, and a variety of analyses are possible. Much will be left to the reader's creativity. A few simple plots will reveal much. Here are a few suggestions to get you started:

- Begin with a matrix scatter plot (as in Figure 5.1) to reveal any obvious strong pairwise relationships.
- The quarter-mile times have outliers at both the high and low ends. What are the characteristics of cars that exhibit these extremes?
- A plot of `disp` against `rar` reveals two distinct groups of cars. How can these be distinguished?
- A plot of weight and displacement reveals either three very influential observations, or possibly three distinct groups of cars.
- Miles per gallon are negatively correlated with horsepower, but note that there are a few exceptions to the overall pattern.

Table 5.10. Characteristics of cars in 1974.

Make and Model	mpg	cyl	disp	hp	rar	wt	qsec	V/S	T	G	C
Mazda RX4	21.0	6	160.0	110	3.90	2.620	16.46	0	1	4	4
Mazda RX4 Wag	21.0	6	160.0	110	3.90	2.875	17.02	0	1	4	4
Datsun 710	22.8	4	108.0	93	3.85	2.320	18.61	1	1	4	1
Hornet 4 Drive	21.4	6	258.0	110	3.08	3.215	19.44	1	0	3	1
Hornet Sportabout	18.7	8	360.0	175	3.15	3.440	17.02	0	0	3	2
Valiant	18.1	6	225.0	105	2.76	3.460	20.22	1	0	3	1
Duster 360	14.3	8	360.0	245	3.21	3.570	15.84	0	0	3	4
Mercedes 240D	24.4	4	146.7	62	3.69	3.190	20.00	1	0	4	2
Mercedes 230	22.8	4	140.8	95	3.92	3.150	22.90	1	0	4	2
Mercedes 280	19.2	6	167.6	123	3.92	3.440	18.30	1	0	4	4
Mercedes 280C	17.8	6	167.6	123	3.92	3.440	18.90	1	0	4	4
Mercedes 450SE	16.4	8	275.8	180	3.07	4.070	17.40	0	0	3	3
Mercedes 450SL	17.3	8	275.8	180	3.07	3.730	17.60	0	0	3	3
Mercedes 450SLC	15.2	8	275.8	180	3.07	3.780	18.00	0	0	3	3
Cadillac Fleetwood	10.4	8	472.0	205	2.93	5.250	17.98	0	0	3	4
Lincoln Continental	10.4	8	460.0	215	3.00	5.424	17.82	0	0	3	4
Chrysler Imperial	14.7	8	440.0	230	3.23	5.345	17.42	0	0	3	4
Fiat 128	32.4	4	78.7	66	4.08	2.200	19.47	1	1	4	1
Honda Civic	30.4	4	75.7	52	4.93	1.615	18.52	1	1	4	2
Toyota Corolla	33.9	4	71.1	65	4.22	1.835	19.90	1	1	4	1
Toyota Corona	21.5	4	120.1	97	3.70	2.465	20.01	1	0	3	1
Dodge Challenger	15.5	8	318.0	150	2.76	3.520	16.87	0	0	3	2
AMC Javelin	15.2	8	304.0	150	3.15	3.435	17.30	0	0	3	2
Camaro Z28	13.3	8	350.0	245	3.73	3.840	15.41	0	0	3	4
Pontiac Firebird	19.2	8	400.0	175	3.08	3.845	17.05	0	0	3	2
Fiat X1-9	27.3	4	79.0	66	4.08	1.935	18.90	1	1	4	1
Porsche 914-2	26.0	4	120.3	91	4.43	2.140	16.70	0	1	5	2
Lotus Europa	30.4	4	95.1	113	3.77	1.513	16.90	1	1	5	2
Ford Pantera L	15.8	8	351.0	264	4.22	3.170	14.50	0	1	5	4
Ferrari Dino	19.7	6	145.0	175	3.62	2.770	15.50	0	1	5	6
Maserati Bora	15.0	8	301.0	335	3.54	3.570	14.60	0	1	5	8
Volvo 142E	21.4	4	121.0	109	4.11	2.780	18.60	1	1	4	2

Don't aim for a complete and thorough analysis of these data – that could take a very long time. It is better to concentrate on some aspect and write a clear story that conveys both your understanding of the data and the statistical methods.

5.7.5 Statistics in Advertising: Wine Prices

For those of us whose expertise at wine consists of being able to tell reds from whites, there are experts who rate wines and give them a score. Higher scores are better, and 99 or 100 is the maximum. Naturally, merchants will advertise high scores in an attempt to charge higher prices.

Here is a list of wines from an advertisement appearing in the *New York Times*, May 1, 2005. The prices in Table 5.11 are per bottle and are probably paid by people who can afford it but would not be caught drinking anything with a rating below 90. That is, the advertisement ends at this value. Such data is called *censored* because certain values are not observed. Recall that the low-birth-weight data of Section 3.1 is also censored. We discuss censored data again when we describe the analysis of survival data in Chapter 11.

Three columns are in Table 5.11: points, year of vintage, and price. In every case, the sale price is one cent less than the value listed here, so the first item sells for $599.99 instead of the $600 listed here. The one bottle with a $1,400 price is not an error. Really. There are four items per line, so remember to use the `@@` option on your `input` statement in SAS.

The vintage years omit the century number, and you will need to fix this before you fit any regression models. For example, subtract 100 for all year values greater than 10. Then 2000 becomes a reference year with value zero; 1999 corresponds to −1; 1998 becomes −2; 2001 is +1; and so on. Similarly, you might subtract 90 or 95 from all ratings to make them easier to compare.

Perform a linear regression using only year and point score to explain the price. Look at the regression coefficients and interpret these. How much of a price difference is one year worth? Explain why one of these regression coefficients is positive and the other is negative.

Which is more important in determining price: older vintage or better rating? What is the tradeoff in price for age and rating: how many years is one point worth? Is the point scale linear in price, or does there appear to be a larger price difference as the points become larger? For example, is the difference in price between 90 and 92 the same as the difference between 96 and 98? Does every year have the same distribution of high and low ranks, or were some years better than others? Can you identify bargains and/or overpriced wines?

Look at the residuals for this model and plot the residuals against the fitted value. Notice how the $1,400 wine distorts the figure. Delete this wine and run the regression again. How does the R^2 change? How do you interpret this? Does the RMS change when you delete the most expensive wine? How do you interpret this? Examine the measures of influence and identify any other unusual observations. Did you notice that there is a wine with a negative estimated price? How do you explain this? *Cheers!*

5.7.6 Statistics in Finance: Mutual Fund Returns

Mutual funds are a convenient way for many investors to pool their savings and participate in the stock market. A manager is hired who invests the money and keeps records. For this work, the manager is paid an annual fee out of the funds being

Table 5.11. Rating points, vintage year and price for bottles of wine in an advertisement.

Pts	Year	Price	Pts	Year	Price	Pts	Year	Price	Pts	Year	Price
99	00	600	99	96	500	99	89	350	99	86	625
99	00	600	99	90	500	99	90	500	99	00	550
99	91	250	99	01	190	99	83	550	99	90	400
99	96	450	99	95	150	99	82	500	98	86	450
98	98	250	98	02	200	98	03	350	98	00	80
98	01	70	97	98	200	97	01	90	97	00	190
97	00	300	97	02	275	96	03	100	96	00	330
96	01	80	96	01	100	96	00	300	96	02	40
95	01	70	95	01	150	95	97	550	95	97	100
95	01	100	95	01	225	95	01	550	95	97	90
95	01	130	95	01	70	95	00	120	95	00	180
95	98	260	95	01	100	95	01	140	95	02	45
95	03	80	95	99	85	95	03	100	95	97	100
95	99	70	95	99	70	95	01	150	95	00	230
95	98	100	94	01	140	94	96	60	94	99	70
94	98	190	94	01	100	94	01	80	94	02	70
94	03	70	94	00	60	94	01	60	94	01	120
94	99	80	94	99	90	94	01	140	94	99	500
94	99	70	94	99	80	94	01	130	94	01	140
94	86	200	94	99	200	94	01	240	94	00	140
94	01	80	93	02	125	93	02	270	93	02	540
93	01	600	93	99	80	93	98	80	93	98	50
93	99	1,400	93	98	125	93	01	130	93	00	55
93	89	150	93	00	140	93	03	30	93	02	100
93	99	60	93	99	130	93	01	50	93	00	40
93	99	50	93	01	75	93	01	240	93	01	100
93	00	30	92	02	65	92	00	50	92	01	35
92	01	60	92	02	40	92	99	90	92	02	27
92	00	400	92	00	70	92	00	120	92	00	60
92	01	75	92	02	53	92	00	70	92	98	70
92	02	80	92	98	60	92	99	50	92	99	60
92	00	100	92	99	60	92	99	50	92	00	70
92	98	60	92	02	28	92	02	22	92	01	35
92	02	70	92	96	60	92	00	70	92	00	48
92	02	28	91	01	35	91	03	30	91	99	80
91	01	25	91	99	50	91	01	35	91	02	18
91	01	50	91	03	16	91	01	30	91	01	27
91	01	130	91	00	75	91	03	19	91	00	275
91	02	37	91	02	50	91	02	50	91	02	35
91	00	19	91	03	40	91	03	27	91	02	60
91	02	40	91	02	50	91	02	35	91	02	20
91	02	40	91	02	50	90	01	10	90	03	13
90	01	18	90	02	13	90	01	40	90	01	20
90	02	17	90	01	24	90	02	19	90	03	13
90	01	40	90	01	45	90	01	19	90	02	18
90	02	20	90	02	30						

Table 5.12. The twenty-five largest mutual funds investing in the stocks of large corporations. The types are Growth, Value, and Blend.

		% Total annual return		Expense	Assets
Name	Type	1 year	5 years	ratio	($ million)
Amer Funds Growth Fund A	G	14.4	15.6	.63	94,406
Fidelity Contrafund	G	20.8	17.7	.89	82,646
Amer Funds Inv Co	V	8.5	13.1	.54	78,309
Amer Funds Washington	V	6.6	12.4	.57	71,169
Dodge & Cox Stock	V	2.9	16.2	.52	68,711
Vanguard 500 Index	B	7.4	12.3	.18	68,416
Vanguard Total Stock	B	7.6	13.6	.19	50,929
Vanguard Inst Indx	B	7.5	12.4	.05	47,686
Fidelity Magellan	G	20.4	11.9	.53	47,337
Fidelity Growth Company	G	23.3	18.4	.96	39,106
Amer Funds Fundamental	B	14.9	18.1	.58	38,851
Vanguard Windsor II	V	6.4	15.2	.33	33,821
Fidelity Equity Income	V	4.2	13.5	.67	32,540
Davis NY Venture A	B	6.4	14.8	.84	32,138
Fidelity Spar US Eq Inv	B	7.5	12.3	.09	24,106
Vanguard PRIMECAP	G	13.5	17.0	.46	23,989
T. Rowe Price Gr Stk	G	12.5	13.6	.70	22,136
T. Rowe Price Eq Inc	V	5.0	13.5	.69	21,977
Fidelity Growth & Income	B	3.1	8.1	.67	21,794
Fidelity Blue Chip	G	13.9	9.6	.59	18,940
Amer Funds Amcap A	G	10.5	12.2	.65	18,913
Amer Funds Amer Mut A	V	6.0	12.1	.55	17,747
Lord Abbott Affiliated A	V	6.2	13.4	.82	16,802
Fidelity Dividend Growth	B	4.6	9.2	.60	16,387
Vanguard Windsor	V	1.9	14.4	.35	14,489

Source: New York Times, November 6, 2007, page C10.

managed. This fee is called the *expense ratio* and is usually a fraction of 1%. The records (at the time of this writing) of the largest mutual funds investing in large corporations are given in Table 5.12.

The two basic approaches to investing in stocks are *growth* and *value.* Growth stocks are in companies that have the potential for new discoveries or products that would lead to large increases in their future income. Value stocks represent bargains in which the price does not fully reflect the true worth of the share of the underlying corporation. In some years one approach may be a much better investment than the other, but over time there is generally little difference in the returns. In the one year leading up to the data in this table, growth stocks performed much better, but in the few years before that, value stocks did better. Blended funds invest in both of these types. Some of the mutual funds in this table emphasize current income, and others look for potential gains at some future date.

What determines the total assets of the fund? We can think of the total assets as a collection of many decisions made by the investors, who could easily move their money elsewhere if they became dissatisfied with the service that the manager is providing. Which is more important in determining the total assets of a fund: the expense ratio, or the return that the fund has experienced? That is, are investors more interested in the history of the fund or the amount they will have to pay for that performance? Similarly, are larger expenses associated with better returns?

Consider other relationships in this data. Do value managers provide lower expense ratios? We might ask if value managers themselves provide value to their investors. Is the one-year return correlated with the five-year return? Why would you expect this to be the case? Is this correlation the same for value and growth managers? Can you identify funds that perform well under all conditions, regardless of whether growth or value stocks provide the best returns?

6

Indicators, Interactions, and Transformations

Linear regression is sometimes more than we really need. A simple rule about whether or not to take a different action is often adequate. When you look at the fuel gauge on your car, at what point do you begin to look for a gas station? An indicator variable takes a continuous measurement and cuts it up into two discrete categories.

We can also transform variables in a nonlinear fashion if this serves to reduce leverage or make the data look more like a straight line. Interactions are variables we use in a regression model to see if the explanatory value of two variables is greater than the sum of their parts. A pizza with two toppings may be much better than two separate halves with the individual toppings. Or perhaps it may be worse.

6.1 Indicator Variables

Water boils at a lower temperature at high altitude, and experienced cooks know that recipes need to be adjusted accordingly. Consider the recipe given in Table 6.1. Most important, notice the footnote about making an adjustment for high altitude. This is expressed in terms of a change that suddenly needs to be made above a critical height above sea level. Ideally, the person preparing this dish should first obtain an accurate measure of the altitude and then use a calculator to determine the precise amount of adjustment that needs to be made. Nobody would consider doing this, of course. Instead we are instructed to use this easily remembered rule that takes effect above a critical level.

Let us take the January temperature data described in the previous chapter and see how to create and interpret an indicator variable. The estimated regression coefficients in Table 5.3 show that temperature drops about two degrees Fahrenheit for every degree latitude north a city is located. Suppose we want to create a simple rule about the temperature in northern and southern cities, much like the one in the recipe. That is, what simple statement can we make about northern and southern cities that does not involve a calculation?

Table 6.1. Recipe for Hamburger Helper Lasagna.

YOU WILL NEED:
1 lb lean ground beef
3 1/4 cups hot water

1. BROWN ground beef in 10-inch skillet; drain.
2. STIR in hot water, Sauce Mix and uncooked Pasta.
   HEAT to boiling; stirring occasionally.
3. REDUCE heat; cover and simmer about 14 minutes, stirring occasionally, until pasta is tender.
   REMOVE from heat and uncover (sauce will thicken as it stands).

HIGH ALTITUDE (3500–6500 ft) Increase hot water to 3 1/2 cups and simmer time to about 15 min.

We can pick any cut point we want, so let us choose Washington, DC, at 38 degrees latitude as the division between northern and southern cities. This choice is intuitive, but it is also arbitrary. We could just as well pick a different division. Notice that we are picking the place to make the cut, and the computer is not estimating it for us. The SAS program that creates the new variable and performs regression using it is given in Table 6.2.

Table 6.2. SAS program to create an indicator variable for latitude north of 38 degrees.

```
data north;                  /* create a new data set */
   set cold;                 /* begin with the original data */
   if lat>38 then DC=1;      /* create indicator variable */
      else DC=0;
   label DC = 'North of Washington';
run;

proc print data=north;       /* always print it out */
   var lat DC maxt city;
run;

proc reg data=north;         /* regression on the indicator variable */
   model maxt = DC;
run;

proc ttest data=north;       /* compare it to a t-test */
  var maxt;
  class DC;
run;
```

Table 6.3. Estimated regression coefficients from the program in Table 6.2.

Parameter Estimates

Variable	Label	DF	Parameter Estimate	Standard Error	t Value	Pr > |t|
Intercept	Intercept	1	57.07692	1.78448	31.99	<.0001
DC	North of Washington	1	-23.04835	2.35582	-9.78	<.0001

The data step in this program begins with the original dataset called `cold` that was created in the program given in Table 5.2. The `data` step creates a new dataset called `north` and adds the new variable DC, which takes on the value 0 for cities south of Washington and 1 for cities to the north. Such a variable is called an *indicator* or *dummy*, because it is not a real observed value, but rather an artificial one that we constructed. It is called an indicator because it operates much like a light switch, with only two positions. The DC variable is created using an `if` and `else` pair of statements. It is very easy to make an error with these, so be sure to print out and check the data after every `data` step.

After creating the new indicator called DC, we are free to use it as we would use any other variable in a linear regression. For simplicity, this is the only explanatory variable in the regression model. Table 6.3 contains the portion of the SAS output with the estimated regression coefficients for this model.

How do we interpret the fitted model and estimated regression coefficients? The estimated intercept is about 57 and the slope is -23, but what does this mean? If we write out the model, then it will become clear.

The fitted regression equation is

$$\text{maximum January temperature} = 57 - 23 \times \text{DC}.$$

When DC $= 0$, we have, on average,

$$\text{maximum January temperature} = 57$$

as the estimate for all cities that are south of Washington.

Similarly, when DC $= 1$, the regression model estimates that

$$\text{maximum January temperature} = 57 - 23 = 34$$

is the average maximum January temperature for cities north of Washington.

In words, the regression slope on the indicator variable DC is the difference of two means. We can verify that the estimated slope is exactly the same as the difference of two means obtained in a Student t-test using the SAS program of Table 6.2. This demonstrates the close connection between the t-test and the use of indicator variables in linear regression.

We can use regression to perform a t-test, but the real benefit of indicator variables is the improved ease of interpretation, as we see in the difference between northern and southern cities as well as in the recipe in Table 6.1. In both of these examples, a continuous variable (latitude and altitude, respectively) has been cut into two categories, resulting in a simple rule that is easy to explain.

How much is lost or gained by creating the indicator variable in this example? At the analytic level, we can show that the residual sum of squares is larger for a regression model with the DC variable than if we regressed directly on latitude. This shows that the model with latitude is more precise and has better explanatory value. There is a price to be paid for this benefit, however.

The first part of the price is the added difficulty we have with the final fitted model. Recall the ease we have with the simple rule about the altitude adjustment in the recipe. The second advantage of using an indicator variable in this example is that the influence of extreme latitude values is eliminated. If we look back at Figure 5.7, we see that the cities at extreme latitudes (Juneau and Honolulu) are also the most influential using the hat matrix diagonal. The use of an indicator variable with only two values will eliminate the influence that results from extreme latitude values. There are advantages and benefits to using either approach, and the user should recognize these.

Let us next create an indicator with more than two categories. Categorical explanatory variables appear often in data analysis. These may be obtained as the unordered categories of race or religion, for example. The categories might also be ordered as in the previous example of latitude, divided up into two or more ordered groups. The use of indicator variables can help in interpreting the data, if performed carefully.

Let us examine the January temperature again and consider dividing the altitude variable into three categories. Many cities are located at or near sea level, so let us define a category for cities at 100 feet or less. Similarly, inland cities and those in the Rocky Mountains tend to be more than 1,000 feet above sea level. These distinctions are somewhat arbitrary but lend themselves to ease of interpretation.

The SAS code that creates the three binary-valued indicators is

```
if alt<100 then sea=1; else sea=0;
if alt<1000 and alt >=100 then mid=1; else mid=0;
if alt>=1000 then high=1;  else high=0;
```

This code creates a variable called `sea` that indicates a city at sea level, a variable called `mid` that identifies cities located between 100 and 1,000 feet, and a variable called `high` that is equal to 1 only for cities above or equal to 1,000 feet. (The characters >= are interpreted as "greater than or equal to.")

We can use these indicators in a regression model, but first let us point out a problem that occurs if we try to use all three in the same model.

If we try to fit the model

```
proc reg;
   model maxt = sea mid high;
run;
```

in SAS, then the mathematical model

$$\mathtt{maxt} = \alpha + \beta_1 \mathtt{sea} + \beta_2 \mathtt{mid} + \beta_3 \mathtt{high}$$

has an inherent ambiguity.

Specifically, this model specifies that every city has a mean temperature of

$$\alpha + \beta_1$$

for sea-level cities,

$$\alpha + \beta_2$$

for medium-altitude cities, or else

$$\alpha + \beta_3$$

for high-altitude cities.

The problem is that there are only three groups of cities, but the model requires us to fit four parameter values. There is no unique value that we can assign to the intercept α for example. We might set $\alpha = 0$ and have each of the βs equal to the mean for that group of cities. We could just as well set the intercept equal to 1 and then set all of the βs equal to 1 less than the averages of the three groups. In this manner, we could assign any value to the intercept.

Such a model is said to suffer from *multicolinearity* or to be *not of full rank*. In multicolinearity, there exists a linear relationship between some of the explanatory variables. SAS will be unable to fit the model with multicolinearity and will give an error message to that effect. The error message will also contain an explanation of the linear relationship.

Specifically, in the example with the three categories of cities, we note that every city has to be in one of these three categories. If we know two of the indicator values for any given city, then we can immediately determine the value of the third, because the three indicator variables for every city satisfy

$$\mathtt{sea} + \mathtt{mid} + \mathtt{high} = 1.$$

The three indicator variables always sum to 1 for every city in the dataset, and this causes the multicolinearity.

We see that with these three categorical indicators, we can use at most two in a linear regression. The use of all three will cause multicolinearity. Notice also, in the previous example of northern and southern cities, that there was only one indicator variable in the model for the two categories. In that example, we used an indicator

Table 6.4. SAS output for the three categories of altitude.

Parameter Estimates

Variable	Label	DF	Parameter Estimate	Standard Error	t Value	Pr > |t|
Intercept	Intercept	1	52.50000	2.82968	18.55	<.0001
mid		1	-14.08333	3.91752	-3.59	0.0007
high		1	-12.63333	4.44419	-2.84	0.0062

for northern cities, but our model did not also include the complementary indicator for southern cities.

How many indicators should be used? The rule is

> Omit one categorical indicator variable from the model.

If we try to fit a model with one indicator variable for every category, then the model will suffer from multicolinearity. We need to leave at least one out of the model.

Having said this, which altitude indicator should we omit? The answer to this question depends on how we want to interpret the fitted regression. The indicator that is omitted becomes the *reference category* because it is associated with the intercept. In most regression models, the intercept is not useful, as we saw in the exercise of Section 5.7.2. In the present example, let us illustrate the use of a reference category by omitting the indicator for sea-level cities.

The SAS program

```
proc reg;
   model maxt = mid high;
run;
```

fits the model

$$\texttt{maxt} = \alpha + \beta_1\,\texttt{mid} + \beta_2\,\texttt{high}.$$

The estimated regression coefficients for this model are given in the SAS output of Table 6.4.

For sea-level cities, both `mid` and `high` are equal to zero, so the average January temperature is equal to the estimated intercept 52.5. The estimated regression coefficients on `mid` and `high` correspond to differences from the average of the sea-level cities, as we see next. This motivates the description of sea level as being the reference category.

For cities between 100 and 1,000 feet, the `mid` indicator is equal to 1 and `high` is equal to 0. The average January temperature for such cities is then estimated as

$$52.5 - 14.08 = 38.42$$

where -14.08 is the estimated regression coefficient for `mid` given in Table 6.4.

The estimated regression coefficient -14.08 on `mid` is significantly different from zero with a p-value of 0.0007. This indicates that such cities are colder than sea-level cities, in line with our intuition.

For cities above 1,000 feet, we estimate the maximum January temperature to be

$$52.5 - 12.63 = 39.87$$

where -12.63 is the estimated regression coefficient for `high` in Table 6.4. The estimated coefficient -12.63 is the difference in average temperature between sea level and high altitude cities.

As with middle-altitude cities, the regression coefficient for high-altitude cities compares these to the cities at sea level. This illustrates how the omitted indicator variable defines the reference category. The estimated regression coefficients of `mid` and `high` correspond to differences with the sea-level cities, justifying our description of `sea` as the reference category.

What is not intuitive is the fact that high-altitude cities are estimated to be *warmer* than mid-altitude cities. This is counter to our understanding of these data. After all, from the estimated regression coefficient on `alt` in Table 5.3, we see that cities at higher altitude are supposed to be colder.

The explanation of this curious conclusion is that cities at higher altitude generally are cooler, but this relationship is not linear. If we only looked at the output of Table 5.3, then we might be led to believe that cities at higher altitudes are colder at a constant change in temperature per foot above sea level. A quick examination, however, of the scatter plot of maximum January temperature by altitude in the extreme upper right-hand corner of Figure 5.1 shows that this relationship is not linear at all. The sea-level cities experience a very wide range of climates, but the highest altitude cities are colder than average. From the estimated regression coefficients in Table 6.4, we see that much of the drop in average temperature occurs between sea-level and mid-altitude cities. The difference in average temperature between mid-altitude and high cities is small. See Exercise 6.2 for more on this.

If the use of a single indicator variable (such as `DC`) in a regression model mimics the t-test, then what is the analogous interpretation of several indicators, such as `sea`, `mid`, and `high`? This generalization of the t-test to comparisons of several groups is called a *one-way ANOVA*. There are often settings where more than two groups of data values need to be compared. Another example involving a comparison of three groups is given in Table 7.8 in the following chapter. A SAS program that performs the one-way ANOVA is described in Section 7.4. Exercise 6.6 examines the assumptions of the one-way ANOVA.

In this section we have seen that, in some cases, linear regression can be more than what we really need. Indicator variables can provide us with a simplified description of the data if we use them carefully and then interpret the results. An easily remembered rule about altitude can be helpful in a recipe and also when explaining temperatures. When it comes time to explain a complicated dataset, your audience will often appreciate simplicity rather than a surfeit of precision.

When we omitted the indicator for sea-level cities, these cities became the intercept or the reference category. The indicator variables that remain in the model act as comparisons with the reference in the sense that their estimated regression coefficients are differences of averages with the reference category. Specifically, in Table 6.4 we see that the intercept is the average temperature of sea-level cities. The regression "slopes" on `mid` and `high` are the differences in average temperatures between mid-altitude and high-altitude cities, respectively, and the cities at sea level.

> The category of the omitted indicator becomes the reference. Estimated regression slopes are differences of averages with to this reference.

Next we see that indicator variables can be combined in more involved settings. These techniques have useful interpretations as well.

6.2 Synergy in the News: Airline Mergers

Sometimes the total is more than the sum of its parts. Sometimes it is less. Think of a great time based on a good meal with old friends. The experience is enhanced by these individual components, but somehow the evening is even more magical as the pieces all fit together nicely. We can also test for *synergy* in regression. Synergy is when $1 + 1$ results in something different from 2.

At the time that Figure 6.1 appeared, there was much speculation about possible mergers of major U.S. airlines. The airlines were suffering from financial problems and there was much talk that a merger was going to be announced.

A merger would likely result in a reduction in labor costs and the elimination of redundant routes because of the duplication of effort. A lot of excess equipment would be sold off, and there would be layoffs as well. This would result in a reduced market share for the resulting company. As an example, United had 16% of the market share and Delta had 14%. Together, this figure estimated their combined market share to be only 27% instead of the 30% we would get by adding their separate parts together. Other potentially merged airlines are similarly estimated in this figure to have a reduced combined capacity.

Airline Merger Match-Up

Delta is mulling an acquisition of either Northwest or United. Here is how some mergers among the network carriers would compare in terms of 2007 capacity.

MARKET SHARE

Each airline's share of the industry's total available seat miles in 2007 and what it would be if they merged, which assumes about a 9 percent reduction in capacity

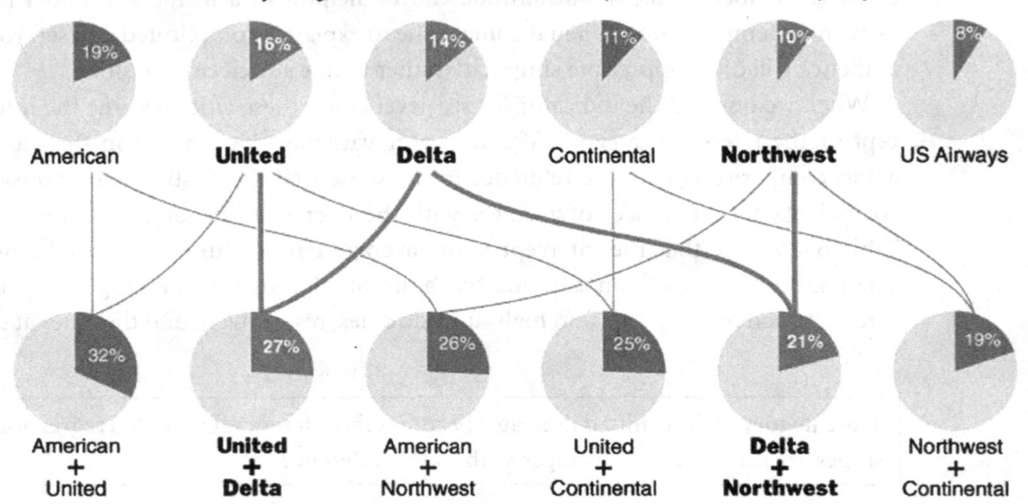

Figure 6.1 Possible mergers of major airlines and the resulting market share. *Source: New York Times*, January 17, 2008, page C12.

6.3 Interactions of Explanatory Variables

Northern cities are colder than average, as are cities situated at high altitude. What can we say about northern cities at high altitude? Are these even colder than expected? What is the combined effect of altitude and latitude?

We can measure the combined or synergistic effects by creating additional variables in the data step. In Section 6.1 we created the indicator DC for northern cities and mid and high for medium- and high-altitude cities. We can create indicators for the combined effects of high altitude and northern latitude by creating an indicator variable that is equal to 1 for cities that have both of these attributes. An easy way to do this is by multiplying these separate indicators together to form new indicators.

If we add the lines

```
hinorth = DC*high;
midnorth = DC*mid;
seanorth= DC*sea;
```

to the data step, then we have created three interaction effects. As an example, hinorth is equal to 1 for cities that are both at high altitude and located north of Washington but equal to 0 for other cities.

Table 6.5. SAS output for the program with interactions.

```
                          Parameter Estimates

                                      Parameter    Standard
Variable    Label                      Estimate       Error  t Value  Pr > |t|

Intercept   Intercept                  51.37500     2.79049    18.41    <.0001
DC          North of Washington?      -19.43750     3.41764    -5.69    <.0001
high                                   -1.37500     4.26255    -0.32    0.7482
sea                                    13.04167     3.60251     3.62    0.0006
hinorth                                 2.54861     5.38372     0.47    0.6378
seanorth                               -6.77917     4.80635    -1.41    0.1640
```

In Section 6.1 we saw that the temperatures of sea-level cities are different from those at medium and high altitudes. In Figure 5.1 we saw a large amount of climate variability among the sea-level cities. Perhaps we can use the `seanorth` indicator variable to separate and explain some of this variation in the cities situated at or near sea level. Notice that `seanorth` is equal to 1 for sea-level cities north of Washington, but 0 for all other cities.

These three interactions can be included with other indicators in a model statement as follows:

```
proc reg;
   model  maxt  =  DC  high  sea  hinorth  seanorth;
run;
```

Recall the discussion of multicolinearity in Section 6.1. In this program, we cannot include the three indicators for altitude: `sea`, `mid`, and `high`. In this example we chose to omit the middle category of altitude. Similarly, we cannot fit a model with all three interactions of altitude and north/south, because the sum of these three will be the same as the `DC` indicator variable. Again, we chose to omit the middle interaction denoted by `midnorth`, and this will define our reference category.

This regression model contains two types of indicators: those for the north/south cities (`DC`), indicators for altitude; and those that make up the interactions (`hinorth` and `seanorth`) of these. Terms such as `DC` and `high` and `sea` are usually referred to as *main effects* in the model, because the interactions are products of these. It is good statistical practice to include the main effects of all interactions in order to facilitate their interpretation. Without both of the the main effects in the model, the interaction would model a combination of both the underlying main effect and the interaction. As a result, the interpretation of such an interaction could be difficult to describe.

A portion of the output from this program is contained in Table 6.5. The largest effect is that of latitude, and cities north of Washington are estimated to be more than

Table 6.6. Model parameters for the six different types of cities.

City location		
Latitude	Altitude	Parameters in model
South of DC	Sea-level	$\alpha + \beta_{\texttt{sea}}$
South of DC	Mid-altitude	α
South of DC	High-altitude	$\alpha + \beta_{\texttt{hi}}$
North of DC	Sea-level	$\alpha + \beta_{DC} + \beta_{\texttt{sea}} + \beta_{\texttt{seaN}}$
North of DC	Mid-altitude	$\alpha + \beta_{DC}$
North of DC	High-altitude	$\alpha + \beta_{DC} + \beta_{\texttt{hi}} + \beta_{\texttt{hiN}}$

19 degrees colder than those to the south. We omitted the indicator for mid-altitude, southern cities, and as a result, these cities correspond to the intercept of the model. Before we try to interpret the values in Table 6.5, it is useful to write out all of the parameters in the model and see how they all fit together.

The model being fitted by SAS is

$$\texttt{maxt} = \alpha + \beta_{\texttt{DC}}\,\texttt{DC} + \beta_{\texttt{hi}}\,\texttt{high} + \beta_{\texttt{sea}}\,\texttt{sea} + \beta_{\texttt{hiN}}\,\texttt{hinorth} + \beta_{\texttt{seaN}}\,\texttt{seanorth}.$$

The estimated regression coefficients appear in Table 6.5. In order to interpret these, we first write out which parameters go with which cities. This is given in Table 6.6.

There are a total of six types of cities being modeled: north or south and three categories of altitudes (sea level and mid and high altitude). The intercept α appears in the model for all six types of cities. We omitted indicators for southern cities and mid-altitude cities, so this type of city becomes the reference category. Specifically, we see that the intercept alone appears in the model for southern, mid-altitude cities.

All southern cities have $\texttt{DC} = 0$, so the regression coefficient $\beta_{\texttt{DC}}$ appears only in the three categories of northern cities. Similarly, $\texttt{sea} = 1$ only for sea-level cities, and $\beta_{\texttt{sea}}$ appears only in models for sea-level cities. The main effect for high altitude and its regression coefficient $\beta_{\texttt{hi}}$ appears only in the model for high-altitude cities.

A good interpretation of these main effects is to say that they *correct* for the effects of latitude and altitude. These main effects suggest that the maximum January temperature of each of the six groups of cities can be expressed as a latitude effect (north or south of Washington) plus an effect due to altitude (in one of three categories). That is, we are expressing the maximum January temperature as

$$\text{Max January temperature} \;=\; \text{Latitude effect} \;+\; \text{Altitude effect}, \tag{6.1}$$

or as the sums of its two component parts.

The estimated coefficient for $\texttt{high}$ is -1.375 and is not statistically different from zero. Consequently, we conclude that cities at high altitude are not significantly colder than cities at mid-altitude. This conclusion is consistent with the earlier output in

Table 6.4. Cities at sea level are much warmer than mid-altitude cities. The estimated regression coefficient on `sea` is 13.0 and is statistically significant. Perhaps we can simplify the altitude effect into two component values, near sea level and more than 100 feet above sea level; because there appears to be negligible difference between mid-altitude and high-altitude cities.

Interactions are concerned with exceptions to the model in (6.1). The interaction called `seanorth` is only equal to 1 when the city is located both in the north and at sea level. The corresponding regression coefficient $\beta_{\mathtt{seaN}}$ only appears in the model for such cities. Similarly, the interaction `hinorth` is only equal to 1 for high-altitude, northern cities. The corresponding parameter $\beta_{hi\,N}$ only appears in Table 6.6 for such cities.

When we look at the estimated interactions in Table 6.5, we see that sea-level cities in the north are 6.8 degrees colder than we would expect them to be based only a model with main effects. These main effects include the separate effects of being in the north and being at sea level. Without these two main effects, it would be difficult to interpret the estimated regression coefficient of `seanorth` in this model. The regression coefficient for this interaction is not statistically significant, but we see that these cities are colder than expected. Similarly, northern cities at high altitudes are not statistically colder than expected. In fact, such cities are estimated to be about 2.5 degrees warmer than expected, after including the separate main effects of being at high altitude and being located in the northern half of the country.

Let us make one final point for this example. In the SAS output of Table 6.5, we see that the estimated effect of being located north of Washington is estimated as 19.43 degrees colder, on average, than cities south of Washington. In Table 6.3 of the previous section this effect is measured to be -23.05. Although these two estimates are close and are both negative, as we would would expect, how do we account for the difference in values?

The answer is that the indicator variables `high` and `sea` are correlated with `DC`. There is not an even balance of U.S. cities located at different altitudes and latitudes. The effects of the indicators overlap slightly and attempt to measure the same attributes in the data. Recall in Section 5.5 how we tried to accurately measure the effect that an infant's length had on its weight. Many of the variables in the low-birth-weight infant dataset are mutually correlated, and it is sometimes difficult to distinguish the effects of any one of these on the weight outcome. A similar situation occurs when we create indicators for altitude and latitude. These are also correlated with each other, and their explanatory values overlap in a regression model.

In general, it is a good idea to examine the interactions of variables that we find to be statistically significant in our models. If the variables are separately important in explaining the outcome, then their interaction may provide even more value. Interactions are generally harder to find statistically significant because the power to detect them is lower than for the main effects. Always include the original main effects in order to facilitate the interpretation of the regression coefficients. Finally,

Table 6.7. For several countries listed, the price of a gallon of gasoline and the average daily consumption per person.

Country	Price in U.S. dollars	Consumption per person
Norway	6.66	1.9
Netherlands	6.55	2.3
Britain	6.17	1.2
Germany	5.98	1.4
Italy	5.94	1.4
France	5.68	1.4
Singapore	3.50	7.3
Brazil	3.35	0.5
India	3.29	0.1
Mexico	3.20	0.8
South Africa	3.13	0.4
United States	2.26	2.9
Russia	2.05	0.8
China	1.78	0.2
Nigeria	1.48	0.1
Iran	0.47	0.8

Source: Reuters; Energy Information Administration.

interactions need not be constructed only from indicator variables. The interaction of any two variables (either continuous or discrete valued) can be constructed as the product of the two.

> An interaction variable is constructed as the product of any two explanatory variables.

If you accidentally include variables that result in multicolinearity, this is not a great problem. SAS will give you an error message and may even try to identify the linear combination of explanatory variables in your model. You will need to omit variables from the `model` statement until SAS is able to fit the model without an error message. Remember that depending on which ones you remove, the interpretation of the intercept and reference category will change.

6.4 Transformations

Table 6.7 presents the 2005 average price of gasoline (in U.S. dollars) and average daily consumption per person for several different countries.[1] What determines the

[1] Available online at http://www.nytimes.com/2005/04/30/business/worldbusiness/30norway.html.

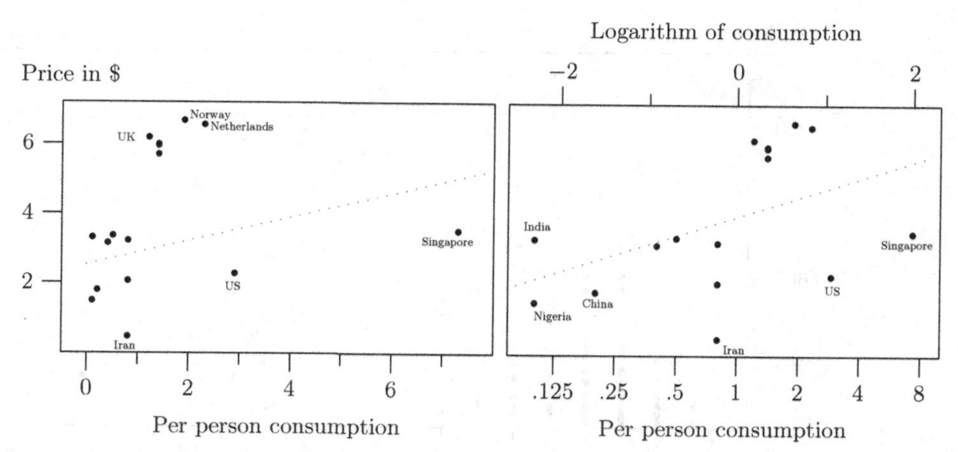

Figure 6.2 **Observed data and fitted regressions of gasoline price using consumption and log consumption.**

price: how much it is taxed, the rate of consumption, or whether the country produces and exports oil? Both Norway and Iran export oil, but Iran has very low consumption per person. Norway has higher consumption and also very high taxes on gasoline. The economy of Singapore relies heavily on shipping and the petrochemical industry, including refining. All of these consume a lot of oil. Given the data in this table, how can we make convincing argument that per-person consumption plays a large role in the price of gasoline?

The graph on the left half of Figure 6.2 plots the raw data including the fitted regression line. The slope of this line is 0.22 with an estimated standard error of 0.30. (See Exercise 6.8 for more on interpreting this slope.) The statistical significance level is $p = 0.49$, indicating a weak linear relationship between price and consumption. In this graph we see that Singapore has a large influence in this regression model because its consumption is so much greater than that of any other country in the dataset. A number of low-price and low-consumption nations (including Iran) are clustered in a tight bunch at the lower left of this figure. It is not clear whether a linear regression is even appropriate from this scatter plot.

Instead of examining per-person consumption, suppose we examine the log (base e) of consumption. This is a new variable created by inserting the line

```
logcon = log(consume);
```

into the `data` step of the SAS program. Again, we should remember to print out the data to make sure that this was programmed correctly.

The right-hand graph in Figure 6.2 shows that this log transformation spreads apart the data on the group of low-consumption and low-gasoline-price countries. We are able to identify the data values for India, Nigeria, and China, for example. This log transformation also pulls in the observation for Singapore and makes it much less influential in the fitted regression. The log consumption values used in

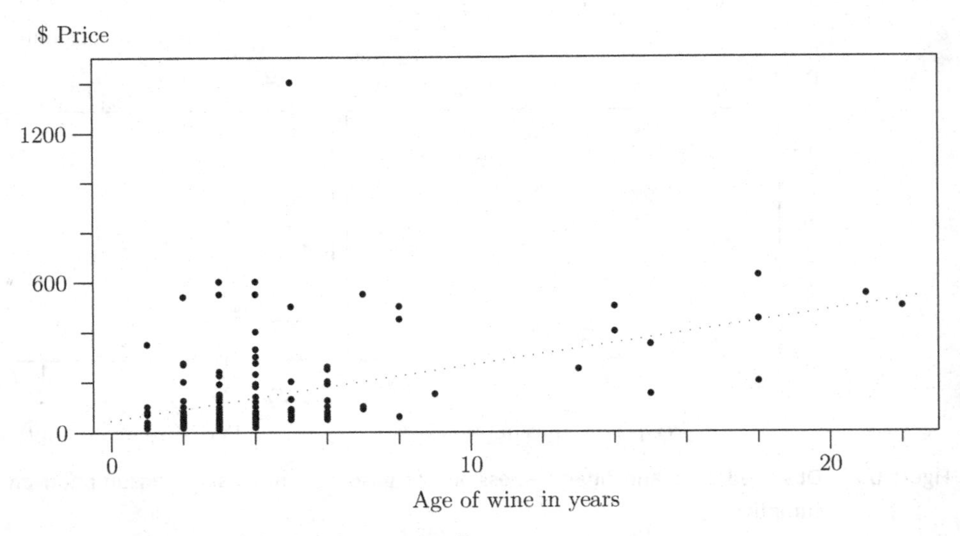

Figure 6.3 Wine price by age and the fitted regression line.

the linear regression are listed along the top of the figure. The values on the original scale are listed at the bottom.

The slope for this new fitted regression on log-consumption is 0.79 with a standard error of 0.41 and statistical significance $p = 0.07$. (See Exercise 6.8 for interpreting this slope.) This improved statistical significance provides a better measure of the effect that consumption has on the price of gasoline. The overall regression influence is more evenly spread among all nations in the dataset after we take the logarithm of the consumption values.

> The logarithm transformation of any variable will pull in large values and spread apart the low values.

Let us consider another example of transformations in regression. Table 5.11 listed the prices of wine in an advertisement. In this example we want to examine the relationship between the age and the price of the wine.

A scatter plot of price by age is given in Figure 6.3. In this figure, we cannot see much if any relationship between these two variables. The prices are mostly bunched up in the lower left corner. There is one extreme price near the top. Many of the wines are fairly new, but there are a few older than ten years. The vertical stripes occur because vintage years are discrete valued. Sometimes jittering the age values can help the display in a figure like this.

The linear regression is statistically significant and $R^2 = 0.2$. The estimated slope is about 22, indicating that the wine appreciates at $22 per year. The relatively small value of R^2 and this figure do not provide very convincing evidence of a linear relationship between wine price and its age. The exercise of Section 6.6.1 asks you to see how much influence the very oldest wines contribute to the linear regression.

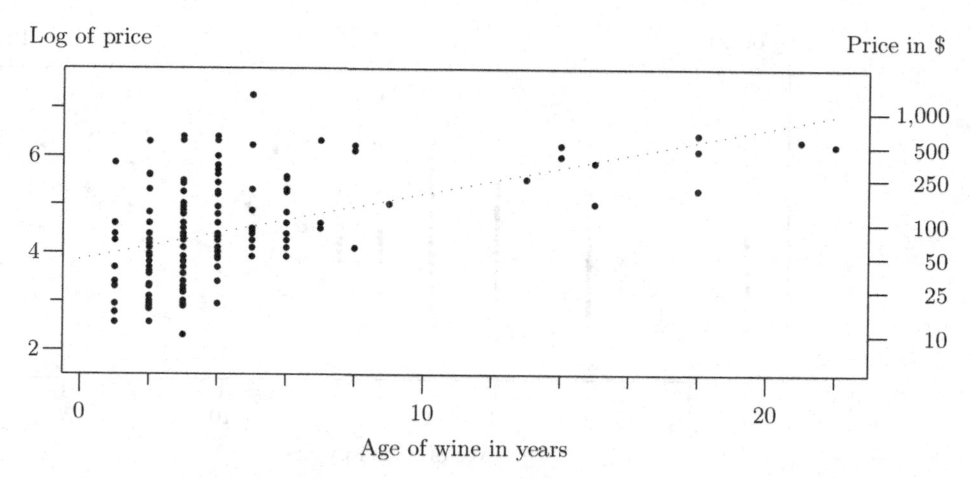

Figure 6.4 Log of wine price by age and the fitted regression line.

In Figure 6.2 we saw that taking logarithms of the gasoline consumption values pulled apart the group of tightly clustered low values and also reduced the effect of the extremely high values. Let us try this with the wine data. In Figure 6.4 we see that taking logs of price has a similar effect. A price in log-dollars may not make sense to most people, so it often helps to include the axis on the right side of this figure, which provides the corresponding values in dollar amounts. Recall that the log scale is multiplicative, so the "doubling" distance from 25 to 50 is the same as from 50 to 100 and the same as from 250 to 500.

The effect of taking logs of price is to break up the tight cluster of values in the lower left corner of the original data plotted in Figure 6.3. By taking logs of price, we can more clearly see individual data points in Figure 6.4. The one very high priced wine is no longer such an extreme outlier.

The linear regression on log price has an improved $R^2 = 0.245$ as well. Wines younger than ten years have a wide range of prices. Wines older than ten years have a smaller variation in relative price. These older wines are more expensive than the average younger wines, but this difference is not dramatic. This difference is probably the largest contributor to the statistical significance of the fitted regression model. See Section 6.6.1 for an examination of this claim.

This regression has a slope of 0.136. Taking logs of the response variable puts the regression on a multiplicative scale. Comparing one year to the next, this model suggests that prices will be in the ratio of

$$\exp(0.136) = 1.146$$

to 1. That is to say, this model estimates that, on average, these wine prices will increase by 14.6% for every year of age.

In Figure 6.4, we also see that the older wines are separated from the others along the age axis, and a few of these influential observations are older than ten years. We

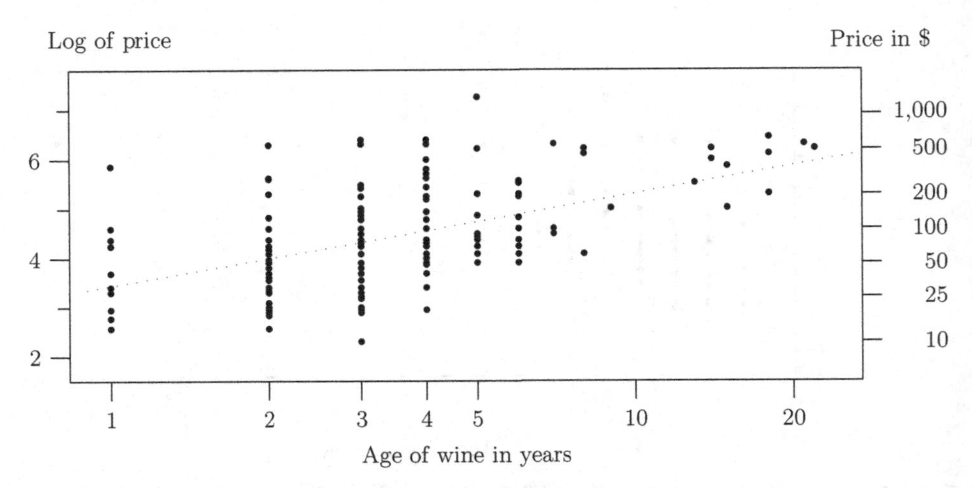

Figure 6.5 **Wine price by age, both on a log scale, and the fitted regression line.**

can take logs of the age values as well as price. This is plotted in Figure 6.5. As with the price values, it is often helpful to the reader if you provide the actual values rather than the transformed values.

In Figure 6.5, we can see the age values more evenly spread out, without the oldest ages exerting great influence. The linear regression in this figure has $R^2 = 0.27$, and the figure provides good evidence of a linear fit to the data. There are no apparent outliers on the log-price scale, and the oldest ages also on a log scale, are not influential. There appears to be larger variation in price at younger ages than among the older wines, but otherwise this appears to be a good application of linear regression.

The estimated regression slope for the transformed data in Figure 6.5 is 0.812. Because both price and age are measured on a log scale, both of these have to be interpreted in a multiplicative fashion. Specifically, the estimated ratio of the average price of one wine is

$$2^{0.812} = 1.756$$

times as great as that of another wine with half the age. At twice the age, then, a wine should cost 75.6% greater, on average.

In this section, the two examples demonstrated that taking logs may sometimes remove influence and reduce the appearance of outliers. Logarithms also pulled apart tight clusters of data points, allowing these to be more clearly seen and to contribute equally to the fitted regression model. Exercise 6.1 provides another example of this. The square root transformation is sometimes used as well. This transformation is not as extreme as the logarithm and has a more subtle effect. See Exercise 6.4 for an example.

There are other important instances in which we might want to transform one or more variables in a linear regression. Sometimes the scatter plot suggests that

Table 6.8. Percent favorable attitudes toward the United States by country.

	1999–2000	Summer 2002	March 2003	June 2003
Israel	–	–	–	79
Great Britain	83	75	48	70
Kuwait	–	–	–	63
Canada	71	72	–	63
Nigeria	46	77	–	61
Australia	–	–	–	60
Italy	76	70	34	60
South Korea	58	53	–	46
Germany	78	61	25	45
France	62	63	31	43
Spain	50	–	14	38
Russia	37	61	28	36
Brazil	56	52	–	34
Morocco	77	–	–	27
Lebanon	–	35	–	27
Indonesia	75	61	–	15
Turkey	52	30	12	15
Pakistan	23	10	–	13
Jordan	–	25	–	1
Palestian Auth.	14	–	–	1

Source: Pew Research Center.

the data are related, but not in a linear fashion. In the exercise of Section 6.6.4, we examine tumor growth rates in mice. These sometimes grow at an exponential rate, and a log transformation may be appropriate in order to apply a linear regression model. In other settings we might accept the nonlinear relationship and try to model it. In Exercise 6.6.8 we describe how to fit a nonlinear relationship with a model containing both the explanatory variable and the square of this variable.

6.5 Additional Topics: Longitudinal Data

As part of a survey conducted by Pew,[2] Table 6.8 summarizes the attitudes toward the United States held by citizens of several other countries at up to four different time points. What is the best way to use regression to analyze this data?

Longitudinal data is the study of observations taken over time. In this example, different people were surveyed at two different times. This is sometimes called *panel data*, in which a cross-section of the population is examined. Similarly, we might ask how individual countries' attitudes change. Such a study is called *transitional.*

[2] Available online at http://people-press.org/reports/pdf/185.pdf.

Longitudinal data is commonly collected in health studies where a change is only apparent over a period of observation. In medical studies, we might follow and collect data on the same subject over a period of time. We might ask whether individuals with poor initial conditions improve over time. This is the transitional approach to examining longitudinal data. Random effects models (see also Section 6.6.4) are useful for this type of modeling, where every subject is measured several times. In public health we might ask whether the average for the whole population changes at each time point. This is the marginal approach. An analysis of the longitudinal data in Table 6.8 is given in Exercise 6.7. Another examination of longitudinal data appears in Exercise 9.4.2.

One of the difficulties that occur when subjects are measured more than once is called *regression to the mean.* Suppose there was no difference in attitudes between the various countries at two different time points. In this case, we would expect that those surveys that were more favorable than average at the first interview time would tend to be more like the average on the second survey. Similarly, those that were most unfavorable at the time of the first interview should look more favorable at the next survey. This property is called regression to the mean, because extremes above and below the average will look more like the average when measured a second time. An example of this behavior is examined in Exercise 6.5.

Another difficulty with longitudinal data is the presence of missing data. Missing data is very common in longitudinal medical and social data, where subjects are asked to return for periodic reexaminations. There can be many reasons for missing data. As an example, did individuals with extreme attitudes refuse to answer the U.S. attitude survey? In this case, there would be a bias in the observed data, because whether or not a data point was missing would be related to what its value might have been had it been observed.

One quick fix for missing data in longitudinal surveys is to use the last observed value. This approach of *last observed value carried forward* is a simple and well-accepted approach to filling in most of the missing values in a longitudinal survey. Clearly this technique would not work for Israel, Kuwait, or Australia, which have no earlier observations, but many of the other missing values in this table could be replaced in this manner.

6.6 Exercises

6.1 Notice how skewed the altitude values are in Figure 5.1. Plot the `dfbeta` for altitude and then again in the model with log altitude. Does this logarithmic transformation reduce the influence of cities at the highest altitudes?

6.2 Examine the three indicator variables for city altitude described in Section 6.1. Use indicator variables in linear regression to show that the difference in maximum January temperature between medium-altitude and high-altitude cities is not statistically significant. *Hint:* Use either the mid- or high-altitude cities as the reference category.

6.3 In Table 3.3 we have the win/loss record of the Baltimore Orioles in addition to the average attendance per home game. If we use both the number of games won and the number of games lost every year, would these two numbers provide more explanatory value than using just one of them? Verify that the number of games played every year is almost the same. Describe the role that multicolinearity plays in fitting a regression model with both the number of games won and the number of games lost as separate explanatory variables. Other analyses of these data appear in Exercises 3.8 and 5.4.

6.4 Reexamine the gasoline consumption data of Table 6.7. Consider the square root of the consumption values. This is done by creating a new variable in the data step using the `sqrt` function in SAS. Specifically, the line in the program might look like this:

```
sqcons = sqrt(consume);
```

Does this transformation provide a better linear regression than the original data? Look at the hat matrix diagonals to see if the highest-consuming countries are as influential as they were in the original data. Compare the square root transformation to the log transformation for these data. Which of these two depictions of the data do your prefer?

6.5 Let us ask all members of the class to predict the order in which heads and tails appear in the course of ten successive tosses of a coin. Some people will be very good at this and can take the rest of the day off. Those who lack this skill are required to watch a movie about how coins are minted and then review Section 2.1 on the binomial distribution. This must be a good strategy, because the next day, the former poor predictors do much better on average. Unfortunately, however, those who took the afternoon off failed to do as well as they did the day before. What happened?

6.6 The one-way ANOVA is the generalization of the t-test to more than two groups of subjects. This is described at the end of Section 6.1, comparing cities at one of three different altitudes. In general, what are the assumptions of Section 4.4 that need to be met when we perform a one-way ANOVA?

6.7 Consider a marginal analysis of the attitude survey given in Table 6.8. To compare the mean attitude at the time of any two surveys, we can perform a t-test. Because each of the countries is compared at two different times, we should perform a *paired t-test.* The paired t-test is the same as a one-sample t-test performed on the column of difference values. We want to test the null hypothesis that the mean difference is equal to 0. Is there a downward trend in the means? Is there evidence that the survey favored countries with a higher initial attitude?

There are several different ways to perform a transitional analysis. We might begin by plotting the attitude values (on the vertical scale) against time of the survey and drawing a line connecting the values for the same country. This mix of lines is called a *spaghetti plot* for obvious reasons. Spaghetti plots will often reveal the general trend of the individuals. Construct the spaghetti plot for the data in Table 6.8. In this figure, do the low initial attitudes tend to become lower in the later survey, or are these more likely to increase? That is, does there appear to be a regression to the mean? What can be said about countries with high initial attitudes toward the United States?

6.8 The estimated slope of the data on the left half of Figure 6.2 is 0.22. Interpret this value.

If consumption is measured on a log scale, the estimated slope is 0.79. Show that if consumption is doubled, this model estimates that the price per person should increase $0.79 \log(2) = \$0.55$ per person, on average.

6.6.1 More on Wine Prices

Let us reexamine the wine price exercise of Section 5.7.5. We can make use of methods described in this chapter, specifically, transformations and interactions of variables. The data was given in Table 5.11.

1. Examine the difference in prices between wines older and younger than ten years using a t-test. Is the comparison stronger if price is measured on a log scale or a linear scale?
2. How do the experts' points relate to price? Is there a benefit in transforming the points as well as price values?
3. Repeat some of the analysis performed in Section 5.7.5 for these data using transformed values. Do you identify the same wines as bargains or overpriced that you identified in the earlier examination of this data?
4. Is there a synergistic interaction between experts' points and old vintage when it comes to modeling the price of a wine? That is, do old wines with high points command a much higher premium than what we might expect from these two factors alone?

6.6.2 Statistics in the News: Nicotine Levels in Cigarettes

Table 6.9 presents data[3] on the cigarettes with the highest nicotine content. A number of comparisons can be made. For example, we can compare the nicotine contents of Lorillard versus all other manufacturers, menthol versus nonmenthol cigarettes, and filter versus nonfilter brands. All of these can be done using separate t-tests. A better analysis plan is to create a series of 0–1 indicators and use these simultaneously in the same regression model. What do these simultaneous comparisons provide that is different from running three separate t-tests?

Examine the interactions among the three indicator variables. How do you interpret these? Should the nicotine levels be transformed? Apply other lessons from this and the previous chapter. Look for influence and outliers.

[3] Source: Massachusetts Department of Public Health.

Table 6.9. Cigarettes and their nicotine content.

Brand	Menthol?	Length	Filtered?	Manufacturer	Nicotine
Old Gold		85	non-filter	Lorillard	4.1
Max		120	filter	Lorillard	3.4
Newport	M	100	filter	Lorillard	3.2
Camel		70	non-filter	RJ Reynolds	3.0
Doral		85	non-filter	RJ Reunolds	3.0
Newport	M	85	filter	Lorillard	2.8
Maverick	M	100	filter	Lorillard	2.7
Camel		100	filter	RJ Reynolds	2.6
Maverick		100	filter	Lorillard	2.5
Kool	M	100	filter	RJ Reynolds	2.5
Newport		100	filter	Lorillard	2.5
Marlboro		100	filter	Phillip Morris	2.4

6.6.3 The Speed of a Reaction

The data in Table 6.10 provides a summary of experiments measuring the speed of an enzymatic reaction both with and without addition of the enzyme puromycin. The reaction depends on the initial concentration (in parts per million), and its rate is measured in radioactive counts per minute.

Plot the rate (y) as a function of initial concentration (x) and describe the relationship. The authors of these data had theoretical evidence for a specific nonlinear

Table 6.10. Data on the speed of an enzymatic reaction both with and without addition of the enzyme puromycin.

Initial concentration	Rate	Puromycin?	Initial concentration	Rate	Puromycin?
0.02	76	Y	0.02	47	Y
0.06	97	Y	0.06	107	Y
0.11	123	Y	0.11	139	Y
0.22	159	Y	0.22	152	Y
0.56	191	Y	0.56	201	Y
1.10	207	Y	1.10	200	Y
0.02	67	N	0.02	51	N
0.06	84	N	0.06	86	N
0.11	98	N	0.11	115	N
0.22	131	N	0.22	124	N
0.56	144	N	0.56	158	N
1.10	160	N			

Source: Bates, and Watts (1988). Appendix A1.3.

Table 6.11. Tumor volumes (in mm^3) in ten mice.

Mouse	Days after injection			
#	11	13	15	17
1	157.1	217.6	379.0	556.6
2	152.2	176.6	317.9	356.4
3	122.4	196.1	388.9	496.3
4	95.0	205.9	307.3	405.1
5	168.8	196.0	340.4	507.3
6	85.0	225.1	289.0	317.9
7	129.8	274.7	340.3	507.2
8	157.0	202.5	307.2	320.1
9	129.7	205.8	419.1	421.2
10	156.9	225.0	372.6	379.2

Source: Koziol *et al.* (1981).

relationship between these variables. Try a log or square-root transformation of the rate. Does this produce a better linear relationship?

What effect does addition of puromycin have on the rate of the reaction? Propose a model and fit it in SAS. After transforming the rate, is there evidence of a nonconstant variance? Are there outliers that need to be pointed out?

6.6.4 Tumor Growth in Mice

In a commonly conducted experiment, a small piece of a human tumor is injected under the skin of a mouse. If the tumor successfully implants and continues to grow, a palpable lump will be felt under the mouse's skin. The volume of this lump can be measured, and changes in its size over time are indicative of the virulence of the tumor. An example of such an experiment is given in Table 6.11 for ten mice.

Draw the spaghetti plot for these data. Perform a linear regression modeling tumor size by date for these ten mice. Check the residuals of this model. Does the regression look linear? Try jittering the dates in the graph to improve the appearance. Of course, you don't want to jitter the dates that you use in the regression model.

Consider a log transformation of the size values. Does this improve the linearity of the model? Taking logs is a reasonable approach if you think that tumor growth is exponential in time. What is wrong with assuming that the exponential growth will continue?

Notice that every mouse is measured four times. Is the linear regression approach valid? Recall the four assumptions we made about linear regression in Section 4.4. One approach that takes into account the multiple observations on the same individual is called *random effects*.

In a random-effects model, we might assume that every mouse has its own intercept and slope, but that collectively all of these intercepts and slopes are not

Table 6.12. Prices of used cars from an advertisement appearing in the *New York Times* on August 5, 2007.

Year	Class	Color	Mileage	Price	Year	Class	Color	Mileage	Price
04	E	black	22	30	04	E	grey	25	32
05	E	black	28	34	04	E	blue	35	36
04	E	grey	19	37	05	E	grey	18	40
05	E	grey	30	42	05	E	grey	16	48
05	E	black	40	57	00	S	black	38	30
01	S	grey	17	35	03	S	black	64	36
05	S	grey	36	49	06	S	black	27	53
04	S	grey	14	55	06	S	grey	30	58
06	S	black	18	58	04	S	black	41	62
07	S	blue	12	75	04	CLS	grey	30	53
03	CLS	black	43	58	06	CLS	blue	9	60
04	CLS	blue	32	65	06	CLS	black	20	70
03	CLK	white	35	29	02	CLK	grey	20	32
04	CLK	red	30	33	03	CLK	black	12	36
06	CLK	grey	9	45	04	M	grey	26	28
04	M	grey	13	28	04	M	grey	28	29
05	M	grey	40	30	05	M	grey	23	34
05	M	black	36	34	05	M	grey	20	36
06	M	white	20	39					

very different from each other. Biologically, each individual intercept and slope may depend on each of the experimental conditions experienced by each mouse, such as the size of the tumor injected or differences in the way it was injected. Random effects models for longitudinal data are described in Section 6.5. Is there evidence that the slopes or intercepts are very different for each mouse?

6.6.5 Statistics in Advertising: Used Car Prices

Table 6.12 gives the prices of used Mercedes in an advertisement from a car dealer. For each car, we have the year, class, color, mileage (in thousands) and price (in thousands of dollars). Mercedes produces various models that are grouped together into larger classes. Cars are listed with two or more colors, and the color listed here is the first color mentioned. Grey includes silver, tan, and pewter; black includes charcoal.

Show that, marginally, across all model classes, the year is very important in determining the price, but the mileage is not. How do you explain this? Interpret the slope of the year in this regression.

When we perform a regression separately for each model class, we see that either the year or the model may be statistically significant, sometimes both are, and sometimes neither is. Why, do you think, this is the case? Notice that the intercepts

Table 6.13. A portion of the body fat dataset.

1.0708	12.3	23	154.25	67.75	36.2	93.1	85.2	94.5	59.0	37.3	21.9	32.0	27.4	17.1
1.0853	6.1	22	173.25	72.25	38.5	93.6	83.0	98.7	58.7	37.3	23.4	30.5	28.9	18.2
1.0414	25.3	22	154.00	66.25	34.0	95.8	87.9	99.2	59.6	38.9	24.0	28.8	25.2	16.6
							.....							
1.0399	26.0	72	190.75	70.50	38.9	108.3	101.3	97.8	56.0	41.6	22.7	30.5	29.4	19.8
1.0271	31.9	74	207.50	70.00	40.8	112.4	108.5	107.1	59.3	42.2	24.6	33.7	30.0	20.9

may be either positive or negative in each of these separate regressions. How do you account for this? What does the intercept represent? Is it meaningful?

Is the color important? Create an indicator variable to identify black and nonblack colors. Use this indicator in your regressions to see if the color of the car influences the price.

Look for outliers and influential observations. Are there bargains or overpriced cars in this dealer's lot? Is there evidence that the regression on year is linear? Do these cars appear to depreciate a constant amount every year, or is there evidence that the largest depreciation occurs earlier?

6.6.6 Percent Body Fat

Accurate estimates of total body fat are inconvenient because these involve weighing a subject who is submersed in a tank of water. This yields a measure of total body density, relative to an equal volume of water. A number of different methods have been suggested over the years to facilitate this computation. Some recent alternative proposals available include the use of a caliper to measure the thickness of a skin fold. These methods too, have their shortcomings. Can you help find a relatively easy way to measure body fat?

The data[4] includes the body fat measurements of 252 male volunteers, along with a number of other physical attributes. The website includes a full explanation of the mathematical relationship between density and body fat, along with many useful references. A small portion of the data is given in Table 6.13. A complete list of the fifteen variables measured on each subject is given in Table 6.14.

See if you can build a good linear model of percent body fat using any of the regression tools we have learned so far. The percent body fat is computed from underwater density, so your regression model should not include the density information. Some of the physical measurements are highly correlated with each other, and not all may be useful. Be sure to examine your residuals and check for influential observations using diagnostics such as `dffits` and Cook's D. It is equally acceptable to find a good model that explains density. Percent body fat can be derived from density, so the model for density should not include body fat, and *vice versa*.

[4] Available online at http://lib.stat.cmu.edu/datasets/bodyfat.

Table 6.14. List of variables in the body fat dataset.

- Density determined from underwater weighing
- Percent body fat
- Age (years)
- Weight (lb)
- Height (inches)
- Neck circumference (cm)
- Chest circumference (cm)
- Abdomen circumference (cm)
- Hip circumference (cm)
- Thigh circumference (cm)
- Knee circumference (cm)
- Ankle circumference (cm)
- Biceps (extended) circumference (cm)
- Forearm circumference (cm)
- Wrist circumference (cm)

Here are some things to look for. Cook's D indicates some very influential observations. One of these is the man with the greatest weight. That observation should be easy to find. The others are not as easy to identify.

In model building we need to make a general statement for most of the population, but we must also include provisions for such exceptions to the rule. Remember the carnival act in which they guess your weight? Most individuals will follow the general pattern, so this is not as remarkable as it first appears. The real test of the model is to see how general it is. Does it include most of the observed data, or are there many outliers that fail to follow the pattern?

6.6.7 Fertility Rates in Switzerland

In 1888, Switzerland began a transition period of reduced birth rates that are close to what they are today. Higher fertility rates before this time are usually associated with those of underdeveloped countries today. This transition is studied by demographers, who note that it is associated with the simultaneous rise in life expectancy, drop in birth rate, and rise in incomes. This has led to the *demographic-economic paradox*, in which the richer nations can support more children, yet tend to have lower birth rates. The fertility rate given in Table 6.15 is a standardized rate I_g widely used by demographers.

The columns in this table are:

- The name of the province
- The standardized fertility rate
- The percent of the population with an agricultural occupation
- The proportion of military "draftees" who scored high on an army examination
- The percent of the population with more than a primary school education

Table 6.15. Fertility rates in forty-seven French-speaking provinces of Switzerland in 1888.

Province	Fertility rate	% Population in agriculture	% High exams	% High education	% Catholic	Infant mortality
Courtelary	80.2	17.0	15	12	9.96	22.2
Delémont	83.1	45.1	6	9	84.84	22.2
Franches-Montagnes	92.5	39.7	5	5	93.40	20.2
Moutier	85.8	36.5	12	7	33.77	20.3
La Neuveville	76.9	43.5	17	15	5.16	20.6
Porrentruy	76.1	35.3	9	7	90.57	26.6
Broye	83.8	70.2	16	7	92.85	23.6
Glâne	92.4	67.8	14	8	97.16	24.9
Gruyére	82.4	53.3	12	7	97.67	21.0
Sarine	82.9	45.2	16	13	91.38	24.4
Veveyse	87.1	64.5	14	6	98.61	24.5
Aigle	64.1	62.0	21	12	8.52	16.5
Aubonne	66.9	67.5	14	7	2.27	19.1
Avenches	68.9	60.7	19	12	4.43	22.7
Cossonay	61.7	69.3	22	5	2.82	18.7
Echallens	68.3	72.6	18	2	24.20	21.2
Grandson	71.7	34.0	17	8	3.30	20.0
Lausanne	55.7	19.4	26	28	12.11	20.2
La Vallée	54.3	15.2	31	20	2.15	10.8
Lavaux	65.1	73.0	19	9	2.84	20.0
Morges	65.5	59.8	22	10	5.23	18.0
Moudon	65.0	55.1	14	3	4.52	22.4
Nyon	56.6	50.9	22	12	15.14	16.7
Orbe	57.4	54.1	20	6	4.20	15.3
Oron	72.5	71.2	12	1	2.40	21.0
Payerne	74.2	58.1	14	8	5.23	23.8
Paysdénhaut	72.0	63.5	6	3	2.56	18.0
Rolle	60.5	60.8	16	10	7.72	16.3
Vevey	58.3	26.8	25	19	18.46	20.9
Yverdon	65.4	49.5	15	8	6.10	22.5
Conthey	75.5	85.9	3	2	99.71	15.1
Entremont	69.3	84.9	7	6	99.68	19.8
Herens	77.3	89.7	5	2	100.00	18.3
Martigna	70.5	78.2	12	6	98.96	19.4
Monthey	79.4	64.9	7	3	98.22	20.2
St Maurice	65.0	75.9	9	9	99.06	17.8
Sierre	92.2	84.6	3	3	99.46	16.3
Sion	79.3	63.1	13	13	96.83	18.1
Boudry	70.4	38.4	26	12	5.62	20.3
La Chaux-de-Fronds	65.7	7.7	29	11	13.79	20.5
Le Locle	72.7	16.7	22	13	11.22	18.9
Neuchâtel	64.4	17.6	35	32	16.92	23.0
Val de Ruz	77.6	37.6	15	7	4.97	20.0
Val-de-Travers	67.6	18.7	25	7	8.65	19.5
Val de Geneve	35.0	1.2	37	53	42.34	18.0
Rive Droite	44.7	46.6	16	29	50.43	18.2
Rive Gauche	42.8	27.7	22	29	58.33	19.3

Source: Mosteller and Tukey, 1977, pp. 549–51.

- The percentage of the population who are Catholic
- The fraction of births in which the infant does not survive one year

What are the determinants of the fertility rate? Model the fertility rates of the different provinces using methods described in this chapter. The percentage of the population with high education, for example, is highly skewed, and the few provinces with high rates have large influence. Try taking logs of the education variable to even out this effect.

Several of the explanatory variables are correlated with each other. For example, in 1888, agriculture was a labor-intensive effort, and large families were generally more successful. Similarly, higher education was a luxury. Lifespans were much shorter than they are today. Additional offspring would be needed to offset a high infant mortality. Identify any strong relationships between the explanatory variables in your model.

See Exercise 7.9 for additional models of this data. More data from this series as well as other historic demographic datasets are available through the Office of Population Research at Princeton University.[5]

6.6.8 ELISA

ELISA (or enzyme-linked immunosorbent assay) is a technique in biochemistry for detecting an antibody. There are many variants of this popular laboratory method. Essentially, a known concentration of an antigen is put in contact with a serum sample. If there is a match, then the specific antibody will bind to the antigen. This is detected through a change in color or through the use of a fluorescent dye. ELISA is commonly used to detect HIV or West Nile virus for example. Many ELISA experiments are run simultaneously under identical conditions using an array of small test tubes called *wells.*

The data[6] in Table 6.16 summarizes one such experiment that was part of the development of an assay for detecting the recombinant protein DNase in rat serum. There were eleven different "runs" of the experiment. Each run consisted of eight different concentrations of the antigen, and each of these was replicated for a total of sixteen paired observations in each run.

Plot the concentration on the X axis and the density on the Y axis. Does a transformation of the concentration seem appropriate to reduce the influence of higher concentrations? Is there a linear relationship with the optical response? Notice that the plot of density by concentration curves in one direction, but the plot with log concentration curves in the other direction. Consider a model that contains both log concentration and the square of log concentration. Does this improve the fit?

[5] Available online at http://opr.princeton.edu/archive.
[6] Source: Davidian and Giltinan (1995), p. 134.

Table 6.16. A portion of the ELISA data.

Observation number	Run number	Antigen concentration	Optical density
1	1	0.04882812	0.017
2	1	0.04882812	0.018
3	1	0.19531250	0.121
4	1	0.19531250	0.124
5	1	0.39062500	0.206
6	1	0.39062500	0.215
7	1	0.78125000	0.377
8	1	0.78125000	0.374
9	1	1.56250000	0.614
10	1	1.56250000	0.609
11	1	3.12500000	1.019
12	1	3.12500000	1.001
13	1	6.25000000	1.334
14	1	6.25000000	1.364
15	1	12.50000000	1.730
16	1	12.50000000	1.710
17	2	0.04882812	0.045
18	2	0.04882812	0.050
19	2	0.19531250	0.137
		...	
174	11	6.25000000	1.385
175	11	12.50000000	1.715
176	11	12.50000000	1.721

Are there differences in the eleven runs? Suppose we want to fit a model with eleven different intercepts, for example. To do this, we need to create eleven indicator variables. A `data` step that does this is appears in Table 6.17.

The `array` statement creates eleven variables corresponding to the `run` values. These indicators can be referred to as `runind(1), ..., runind(11)`, or else by the names `runind1, ..., runind11`. The `do; ...end;` statements create a loop that initializes all of these equal to 0, and the `runind(run)=1;` sets one indicator equal to 1 for each value of `run`. It is a good idea to run this program followed by a `proc print;` statement to verify that your program works correctly.

The `model` statement can refer to all eleven indicators if we write

```
model dens = logc runind2-runind11;
```

Table 6.17. The `data` step to read the ELISA data.

```
data ELISA;
   infile 'ELISA.dat';
   input count  run  conc dens;
   logc=log(conc);
   array runind(11) runind1-runind11;
   do i=1 to 11;
   runind(i) = 0;
   end;
   runind(run)=1;
run;
```

and we leave out the indicator corresponding to the first run in order to avoid multicolinearity. This statement will fit a model with eleven separate intercepts, using the first run as the reference category.

Fit a model with eleven slopes? *Hint:* Think of these as the interaction between the intercepts and the slope.

7

Nonparametric Statistics

Do you remember all of the assumptions that have to hold in order for statistical inference to be valid when we perform a t-test? What happens if the variances aren't equal in the two groups? Do you need to test for this? What happens if the data is not normally distributed? How can you tell when it is? What happens if there are outliers? How do you know for sure whether a given data point is an outlier? Statisticians tend to be a cautious bunch, but there is no need for you to be overly concerned. Nonparametric statistics are just the cure for messy data where outliers and highly skewed distributions would plague most analyses.

In a motivation for this chapter, suppose you learn that the average salary at a company has increased but at the same time the median income is unchanged. This means that most of the benefits were accrued by a few individuals, either at the top or at the bottom. In this example, is the average or the median more representative of the typical individual? We would like to cite a *robust* estimator that is not sensitive to a small number of unusually large or small values. In this example we see that the median remains unchanged if some of the largest or smallest values are altered.

Nonparametric methods are used for continuous, but not necessarily normally distributed data, with possible outliers.

Nonparametric statistics are a whole different approach to statistics. These include a wide variety of methods for the analysis of data with a minimum of assumptions about the underlying population. As an example, we might be able to rank different flavors of ice cream but would not be able to assign a quantitative value to those preferences.

7.1 A Test for Medians

Let us begin with an example from agriculture. Table 7.1 lists the dried weights of plants grown under either a control or a treated setting. The question to answer is to determine whether the treatment increases the dried plant weights.

Table 7.1. Dried weights of 20 plants grown under separate conditions.

Control:	4.17	5.58	5.18	6.11	4.50	4.61	5.17	4.53	5.33	5.14
Treated:	6.31	5.12	5.54	5.50	5.37	5.29	4.92	6.15	5.80	5.26

	Control	Treated
Means:	5.03	5.53
St. Dev.:	0.583	0.443

Stem and leaf plot

Control		Treated	
4	2556	4	9
5	12236	5	1334558
6	1	6	23

Source: Dobson (2002), Table 6.6, p. 96.

The data in Table 7.1 is followed by a *stem and leaf plot.* The stem and leaf is like a histogram, but instead of boxes to represent numbers, we let the numbers represent themselves. The vertical lines represent the decimal points in this figure. Looking at the stem and leaf, we see that the four smallest numbers in the control group of plants include the numbers 4.2, 4.5, 4.5, and 4.6 rounded to a single decimal point. From the stem and leaf we can see that the plants grown under the control conditions tend to be lighter and also have greater variability when compared to the treated plants. These conclusions are confirmed by looking at the means and standard deviations of the two groups.

One way to compare the two groups of plants is to compare their *medians.* Recall that the median is the number that evenly divides the sample. Half of the observations are either above or below the median. In the present example, when we sort all 20 observations in the combined or *pooled* sample of both groups, we find that the median of all observations falls between 5.26 and 5.29, both from the treated group. With an even number of observations we average the two middle values, giving 5.275 as the pooled median.

We can verify that of all 20 observations in the pooled sample, exactly half are above and half are below this value. If this median value of 5.275 is truly representative of the combined sample, then we would expect that this statement will also be approximately true within each of the two groups of plants as well. That is, about half of the controls and half of the treated plants should also be above or below this value. Let us see if this is the case.

Among the control plants, 3 had values above 5.275 and 7 were below this value. Similarly, among the treated plants, 7 were above 5.275 and 3 were below. We can

Table 7.2. The plant growth data summarized for the median test. The median is for the pooled sample.

	Control	Treated	Totals
> median	3	7	10
< median	7	3	10
Totals	10	10	20

summarize this finding in a 2 × 2 set of frequencies given in Table 7.2. Exercise 7.2 asks the reader to verify some properties of this table.

> The medians test examines the number of observations within each group that are above and below the pooled median.

We should immediately recognize that the next step is to compute a Pearson chi-squared test on the data in Table 7.2. The value of the statistic is 3.2 (1 df) and p-value of .074. The presence of very small counts in this table suggests that the chi-squared approximation might not be very accurate. The continuity-adjusted chi-square is 1.8 with $p = .18$, and the exact test also gives us $p = .18$, suggesting that there is little difference in the weights of the two plant groups. (See Section 2.6 for a discussion of these different methods for examining the counts in a 2 × 2 table.) In the present case, the p-value of .18 seems more accurate.

Before we interpret the p-value for this table, we need to ask what are the hypotheses that we are testing. The chi-squared statistic tests independence of rows and columns in this table, but how does independence relate to the problem of medians? The answer is that if the rows are independent of the columns, then the distribution of the numbers of data points above and below the pooled median should be about the same for both groups of plants we are discussing. In other words, independence means that the medians of separate plant groups should be close in value.

Suppose we went ahead and examined the usual Student t-test for this example. In such an examination of these data, we have $t = 2.13$ and $p = .048$. In words, the t-test provides strong evidence that the treatment and control are different, but the medians test does not. Which approach is correct? Unfortunately, the answer is not so simple. If we are willing to assume that the two populations of plants are normally distributed with the same variances, then the t-test is the correct way to proceed.

On the other hand, the medians test is very *robust* against misspecification of assumptions such as whether or not the data are normally distributed. The word *robust* is often used, when describing a statistical procedure, to mean that it is insensitive to incorrect specifications or even gross outliers.

To convince ourselves about the robust properties of the medians test, suppose the value of the first treated plant was recorded as 7.31 rather than as 6.31. Such errors are more common than you might expect. If this were the case, then the frequencies in Table 7.2 would remain unchanged. Some might argue that the value of 7.31 is still a valid data point. Suppose the value was recorded as 63.1 rather than 6.31. In this case the median test would again remain unchanged, but this extreme value would have a great effect on the t-test. The t-test would reject the null hypothesis of no treatment difference.

The point here is that some outliers might not be recognized as such and could produce some very misleading results. Of course, if there are no outliers, we pay a price for our caution. As we see in this example, the medians test is unable to detect an alternative hypothesis that the t-test finds statistically significant. Notice also that the t-test compares the two means, but the medians test compares the medians. In symmetric distributions, such as the normal, these two measures will coincide. If the data is skewed, then these will be different.

> Nonparametric methods are insensitive to model assumptions and outliers but have reduced power.

So, in conclusion, are the treated plants heavier than the control plants? In this example there do not appear to be large departures from the assumptions of equal variances and normally distributed data, so the t-test seems appropriate. Inference based on the t-test indicates that the treated plants are heavier, and this appears to be a reasonable conclusion. Perhaps our use of the medians test was overly cautious. There is no telling what might happen the next time we are faced with a similar situation, of course. The medians test is a good tool to remember just in case the data do not confirm to the assumptions as well as in this example.

In a critical situation where the statistical significance is very important to us, the only fair approach is to specify the statistical analysis before we are able to observe the data. Otherwise we might be accused of fishing for the statistical method that achieves the most extreme level of significance, hence distorting its interpretation. Although such a level of caution is unnecessary in the present example involving plant weights, there are times when an honest and unbiased assessment of statistical significance is essential. Such an example might include a clinical trial of a new experimental drug in which we need an accurate measure of its efficacy.

This plant data example is continued in Exercise 7.8. There were two treatment groups in addition to the control group of plants. Simultaneous comparisons of more than two groups can be done in the `npar1way` procedure in SAS. This is illustrated in Section 7.4.

7.2 Statistics in the News: Math Achievement Scores

As a part of federal funding provided by the No Child Left Behind Act, there were great efforts to document progress in reading and math skills of elementary school students. This progress was measured by standardized tests given by the schools to

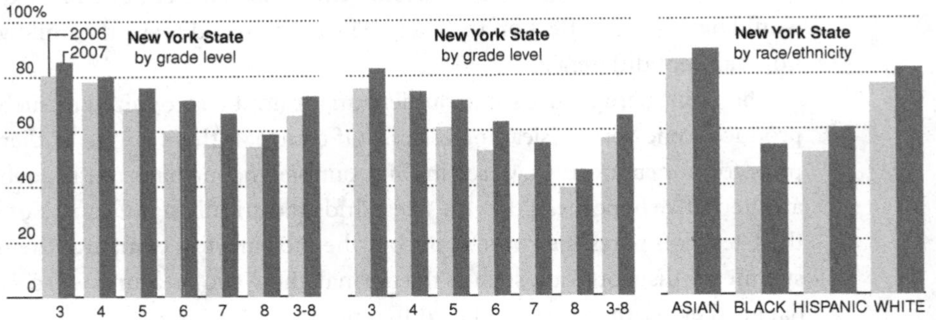
Improvement in Math
Math achievement in grades 3 to 8 improved this year in every grade and among all ethnic and racial groups in New York State and New York City. Below, the percentage of students performing at or above grade level in math.
100%
80
60
40
20
0
2006
2007
New York State
by grade level
3 4 5 6 7 8 3-8
New York State
by grade level
3 4 5 6 7 8 3-8
New York State
by race/ethnicity
ASIAN BLACK HISPANIC WHITE

Figure 7.1 Math achievement scores among elementary school students. *Source: New York Times*, June 13, 2007, page B8.

the children. The tests were designed to identify poor or failing schools. Among many criticisms of the program were claims that teachers were coaching their students in test-taking skills rather than covering subject-matter material. Nevertheless, schools with improving records were quick to publicize their results. One example from New York City and state school systems appeared in the summary in Figure 7.1.[1] Results for the year 2006 appear in lighter gray, and the 2007 results are in the darker color.

Without exception, in every possible category of age and race, in both the city and the state, there was an improvement. How is it possible that every grade in both New York City and state and every racial/ethnic group shows an improvement in math scores? Can we assign a p-value to this outcome?

We could use a Student t-test to compare differences in the two years' results, but the figure is missing the numerical values of both the means and standard deviations. Instead, we can simply use the increase or decrease as a binary-valued outcome, regardless of the actual amount of change. If each year's test scores are comparable to the previous year's, then it should be equally likely to rise or fall.

Consider tossing a coin six times, corresponding to whether there was an improvement in each of the grades 3 through 8. What is the probability of observing six heads in six tosses of a fair coin? The answer is

$$\frac{1}{2^6} = \frac{1}{64} = .015625.$$

Remember that the fifth graders in 2006 became the sixth graders in 2007, so maybe the "coin tosses" are not quite independent. But then again, test scores improved in both the city and also in the state. These outcomes are also not independent, because the city is included as part of the state. The improvement also appears across all ethnic/racial groups, and these are also included in the city and state data.

[1] Available online at http://www.nytimes.com/2007/06/13/education/13math.html.

Perhaps we should consider a two-tailed test for this outcome. That would have us ask the question, "What are the chances that the change is in the same direction for all grades 3 through 8?" In terms of nonparametric statistics, this is also expressible as the probability of either 6 heads or 6 tails in 6 tosses of a fair coin. In this case, the probability is .03125. In either the one- or two-tailed test, these probabilities are still small.

How can we explain this finding? Did large numbers of underachievers drop out each year, resulting in better scores year after year? Are the tests comparable in different years? We appear to reject the hypothesis that 2006 and 2007 tests are comparable in favor of some other explanation. Maybe teachers and teaching methods suddenly became much better. We cannot claim that the students suddenly became smarter, because they appear more than once in this table. Standardized tests such as the GRE and the SAT are said to be "equated" by the administrators so that the results can be compared from one year to the next. Was this done with the test values summarized in this figure? There are conferences among educators and statisticians that discuss how and whether this should be done.

The nonparametric analysis of these data reduces the year-to-year comparison of math scores to the results of a simple coin toss. The actual magnitudes of the differences might be compared using a t-test. Instead, in this statistical analysis, we are only looking at the *direction* of change, not the actual amount.

7.3 Rank Sum Test

The medians test and the examination of the math test scores in Section 7.2 reduce every observation to a coin toss. Specifically, the medians test judges every observation as being either above or below the pooled sample median. The actual magnitude of every observation is lost. It does not matter how far above or below the median an observation is. Does this seem like a tremendous loss of information? Rank methods meet this loss halfway: Instead of reducing all observations to binary above/below status, rank methods replace the actual observations with their order when the data is sorted.

To illustrate this method, consider the plant growth data from Table 7.1. All 20 of the pooled sample values are sorted in Table 7.3 from smallest to largest and identified as belonging to either the control or the treated groups. Each observation is also identified with its rank or order number, from 1 to 20 in terms of the pooled sample. So, for example, the four smallest observations (ranked 1–4) are associated with the control group, and then the next two smallest observations (ranked 5 and 6) are in the treated group.

In rank statistical methods, the original observations are replaced by their ranks when the values are sorted.

Table 7.3. The plant growth data from Table 7.1 converted to ranks.

Control	4.17	4.50	4.53	4.61			5.14	5.17	5.18	
Treated					4.92	5.12				5.26
Rank	1	2	3	4	5	6	7	8	9	10

Control		5.33				5.58		6.11		
Treated	5.29		5.37	5.50	5.54		5.80		6.15	6.31
Rank	11	12	13	14	15	16	17	18	19	20

In rank methods, we replace the observations by their ranks. A large observation achieves a high rank, unlike the medians test where all observations larger than the median are treated equally. In Table 7.3, if both the treated and the control plants had roughly the same means, then we would also expect these two samples to have roughly the same average rank values.

We will return to this example and the SAS program for the rank test in Section 7.4. Before we get to that, let us again illustrate the use of ranked data and show that this is a frequently used approach to describing data that is sometimes qualitative, rather than quantitative, in nature.

7.4 Nonparametric Methods in SAS

The program using the SAS procedure `npar1way` given in the program of Table 7.4 examines the plant weight data of Table 7.1 using several different nonparametric

Table 7.4. SAS program to compare the two groups of plants in Table 7.1.

```
title1 'Plant growth using nonparametric statistics';
data grow;
   input weight group $  @@;
   datalines;
      4.17  c   5.58  c   5.18  c   6.11  c   4.50  c
      4.61  c   5.17  c   4.53  c   5.33  c   5.14  c
      6.31  t   5.12  t   5.54  t   5.50  t   5.37  t
      5.29  t   4.92  t   6.15  t   5.80  t   5.26  t
proc print;
run;
proc npar1way data=grow;
   var weight;
   class group;
run;
```

approaches. The variable name in the `var` statement determines the response variable, in this case plant weight. The variable name in the `class` statement contains values identifying the different groups. In this example, the variable `group` contains two values identifying the different treatments. The `npar1way` procedure is not limited to two groups, and more than two groups can be compared simultaneously. In Exercise 7.8, a third group of plants is introduced and compared to the others. The `npar1way` procedure performs a one-way ANOVA for two or more groups in addition to the analogous nonparametric tests.

The `npar1way` procedure produces a large number of comparisons between the two different groups of plants. The first of these is the familiar t-test, produced in an ANOVA table. The t-test material is omitted from Table 7.5. The output from the rank sum and medians tests are included in this table.

The medians test is covered in Section 7.1. The data is reduced to a 2×2 table of frequencies, given in Table 7.2. The `sum of scores` gives the frequencies in the top row of the 2×2 table, namely 3 and 7. The expected counts are both equal to 5, under the null hypothesis of equality of medians. The SAS output provides two different p-values associated with these frequencies corresponding to a one- or two-tailed normal test. There are also chi-squared statistics that can be performed on this 2×2 table. These p-values are either .0406 or .0812. Notice that the lower p-value is half of the larger, corresponding to the two-tailed test. In the present example where no clear alternative hypothesis is apparent, the two-tailed test results should be preferred.

The output for the Wilcoxon rank-sum test is included at the top of Table 7.5. To appreciate the computer output given in the table, refer back to the ranked values in Table 7.3. The sum of ranks for the Control plants is 80 and for the Treated plants, it is 130. The `Mean Score` is the average of these ranks in the two groups, namely 8 and 13, respectively. The sum of all ranks is 210. Both groups have an equal number of plants, so the expected sum of the ranks in both groups should be 105. See Exercise 7.3 for details on these calculations.

The rank sums are compared to these expected sums in SAS using both normal and t-distributed approximations and using both one- and two-tailed tests, resulting in four p-values in Table 7.5. As we pointed out for the medians test, in the present example, a two-tailed test is appropriate. The p-value is then either .0640 or .0796, depending on whether we use a normal or t-distribution approximation. These two p-values are not very discrepant and they indicate a moderate amount of weight differences between the two groups of plants. If the p-values were very different because of a small sample size, then the t approximation should be preferred.

7.5 Ranking and the Healthiest State

Do you feel comfortable with ranked data rather than the actual values? We have all seen rankings of the "best" cities to live in and the "best" universities to attend.

Table 7.5. A portion of the SAS output for the program in Table 7.4.

```
          Wilcoxon Scores (Rank Sums) for Variable weight

                        Sum of      Expected       Std Dev          Mean
group          N        Scores      Under H0      Under H0         Score
------------------------------------------------------------------------
C             10          80.0         105.0     13.228757           8.0
T             10         130.0         105.0     13.228757          13.0

                         Wilcoxon Two-Sample Test

                     Statistic                 80.0000
                     Normal Approximation
                     Z                         -1.8520
                     One-Sided Pr <  Z          0.0320
                     Two-Sided Pr > |Z|         0.0640

                     t Approximation
                     One-Sided Pr <  Z          0.0398
                     Two-Sided Pr > |Z|         0.0796

    Median Scores (Number of Points Above Median) for Variable weight

                        Sum of      Expected       Std Dev          Mean
group          N        Scores      Under H0      Under H0         Score
------------------------------------------------------------------------
C             10           3.0           5.0      1.147079          0.30
T             10           7.0           5.0      1.147079          0.70

                          Median Two-Sample Test

                     Statistic                  3.0000
                     Z                         -1.7436
                     One-Sided Pr <  Z          0.0406
                     Two-Sided Pr > |Z|         0.0812
```

There are popular websites that rank the best (and worst) dressed celebrities. There is even a ranking of the New York City subway lines.[2] The actual ranking depends on how much weight we give to each criteria that goes into the ranking.

As an example of how such a ranking might be conducted, let us take some public health data[3] collected on each of the fifty states and the District of Columbia given

[2] Really. See http://www.straphangers.org/statesub08/table1.pdf.
[3] Available online at http://www.cdc.gov/nchs/data/hus/hus07.pdf.

Table 7.6. Health statistics on the fifty states and the District of Columbia.

	Physicians	Vaccination rate	Prenatal care	Low birth weight	Mortality	
					Age adjusted	Neonatal
Alabama	21.4	79	82.8	10.35	1004.0	5.4
Alaska	24.1	67	80.0	6.02	781.5	2.9
Arizona	22.5	71	76.4	7.05	775.2	4.3
Arkansas	20.4	73	79.5	9.04	934.6	5.2
			. . . .			
West Virginia	25.2	68	85.8	9.16	974.1	4.9
Wisconsin	25.7	81	84.0	6.93	758.3	4.4
Wyoming	19.4	64	82.9	8.71	814.6	4.6
United States	26.9	77%	83.2%	8.07	812.0	4.6

Source: Centers for Disease Control.

in Table 7.6. For each state we have the number of physicians per 10,000 population, the rate of childhood vaccination, the rate of prenatal care, the rate of low-birth-weight infants, and infant and age-adjusted mortality.

Let us see how we might rank the different states on their degree of health. This requires that we construct a scale of "health." This scale is rather arbitrary and depends on what we value most. As an example, we might say that health depends on low infant mortality and high childhood vaccination rates. The first health measure is then defined as

$$\text{Health}_1 = \text{vaccine rate} - 10 \times \text{infant mortality},$$

ignoring all other information available.

Notice that infant mortality rate is given a negative weight because large values are unhealthy. The multiple of 10 in this weighting is arbitrary. The healthiest state using this criteria is Massachusetts, with a "score" of 47. Iowa and Minnesota are both tied for second place with scores of 45. The District of Columbia is worst.

For another example, if we decide that a low mortality rate and a large number of physicians is more important, then we might decide on the second health measure

$$\text{Health}_2 = 100 \times \text{Physicians} - \text{mortality}.$$

If we use this criterion, then Washington, DC, is the healthiest, largely because of a very large number of physicians living in the city. In other words, Washington, DC, is either ranked as the most healthy or the worst, depending on the criteria we use. Watch for similar rankings that are reported in the popular press, and be ready to ask for details about the methodology used to create the rankings. The data from this section is examined in Exercise 7.11

7.6 Nonparametric Regression: LOESS

There are also nonparametric regression methods. Suppose we want to show how the values of an outcome variable y are related to an explanatory variable x, but we are not sure whether a straight-line relationship is appropriate. Maybe the best descriptive relationship is a straight line, or maybe a polynomial, or maybe some transformation of either x or y might be better. This is the spirit of nonparametric statistics: we don't want to make any more assumptions than necessary.

Suppose, however, we are willing to say that the relationship between x and the mean of y at that value of x is "smooth" in some sense but cannot commit ourselves to much more than that statement. LOESS (pronounced and sometimes also written as LOWESS) is the abbreviation for locally weighted scatter-plot smoothing. Very simply, LOESS represents a compromise between minimizing the sum of squared residuals and providing a smooth response model. Too much roughness may produce a smaller sum of squared errors, but a model that wiggles around is not a simple summary of the data. At the other extreme, the ultimate smooth fit says that the best description of the y values is their mean. This flat-line model is usually not of much use to us either, and we should be able to do better.

Let us consider fitting a LOESS model to the gasoline consumption data examined in Section 6.4. In that section we showed that taking logs of the per-person consumption of gasoline was much better than examining the original consumption values.

A SAS program that fits the LOESS curve to these data is given in Table 7.7. In this program, `proc loess` finds an optimal smoothing parameter that makes a good compromise between a good fit and a smooth model. The output from this program includes the fitted values, residuals from the model, and a 95% confidence interval for the fitted model. Although these values are useful, it is much better to see these displayed in a graph, plotted along with the original data. The full program does this, and the result from `proc gplot` appears in Figure 7.2.

The center curve is the LOESS fit, and the outer two represent the 95% confidence interval of the LOESS fit. We can see that the price of gasoline is relatively flat for the lower half of the consumption values, but jumps up corresponding to the higher consuming European nations. The highest consumption and relatively low prices in the United States and Singapore cause the LOESS fit to fall again at the right side of this figure.

Perhaps we may still feel that the low prices in the United States and Singapore provide too much leverage and that the fitted model is not quite smooth enough. It is possible to adjust the LOESS smoothing parameter that determines the compromise between smoothness and good fit. The program in Table 7.7 estimates this smoothing

Table 7.7. SAS program to fit and plot the LOESS curve to the gasoline consumption data.

```
title1 'Gasoline consumption and price in several countries';
data gasoline;
   input price consume name $ 21-32;
   logcon=log(consume);
   datalines;
       6.66    1.9    Norway
       6.55    2.3    Netherlands

        ...           ...

       1.48    0.1    Nigeria
       0.47    0.8    Iran
   run;
proc print;   /* Always a good idea */
run;

proc sort data=gasoline;
   by consume;
run;

title2 'A LOESS smooth fit and CI for these data';
proc loess data=gasoline;
   model price = logcon /
     details(OutputStatistics ModelSummary) clm residual;
   ods output  OutputStatistics = smoothfit;
run;

proc gplot data=smoothfit;
   axis1 label=(angle=90 rotate=0);
   symbol1 color=black value=dot;
   symbol2 color=black interpol=spline value=none;
   symbol3 color=black interpol=spline value=none;
   symbol4 color=black interpol=spline value=none;

   plot (DepVar Pred LowerCL UpperCL) * logcon /
      vaxis=axis1 hm=3 vm=3 overlay name='gasprice';
run;
quit;
```

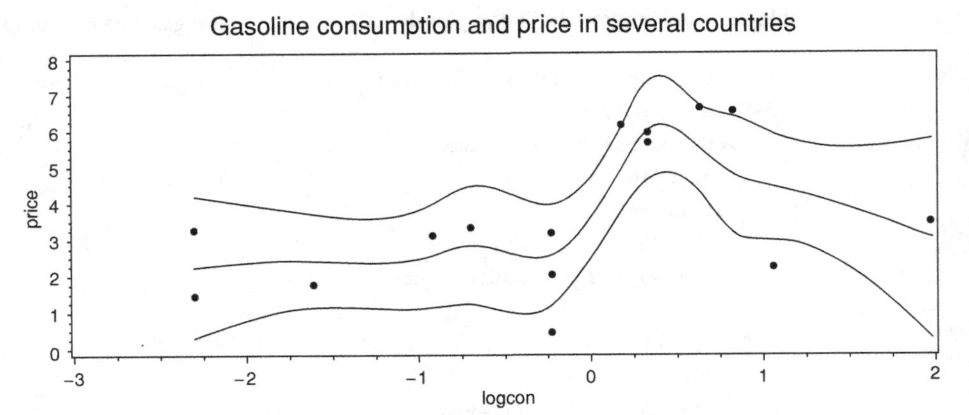

Figure 7.2 LOESS fit and its 95% confidence interval for the gasoline consumption data.

parameter to be .59, but it is sometimes useful to consider other values. We can specify a list of other smoothing parameter values in `proc loess` using the `smooth` option as in this example:

```
proc loess data=gasoline;
   model price = logcon / details(OutputStatistics)
      residual  clm  smooth=.35 .5 .7 .9 ;
run;
```

These four different smoothing parameters produce the models that appear in Figure 7.3. A smoothing parameter of .35 produces a model with several small twists and turns that is trying to fit the observed data too closely. The smoothing value of .5 produces a model that is similar to the value of .59 used in Figure 7.2. A value of .7 produces a much smoother fit, but the model is still trying to drop in order to

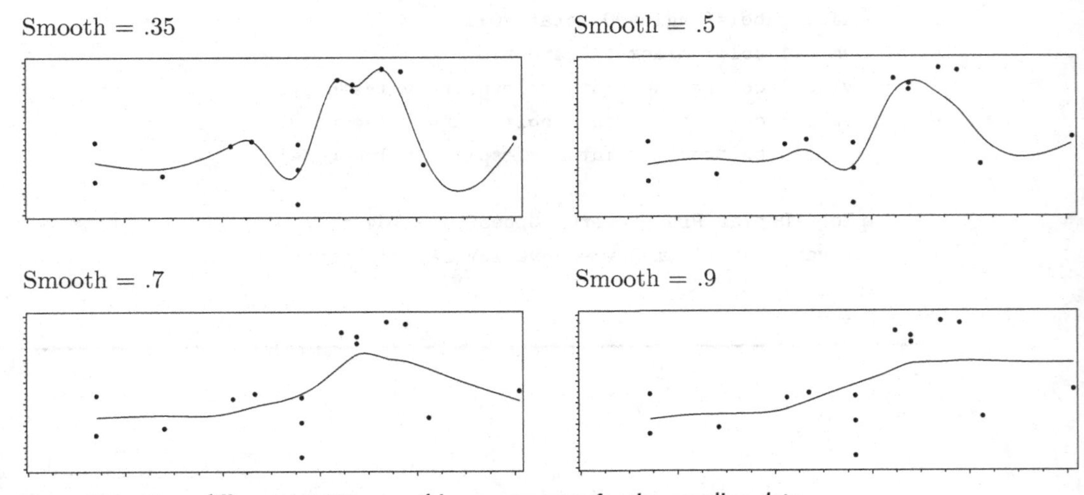

Figure 7.3 Four different LOESS smoothing parameters for the gasoline data.

accommodate the data values from the United States and Singapore. The smoothest graph uses a smoothing value of .9. This graph shows that price is fairly flat across nations with the lowest consumption of gasoline, rises in the middle, and then levels off again. In this example, the smoothest of the four LOESS models seems to provide the best summary of the data on the basis of this simple summary. Letting the computer decide on the model for you may not lead to a useful outcome.

7.7 Exercises

7.1 What are all of the assumptions of a t-test?

7.2 Why are the row and column sums all equal to 10 in Table 7.2? In this medians test, would the results be any different if we took logs of the weight data? Would the results change if we took logs before performing the t-test or the rank sum test? Why? If you can't answer these questions, try it with some data in SAS and see what happens.

7.3 Verify that sum of ranks in Table 7.3 are 80 for the Controls and 130 for the Treated plants. Verify that the sum of all ranks available in 20 observations is equal to

$$1 + 2 + \cdots + 20 = 210.$$

Hint: Write this sum as

$$(1 + 20) + (2 + 19) + \cdots + (10 + 11).$$

7.4 Which of these four smooth fitted models of Figure 7.3 do you prefer: the best-fitting model or the smoothest fit? The smoothest fit also provides a relatively simple description for the data. This is an important goal in statistics.

7.5 The diastolic blood pressures of subjects who were treated and of untreated controls are listed here:

Treated: 92 108 112 90 88

Controls: 83 90 78 90 90 106 92 78 103 98

Compare these two groups using nonparametric methods and the t-test. Do you have more confidence in one or the other of these two methods? Are there any data values that you feel that might provide too much influence on the t-test? Try changing one of the data values to see how much this varies the conclusions of the two different statistical methods.

7.6 Reexamine the fusion time data in Table 2.1. Use both the medians and the rank sum tests to see if there is a statistically significant difference in these two groups. Do the significance levels you find agree with those using a t-test? Suppose we multiply some of the largest observed values by some large number. Does this change our statistical inference based on the t-test? Are the medians

Table 7.8. The full data on plant weights.

Control:	4.17	5.58	5.18	6.11	4.50	4.61	5.17	4.53	5.33	5.14
Treatment 1:	4.81	4.17	4.41	3.59	5.87	3.83	6.03	4.89	4.32	4.69
Treatment 2:	6.31	5.12	5.54	5.50	5.37	5.29	4.92	6.15	5.80	5.26

and rank sum tests changed by this action? What does this say about how robust these different methods are?

7.7 In pharmacokinetics, we often want to know how long it takes for a drug to reach its peak serum concentration. This time is called *Tmax*. The subject's blood is not sampled continuously, but rather at irregular time points following the administration of the drug. Here are the results of Tmax for an experiment comparing two different formulations of a pain reliever, rounded to the nearest 1/4 hour:

Standard formulation: 1.0 1.25 1.5 1.5 1.0 1.25 1.0 1.5

New formulation: 0.5 0.75 0.5 1.0 0.75 1.25 1.0 1.5

Compare the Tmax values for these two formulations using the t-test, the median test, and the rank method. Which of these methods do you feel provides a more reliable conclusion? Explain why.

7.8 The plant growth data in Table 7.1 is part of a larger experiment involving two treatments in addition to a control group of plants. The full dataset is given in Table 7.8. Each of the three groups of experimental conditions contained ten plants. This exercise asks you to develop a generalization of the medians test described in Section 7.1 to test for simultaneous differences between the medians of these three groups.

Begin by finding the median of the sample pooled over all three groups. Within each of the three groups, count the numbers of observations above and below this pooled median. Display these frequencies in a 2×3 table of counts and use `proc freq` to compute the usual 2-df Pearson chi-squared statistic on this table testing for independence of rows and columns. Express the null and alternative hypotheses for this test in terms of the comparisons of the medians. The SAS program will also perform a one-way ANOVA, described in Section 6.1.

7.9 Reexamine the Swiss fertility data in Table 6.15. Consider the relationship between fertility rates and the percentage of population with higher education levels. Use LOESS to show that the smooth, nonparametric relationship between fertility and education is nearly a straight line.

In the exercise of Section 6.6.7, we suggested taking logs of education in order to remove the influence of the few highly educated provinces. Use LOESS to model fertility in terms of log education. Notice that the smooth fit on log education has a very different form. Interpret this model in simple, nonmathematical terms.

7.10 A group of mentally deficient children were enrolled in a speech therapy program. These children were classified as either aphasic or mentally retarded. Their scores on the Vineland Social Maturity Scale were as follows:

Aphasic: 56 43 30 97 67 24 76 49 46 29 46 83 93 38 25 44 66 71 54 20 25

Retarded: 90 53 32 44 47 42 58 16 49 54 81 59 35 81 41 24 41 61 31 20

How do these two groups differ? Compare these two groups using a t-test and nonparametric methods. Plot the data using boxplots and with a jittered group to see if the values appear to be sampled from a normal distribution. (Data source: Glovsky and Rigrodsky, 1964.)

7.11 Examine the data in Table 7.6 and provide your own ranking of the healthiest state. Can you provide an intuitive reason for your ranking method?

7.7.1 Cloth Run-up

The data in Table 7.9 represents the percentage of cloth run up (wasted) by each of five different suppliers to a clothing manufacturer.[4] The values in this table are comparisons to the manufacturer's computer model that suggests how much cloth will be run up. A negative number is possible if the supplier is careful and manages to lose less material than anticipated by this model.

Examine a boxplot for percentage run-up by each of the five suppliers. Is there evidence that all five have the same variability? (See Exercise 6.6 for an examination of the assumptions of a one-way ANOVA.) Is a one-way ANOVA an appropriate way to compare the five suppliers? Is this method affected by the exclusion of any outliers you see?

Does a nonparametric approach reach a different conclusion? Are the five suppliers about the same, or are there real differences? Can you identify good or bad ones? Which is a better property: consistency (i.e., a small variance) or low mean run-up?

7.7.2 Prices of Beanie Babies

Beanie babies are small cloth toys filled with plastic beads. These animal models come in a wide variety of colors, and small variations can result in large differences in their value to collectors. The prices (as of the year 2000) and year of production (often referred to as "birth date") are given in Table 7.10. Also included is an indicator of whether the item is currently being manufactured or retired. The price is often determined by what collectors are willing to pay. As a result, there are some extreme outliers here. Be sure to identify these.

Compare the prices for current and retired items. Begin by examining the means and standard deviations using `proc means`. Plot the data. Does jittering the current/retired status indicator help you see the distribution of values?

[4] Available online at http://lib.stat.cmu.edu/DASL/Datafiles/wasterunupdat.html.

Table 7.9. Cloth run-up from five suppliers.

Supplier				
A	B	C	D	E
1.2	16.4	12.1	11.5	24.0
10.1	−6.0	9.7	10.2	−3.7
−2.0	−11.6	7.4	3.8	8.2
1.5	−1.3	−2.1	8.3	9.2
−3.0	4.0	10.1	6.6	−9.3
−0.7	17.0	4.7	10.2	8.0
3.2	3.8	4.6	8.8	15.8
2.7	4.3	3.9	2.7	22.3
−3.2	10.4	3.6	5.1	3.1
−1.7	4.2	9.6	11.2	16.8
2.4	8.5	9.8	5.9	11.3
0.3	6.3	6.5	13.0	12.3
3.5	9.0	5.7	6.8	16.9
−0.8	7.1	5.1	14.5	
19.4	4.3	3.4	5.2	
2.8	19.7	−0.8	7.3	
13.0	3.0	−3.9	7.1	
42.7	7.6	0.9	3.4	
1.4	70.2	1.5	0.7	
3.0	8.5			
2.4	6.0			
1.3	2.9			

Table 7.10. Value of Beanie Babies with production year and whether current (0) or retired (1).

Name	$ Value	Retired?	Year
Ally, Alligator	30.00	1	1994
Almond, Beige Bear	11.00	0	1999
Amber, Gold Tabby	10.00	0	1998
Ants, Anteater	10.00	1	1997
. . . . . .			
Zero, Penguin	14.00	1	1998
Ziggy, Zebra	15.00	1	1995
Zip, Black Cat w/pink ears, no white paws	900.00	1	1994
Zip, Black Cat white face/belly	350.00	1	1994
Zip, Black Cat, Newly retired	30.00	1	1994

Table 7.11. Subject outcomes and the four cracker diets.

Cracker type	Diet	Subject no.	Calories digested	Bloat?	Cracker type	Diet	Subject no.	Calories digested	Bloat?
control	1	3	1772.84	none	bran	4	3	1752.63	low
combo	3	9	2121.97	med	gum	2	4	2558.61	high
gum	2	1	2026.91	med	bran	4	1	2047.42	low
combo	3	1	2254.75	low	control	1	1	2353.21	med
combo	3	2	2153.36	none	gum	2	2	2331.19	none
bran	4	2	2547.77	none	control	1	2	2591.12	none
gum	2	3	2012.36	low	combo	3	3	1956.18	low
combo	3	4	2025.97	none	bran	4	4	1669.12	none
control	1	4	2452.73	none	bran	4	5	2207.37	low
gum	2	5	1944.48	med	control	1	5	1927.68	low
combo	3	5	2190.1	high	control	1	6	1635.28	none
combo	3	6	1693.35	low	bran	4	6	1707.34	low
gum	2	6	1871.95	high	gum	2	7	2245.03	none
combo	3	7	2436.79	low	control	1	7	2667.14	low
bran	4	7	2766.86	none	bran	4	8	2279.82	none
combo	3	8	1844.77	high	gum	2	8	2002.73	high
control	1	8	2220.22	med	control	1	9	1888.29	low
gum	2	9	1804.27	high	bran	4	9	2293.27	med
bran	4	10	2357.40	none	control	1	10	2359.9	none
combo	3	10	2292.46	low	gum	2	10	2433.46	high
gum	2	11	1681.86	low	control	1	11	1902.75	none
bran	4	11	2003.16	none	combo	3	11	2137.12	med
combo	3	12	2203.07	med	control	1	12	2125.39	low
gum	2	12	2166.77	med	bran	4	12	2287.52	none

Source: Available online at http://lib.stat.cmu.edu/DASL/Datafiles/Fiber.html.

Perform a t-test. Do you have confidence in the assumptions for this method? What do you learn using the median or rank-sum tests? Do the nonparametric methods seem more appropriate? Explain why.

How would you use the production year in a linear regression? Should the slope be positive or negative if older models are more valuable? Is it? Try running LOESS and see if you can make a simple statement about the relationship between age and price.

7.7.3 The Cracker Diet

The manufacturer of crackers thought it would make for good marketing if they could advertise their product as a way to lose weight. An experiment was conducted to see if eating their crackers before a meal would reduce hunger and decrease the urge to consume a higher number of calories. Twelve overweight women were recruited and asked to eat one of four different fiber crackers: a control with none; gum; bran; or a combination of bran and gum. Then they were allowed to eat as much as they wanted in a carefully monitored meal. The number of calories they consumed was carefully measured. An unfortunate side effect of the diet was feelings of gastric upset or bloating reported by many of the subjects. The results from this experiment, including the number of calories consumed, are given in Table 7.11. Subjects were examined once for each of the four different cracker types. In this exercise, let us assume that these multiple measurements on the same person are independent of each other.

Is the feeling of bloat related to the diet? Summarize the data in a 4×4 table of frequencies using the different row and column categories of diet and bloating. Perform a chi-squared test to see if these are independent of each other. The exact test of significance may be a better choice than the chi-squared because of the small counts in this table. You might review the discussion of these methods given in Section 2.6.

In each of the 16 categories, compare the observed and expected counts. Are some of the diets more likely to result in bloating? Can you make a convincing case for this? Consider combining rows and columns in this table to make your argument clearer.

Is there a difference between the four diets with regard to the number of calories consumed? Does a boxplot reveal any outliers? Run `npar1way` and examine the differences using a one-way ANOVA as well as a nonparametric method. Which of these methods seems appropriate to make the comparison? Do these methods come to the same or different conclusions when comparing the four diets?

8

Logistic Regression

Everything we have discussed so far has been concerned with models for the means of normally or, at the least, continuously distributed data. The rest of this book is about models for other distributions. This chapter discusses models for binomial distributed data. (It might be a good idea to review the material in Section 2.1 on this important statistical distribution before going much further.) Logistic regression is the preferred method for examining this type of data. These methods are different from what we have seen so far. At the same time, you will recognize a lot of similar features.

8.1 Example

Let's begin with an example of the type of data that lends itself to this analysis. Consider the experimental data summarized in Table 8.1. There were six large jars, each containing a number of beetles and a carefully measured small amount of insecticide. After a specified amount of time, the experimenters examined the number of beetles that were still alive. We can calculate the empirical death rate for each jar's level of exposure of the insecticide. These are given in the last row of Table 8.1 using

$$\text{Mortality rate} = \frac{\text{Number died}}{\text{Number exposed}}.$$

How can we develop statistical models to describe this data? We should immediately recognize that within each jar the outcomes are binary valued: alive or dead. We can probably assume that these events are independent of each other. The counts of alive or dead should then follow the binomial distribution. (See Section 2.1 for a quick review of this important statistical model.) There are six separate and independent binomial experiments in this example. The n parameters for the binomial models are the number of insects in each jar. Similarly, the p parameters represent

Table 8.1. Mortality of beetles exposed to various doses of an insecticide.

Dead	15	24	26	24	29	29
Alive	35	25	24	26	21	20
Number exposed	50	49	50	50	50	49
Exposure dose	1.082	1.161	1.212	1.258	1.310	1.348
Mortality rate	0.30	0.49	0.52	0.48	0.58	0.59

Source: Plackett (1981), p. 54.

the mortality probabilities in each jar. The aim is to model the p parameters of these six binomial experiments. Any models we develop for this data will need to incorporate the various insecticide dose levels to describe the mortality probability p in each jar. The alert reader will notice that the empirical mortality rates given in the last row of Table 8.1 are not monotonically increasing with increasing exposure levels of the insecticide. Despite this remark, there is no reason for us to fit a nonmonotonic model to these data.

> Use logistic regression to model the p parameter in data from a binomial distribution.

The aim of this chapter is to explain models for the different values of the p parameters using the values of the doses of the insecticide in each jar. The first idea that comes to mind is to treat the outcomes as normally distributed. All of the ns are large, so a normal approximation to the binomial distributions should work. We also already know a lot about linear regression, so we are tempted to fit the linear model

$$p = \beta_0 + \beta_1 \text{Dose} + \text{error}.$$

What is wrong with this approach? It seems simple enough, but remember that p must always be between 0 and 1. There is no guarantee that at extreme values of the Dose, this straight line model would result in estimates of p that are less than 0 or greater than 1. We would expect a good model for these data to always give an estimate of p between 0 and 1. A second but less striking problem is that the variance of the binomial distribution is not the same for different values of the p parameter so the assumption of constant variance is not valid for the usual linear regression.

8.2 The Logit Transformation

We like the idea of fitting straight lines but have not yet encountered a constraint on the fitted model, such as p always remaining between 0 and 1, as in this case.

The solution is to introduce a new class of models. We define the *logit* of p as the logarithm (base e) of the odds. Mathematically,

$$\text{logit}(p) = \log \frac{p}{1-p}. \tag{8.1}$$

The ratio $p/(1-p)$ is the odds, or ratio of the probability of the event (in this case, insect death) to the probability of the complementary event (again, in this case, a living insect). The *odds ratio* is familiar to epidemiologists and horse-race handicappers alike. The logit is the log-odds of an event occurring. In epidemiology we usually talk about the odds rather than the probability of an event, especially when the events are rare.

It does not matter much which event is considered a "success" or "failure" in the binomial distribution. Recall the property of the logarithm of a reciprocal: For any positive number z

$$\log(1/z) = -\log(z)$$

so we have

$$\text{logit}(p) = \log \frac{p}{1-p} = -\log \frac{1-p}{p} = -\text{logit}(1-p). \tag{8.2}$$

That is, the logit of 'success' is the negative of the logit of "failure." We only need to remember which outcome we are calling a "success."

> The logit is the log-odds of the probability.

Let us take a moment to motivate the use of the logit. The p parameter is restricted to values between 0 and 1. The logit transforms p to cover the entire number line. A plot of logit(p) against p is given in Figure 8.1. From this figure we see how values of p are spread out from the interval of 0 to 1 onto the entire number line. As p gets very close to 0 or 1, this transformation takes on extremely large negative and positive values, respectively.

From this figure we can see that logit(p) is 0 when p is 1/2. Similarly, logit(p) is positive for p greater than 1/2, and logit(p) is negative when p is less than 1/2. The plot of logit($1-p$) in this figure demonstrates the relation given at (8.2) namely, the logit of "failure" is the negative of the logit of "success."

Logistic regression is the statistical method in which we model the logit(p) in terms of the explanatory variables that are available to us. In the specific case of the beetle data in Table 8.1, we have

$$\text{logit}(p) = \beta_0 + \beta_1 \text{Dose} \tag{8.3}$$

where the intercept and slope parameters β_0 and β_1 are estimated by the computer.

On the right-hand side of this relationship, we see the familiar linear summary of the explanatory variable that we encountered in linear regression in Chapter 3. The

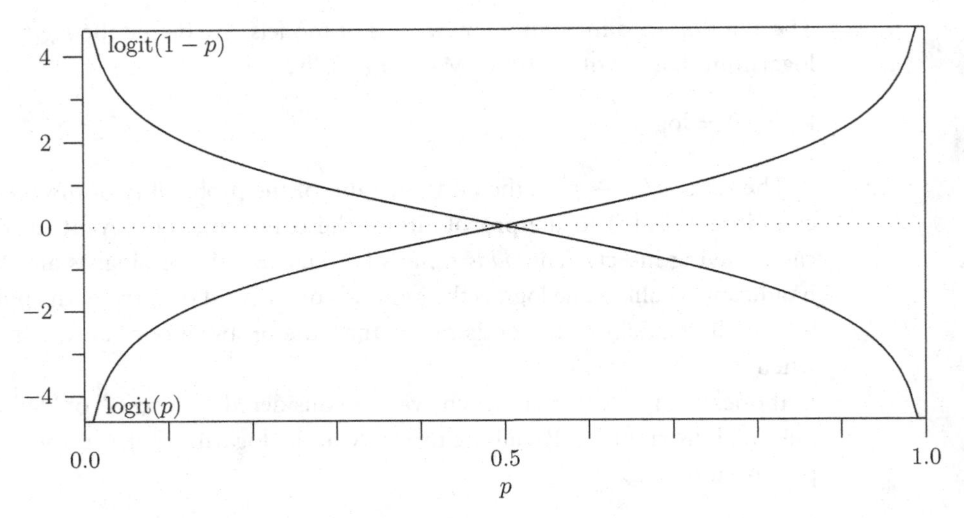

Figure 8.1 Plot of logit(p) and logit($1 - p$) against p.

logit on the left side of this model is the nonlinear transformed value of the binomial p parameter.

Logistic regression specifies that the logit of p is a linear combination of the risk factors.

The relationship in (8.3) can be solved for p in terms of the Dose, giving us

$$p = \frac{\exp\{\beta_0 + \beta_1 \text{Dose}\}}{1 + \exp\{\beta_0 + \beta_1 \text{Dose}\}}. \tag{8.4}$$

The exponential function ($\exp(z) = e^z$) is always positive and the denominator is always 1 more than the numerator. This shows that this model produces values of p between 0 and 1 regardless of the values of the parameters β_0, β_1, and the Dose of the insecticide. The relationships in (8.3) and (8.4) are equivalent. You will see these two different forms equally often in published literature that uses logistic regression.

Let us end this section with a description of another method that is closely allied with logistic regression. The relation at (8.3) is not the only method that can be used to model p in linear terms of the insecticide dose that maintains the restriction of p between 0 and 1. Another popular method that is used to model the p parameter for binomial data is called the *probit* model. The probit of p is related to the area under the normal curve.

More specifically, *probit regression* is the area under the normal curve to the left of

$$\alpha_0 + \alpha_1 \text{ Dose}$$

where the intercept α_0 and slope α_1 are parameters that are estimated by the computer. All normal areas are positive and less than 1, so we are assured that such values of p will always be between 0 and 1.

The parameters β_0 and β_1 of the fitted logistic model and α_0 and α_1 of the fitted probit model will be different but will generally exhibit similar statistical significance levels. The interpretations of the logit and probit models are very different but, as we demonstrate in Figure 8.2 of the following section, the fitted models are usually in close agreement. The reason for this agreement is not obvious, but we might think of the logistic model as a t-distribution with a small number of degrees of freedom. In Figure 2.6 we see that these are not very different from the normal distribution.

We often use the term *link* to describe the connection of the p parameter and the linear function of the Dose. We have just described two link functions for these data: the logistic link and the probit link. There are other link functions available for binary-valued data. These include the complementary log-log link and are described in the SAS help file. The link function also appears in a different context in Chapter 10.

8.3 Logistic Regression in SAS

The SAS program to fit logistic and probit models to the beetle data is given in Table 8.2. A portion of the output from this program is given in Table 8.3. There are also many number of diagnostics and residual plots that are produced by the program. These diagnostic measures of fit and outliers are discussed in Chapter 9. Right now we want to emphasize the computing and interpretation of the models.

In the program of Table 8.2, the `data` step reads the data into a SAS dataset. After every `data` step; always include a `print` procedure to be certain that the data has been read correctly by your program. Both the logistic and probit models can be fitted using `proc logistic` in SAS. Logistic regression is the default for this procedure. The probit model is fitted with the addition of the `link=probit` option. The logistic link is the default if none is specified.

The two `model` statements in Table 8.2 specify the model to be fitted. After the equal sign, we can list any number of explanatory variables we want to put into the model. The program will fit a slope for each variable and an intercept. Notice the syntax when we specify the dependent variable, the number of insects that died. This is written as `died/total`. This notation is not division, as it appears, but is the way we specify the binomial n parameter to the program. In this example, the total number of exposed beetles is the binomial n. If all of the n parameters are equal to 1, then the `/total` portion can be omitted. We will see examples of this. In Chapter 9 we discuss regression diagnostics for logistic (and probit) regression models.

Part of the output from the program in Table 8.2 is given in Table 8.3. There is much more output than this, and it is explained in Chapter 9. The output given in Table 8.3 includes a portion that is very similar to the output we saw in the output for linear regression. Specifically, there are parameter estimates, estimated standard

Table 8.2. SAS program to fit logistic and probit regression models for the pesticide experiment in Table 8.1.

```
title1 'Beetle mortality and pesticide dose';

data beetle;
   input died total dose;
datalines;
          15    50     1.082
          24    49     1.161
          26    50     1.212
          24    50     1.258
          29    50     1.310
          29    49     1.348
run;

proc print;  /* always do this after a data step */
run;

title2 'Logistic dose effect';
proc logistic;
   model died / total  =  dose;
run;

title2 'Probit dose effect';
proc logistic;
   model died / total  =  dose / link=probit;
run;
```

errors for these, tests of statistical significance, and a confidence interval for the slope. Let us go over these before we proceed.

The fitted model in Table 8.3 is

$$\text{logit}(\widehat{p}) = -4.8977 + 3.9639\,\text{Dose} \tag{8.5}$$

or, equivalently,

$$\widehat{p} = \frac{\exp(-4.8977 + 3.9639\,\text{Dose})}{1 + \exp(-4.8977 + 3.9639\,\text{Dose})}.$$

This fitted logistic function of Dose is plotted in Figure 8.2.

Both the intercept and slope have estimated standard errors given in Table 8.3. The Wald chi-squared statistic is the square of this ratio,

$$\text{Wald chi-squared} = \left(\frac{\text{parameter estimate}}{\text{standard error}}\right)^2,$$

Table 8.3. A portion of the output from the program in Table 8.2.

```
                 Beetle mortality and pesticide dose
                        Logistic dose effect

                       The LOGISTIC Procedure

              Analysis of Maximum Likelihood Estimates

                                 Standard          Wald
Parameter    DF    Estimate        Error    Chi-Square    Pr > ChiSq

Intercept     1     -4.8977       1.6451        8.8636        0.0029
dose          1      3.9639       1.3346        8.8219        0.0030


                         Odds Ratio Estimates

                       Point          95% Wald
              Effect   Estimate     Confidence Limits

              dose       52.663       3.850    720.281


                 Beetle mortality and pesticide dose
                         Probit dose effect

                       The LOGISTIC Procedure

              Analysis of Maximum Likelihood Estimates

                                 Standard          Wald
Parameter    DF    Estimate        Error    Chi-Square    Pr > ChiSq

Intercept     1     -3.0632       1.0175        9.0627        0.0026
dose          1      2.4791       0.8258        9.0127        0.0027
```

and behaves as a 1-df chi-squared statistic under the null hypothesis that the underlying parameters being estimated are equal to 0.

That is, the Wald statistic tests whether the parameter is zero or not. The p-value associated with this test is also given in the output of Table 8.3. In this example we see that there is considerable evidence that neither the intercept nor the slope are zero. Inference on the intercept is not particularly useful in this example, but the positive slope on Dose and the corresponding small p-value (0.003) provide

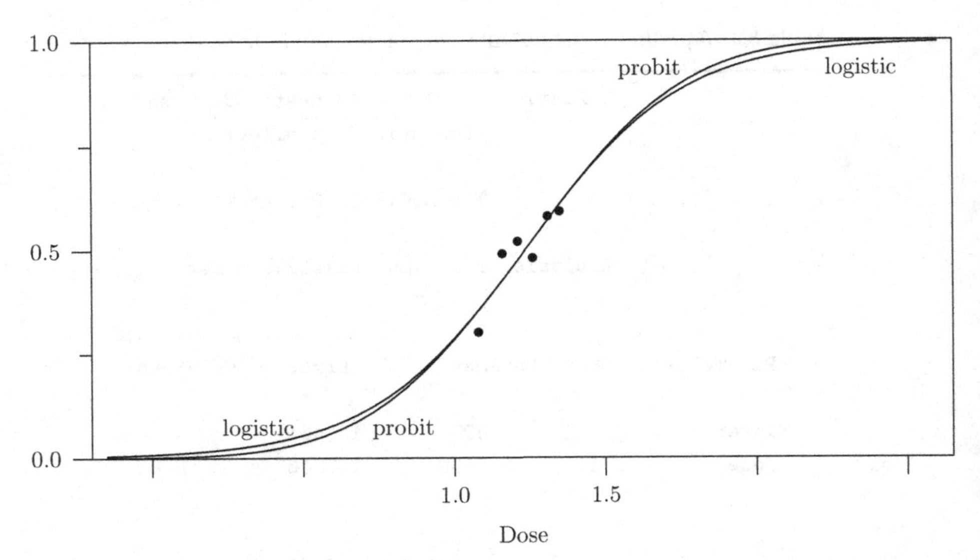

Figure 8.2 Fitted logistic and probit models for the beetle data in Table 8.1. The dots are the empirical rates for each of the six groups.

strong evidence that the insecticide is toxic to these insects, and increasing the exposure level is associated with greater levels of mortality.

The `Odds Ratio Estimates` in Table 8.3 provide an estimate and confidence interval of the slope on a linear, rather than a logarithmic scale. Specifically, the Dose effect is

$$\exp\left(\widehat{\beta}_1\right) = \exp(3.9639) = 52.663.$$

We interpret this number to mean that a 1-unit increase in the dose represents a 52.66-fold increase in the likelihood of insect mortality. This is a huge effect. A 95% confidence interval for this value can be obtained using a normal approximation to the distribution for the estimated parameter. This is calculated as

$$\exp(3.9639 \pm 1.96 \times 1.3346) = (3.850,\ \ 720.281)$$

where ± 1.96 is the 95% confidence interval for the standard normal distribution and 1.3346 is the estimated standard error of the estimated parameter value given in Table 8.3.

Why is this estimated odds ratio so large, and is it relevant to the present experiment? If we refer back to the original data in Table 8.1, we see that the range of insecticide used varied from 1.082 to 1.348 units. The difference in these values provides a range of less than 0.3 units. A 1-unit increase is much larger than the range of the empirical data. In other words, for the present experiment, the odds ratio estimate is not a useful measure because it represents an estimate of an effect that extrapolates beyond the range of the observed data.

The second half of Table 8.3 contains the analogous parameter estimates for a probit regression. The slope and intercept each have estimates, standard errors, Wald chi-squared statistics, and p-values. Again, we see that the slope on Dose is positive and achieves a high level of statistical significance, leading, again, to the conclusion that higher levels of the insecticide are associated with greater mortality. Notice that the estimates are different from those of logistic regression, but in general, the Wald statistics and p-values should be comparable. There is no reason for the estimated slopes and intercepts for probit and logistic regressions to be comparable, because these are very different models for the binomial p parameter. The probit slope does not have the interpretation as a log-odds-ratio, so there is no corresponding odds ratio estimate for the probit regression in Table 8.3.

What is missing in logistic and probit regression is a sense of the overall model being fitted. The p parameter is not itself a linear function of the Dose. To find p for the fitted logistic regression model we need to use the relation in (8.4) with the estimated parameters in (8.5). Figure 8.2 plots the models for both the fitted logistic and probit regressions. This graph includes the empirical mortality rates for each of the six jars of beetles, plotted as dots.

Figure 8.2 shows the overall fitted models for the beetle data. Points to notice are that the fitted binomial p parameter is always between 0 and 1, for all possible exposure levels of the insecticide. We can also see that, at least for the range of exposure levels in these data, there is not much of a difference between the fitted models for logistic and probit regression models, except in the extreme tails of these models. The probit model is associated with the normal distribution and tends to have shorter tails. That is, the logistic model approaches the limits of 0 and 1 more slowly than those of the probit model for extreme levels of exposure.

8.4 Statistics in the News: The New York Mets

Sports reporting of the news probably involves as many numbers as the business news, and these are also examined by many statisticians. Table 8.4 presents the win/loss record on a game-by-game basis of the New York Mets from the beginning of the 2007 baseball season until June 3 of that year.

The news article[1] describes a steadily improving record for this team. Is this actually the case? We can use logistic regression to test for an improving or worsening trend. Each game's outcome is a binary-valued outcome: win or loss. Tied games are a rare possibility, and we might have to make up a rule in order to include these. We can use the number of days since the start of the season as the explanatory variable in the same way Dose of insecticide is used in (8.3). A positive or negative estimated slope would be indicative of an increasing or decreasing trend in the team's record.

[1] Available online at http://www.nytimes.com/2007/06/05/sports/baseball/05mets.html.

Table 8.4. Win/loss record of the NY Mets for the 2007 season up to June 3.

Game number:																			
									1	1	1	1	1	1	1	1	1	1	2
1	2	3	4	5	6	7	8	9	0	1	2	3	4	5	6	7	8	9	0
W	W	W	L	L	W	L	W	W	L	W	W	W	L	W	L	W	W	L	L
2	2	2	2	2	2	2	2	2	3	3	3	3	3	3	3	3	3	3	4
1	2	3	4	5	6	7	8	9	0	1	2	3	4	5	6	7	8	9	0
W	W	L	L	W	W	W	W	L	L	W	W	W	L	W	W	L	W	W	W
4	4	4	4	4	4	4	4	4	5	5	5	5	5						
1	2	3	4	5	6	7	8	9	0	1	2	3	4						
W	L	L	W	L	W	W	W	W	L	W	L	W	L						

Is this a valid use of logistic regression? On the surface, the data appears to take the correct form: binary-valued outcomes and an explanatory variable (game number). A closer examination of the way the teams play each other reveals some potential problems. Remember that not all of these games are played against the same opponents. Baseball teams are usually scheduled to host an out-of-town visiting team for a series of several games and then travel to some distant city for a series of several games with another team. A pitcher needs to rest his arm for a few games after playing, so the same "team" is not made up of the same key players from one game to another. Additional explanatory variables might include whether each of the games played was "at home" or "away" and the strength of the opponent at each game. There are statisticians who analyze sports data very carefully and include all of these factors in their models. Exercise 8.3 asks you to perform your own analysis of this data.

8.5 Key Points

Logistic regression is a useful method for studying binomial or binary-valued data. The logit is not a probability, and this concept takes some getting used to. Epidemiologists talk in terms of a change in the odds (or in our case the log-odds) of some outcome. We are not building a linear model of the probability of the outcome, but rather a linear model of the log-odds.

The probit has the same curved shape as the logit. Both produce approximately the same fitted model although the regression coefficients (betas) will be measured on a different scale. Look back at Figure 8.2 and remind yourself what the model represents. There will not be much difference between the logit and the probit unless the probabilities you are measuring are very close to either zero or one.

Use logistic regression to model the p parameter of binomial data. The probit model is another equally good choice. The model statement in `proc logistic` looks like the one you used to fit linear models but here we model the log-odds of the binomial probability. The y/n notation in the model statement is not division but instead, the way we specify the binomial n parameter to SAS. The iplots and influence options print out a large number of diagnostic measures that are explained in Chapter 9.

Are there times when we need to estimate the n parameter of the binomial distribution as well as p? Sometimes we want to estimate the size of a finite population. In Section 1.1, for example, we discussed problems with the census undercount. As another example, suppose we want to estimate the number of homeless people, or the number of persons with HIV in a city. We might need to estimate the fraction p who routinely visit a shelter or clinic but also want to estimate the number n who are potential users of these facilities. The usual way to do this is to initially identify individuals and then wait until we see them again, if we ever do. Such surveys are sometimes called *mark-recapture* because of their use in wildlife abundance studies. These are specialized statistical methods that are beyond the scope of the present book but have more recently been used in studies of human populations.

8.6 Exercises

8.1 a. Use an e^x function on a calculator (or otherwise) to estimate the fraction of beetles that would be killed if left unexposed to the insecticide. Can you explain why is this value much larger than zero? Look at Figure 8.2 and notice that *negative* dose will also have a nonnegligible proportion of insects killed.

b. Estimate the dose of insecticide that kills 50% of the insects from the output in Table 8.3. *Hint*: What is the logit of 1/2?

c. Estimate the dose of insecticide the kills 0.1% of the insects. Would you judge this to be a "safe" exposure level for humans? Why? For more details on the methods of this exercise, also see Section 8.6.3.

d. If you were to perform this experiment again, how would you choose doses to answer part (c)? Would you select values of the dose between 1 and 1.5, or would you spread the doses over a wider range?

8.2 Suppose we spent a lot of time writing a program to fit a logistic regression to some data. Just when we thought that we were done, we found out that the binomial outcomes that we called "successes" were really "failures." Must we rewrite the program? Must we rerun the program? *Hint*: Compare the log odds of "success" with that of "failure."

8.3 Examine the Mets' record given in Table 8.4. Fit a logistic model with the game number as the explanatory x variable. Does it look as though the Mets are losing more games as the season progresses? Is there trend in the earlier games that is different in the later games?

8.6.1 A Phase I Clinical Trial in Cancer

One of the dangerous side effects of high-dose chemotherapy is the destruction of beneficial neutrophils, resulting in a condition called neutropenia. A cancer patient

Table 8.5. Topotecan dose, G-CSF use, neutropenia cases, and number of treatment courses in a Phase I clinical trial in cancer.

Dose	G-CSF use?	Neutropenia cases	Treatment courses
2.5	no	0	3
3.0	no	0	3
4.0	no	1	6
5.0	no	1	6
6.25	no	0	3
8.0	no	0	3
10.0	no	1	3
12.5	no	2	6
12.5	yes	1	6
15.0	yes	3	5

Source: Abbruzzese *et al.* (1996).

may simultaneously be given granulocyte colony stimulating factor (G-CSF), which encourages neutrophil production and reduces the risk of neutropenia. Abbruzzese *et al.* (1996) report the data in Table 8.5 from cancer patients treated at various doses of topotecan, with and without G-CSF.

Patients may appear more than once in this table because they are typically treated in multiple courses and at different doses. Patients are given sufficient time to recover between courses, so we can usually assume that courses are independent of each other. Each course can result in neutropenia or not, so consider the number of courses as the binomial n. The number of neutropenia cases in each group of courses is the binomially distributed number of "successes." The binomial p will depend on the dose of topotecan and whether or not G-CSF is used.

Fit a logistic model to explain the incidence of neutropenia in Table 8.5. Is there evidence that the risk of neutropenia is nonlinear in the dose of topotecan? Try fitting a logistic regression that is linear in Dose and Dose^2. Is the use of G-CSF beneficial?

One goal of Phase I clinical trials is to estimate a safe dose of the drug being tested. Can you estimate a "safe" dose for topotecan, with and without G-CSF? The word "safe" usually means a probability of 1 (or lower) in 6 of an adverse experience.

Hint: If $p = 1/6$ then the logit of p is

$$\text{logit}(1/6) = \log\left\{\frac{1/6}{5/6}\right\} = \log(1/5) = -1.6094$$

and the logistic model specifies

$$\text{logit}(p) = \beta_0 + \beta_1\text{Dose}.$$

Table 8.6. Toxoplasmosis cases among children in villages in El Salvador.

Cases	Number tested	Rainfall	Cases	Number tested	Rainfall
2	4	1735	3	10	1936
1	5	2000	3	10	1973
2	2	1750	3	5	1800
2	8	1750	7	19	2077
3	6	1920	8	10	1800
7	24	2050	0	1	1830
15	30	1650	4	22	2200
0	1	2000	6	11	1770
0	1	1920	33	54	1770
4	9	2240	5	8	1620
2	12	1756	0	1	1650
8	11	2250	41	77	1796
24	51	1890	7	16	1871
46	82	2063	9	13	2100
23	43	1918	53	75	1834
8	13	1780	3	10	1900
1	6	1976	23	37	2292

Source: Efron (1978).

Given the estimates of the slope β_1 and intercept β_0 for this model, we can then solve for the "safe" dose of topotecan.

8.6.2 Toxoplasmosis in El Salvador

The data in Table 8.6 summarizes the incidence of toxoplasmosis in 11- to 15-year-old children for 34 villages in El Salvador. The table gives the number of children tested (the binomial n parameter), the number of these who were found positive for toxoplasmosis (the binomial response y), and the annual rainfall (in millimeters) for each village. Toxoplasmosis is a disease caused by a parasite. Those with healthy immune systems may experience no ill effects or symptoms.

When the data is arranged with more than one observation per line, as in this example, you should use @@ in your SAS input statement, as in this example:

```
data toxo;
   input positive tested rain @@;
datalines;
   2  4  1735  3  10  1936
   1  5  2000  3  10  1973
   2  2  1750  3   5  1800
      . . .
```

The `@@` at the end of the `input` statement allows you to read more than one set of data from the same input line.

Fit a linear logistic model using annual rainfall to explain the rate of toxoplasmosis. Does the incidence increase or decrease with rainfall? Is there evidence that more children were tested in villages with greater rainfall? What does this say about how the data was collected?

Fit a logistic model with polynomial terms in rainfall up to the third power. That is, for each village,

$$\text{logit}(p) = \beta_0 + \beta_1 \text{rain} + \beta_2 \text{rain}^2 + \beta_3 \text{rain}^3.$$

You should first rescale the rainfall observations by dividing these by 1,000. (What happens if you don't?) Does this cubic model explain the data any better than the model that only has a linear term? What does this tell you about the effect of rainfall on the risk of toxoplasmosis? Does a graph of this fitted cubic function generally increase in rainfall? How does it differ from a straight line?

8.6.3 Estimation of the ED_{01}

Government agencies are charged with identifying safe exposure levels of toxic chemicals in our air and water. Workers who routinely come in contact with these chemicals also have to be protected against toxic levels. Health-care workers usually wear photographic sensitive badges that measure their cumulative exposure to x-ray radiation. How are these safe exposure levels established? The regulatory process is rather lengthy, but we can sometimes provide a rough estimate using simple methods.

The data given in Table 8.7 was generated, in part, to see how well the logit and probit models can be used to estimate extremely low probabilities of developing liver cancer when exposed to a known carcinogen. Very large numbers of female mice were exposed to low levels of the chemical in order to estimate the dose-response at such low levels.

The *effective dose* of a compound that results in 50% of the outcome is abbreviated as ED_{50}. Similarly, the ED_{01} is the exposure level with a 1% effective rate. Sometimes these may be written as the LD_{01} for an estimated 1% *lethal dose*, or even the LD_{001} for a 0.1% lethal dose.

This table summarizes the outcome of a very large number of female mice that were continuously exposed to the carcinogen 2-acetylaminofluorene (2-AAF) at very low doses for long periods of time. The mice were then sacrificed and examined by pathologists for the presence of tumors in their livers.

Use this data to see how well the logit and probit models estimate the cancer rates in mice at extremely low levels of exposure. Notice that the unexposed mice were not entirely disease-free. Does the logit of the cancer rate appear to be linear in dose? Are the effects of dose and duration additive, or does there appear to be an interaction between these two risk factors?

Table 8.7. The upper number is the number of mice that developed liver cancer, and the lower number is the number exposed to that combination of dose and duration.

Months	Dose in parts 10^{-4}							
on study	0.0	0.30	0.35	0.45	0.60	0.75	1.00	1.50
9	0	1	1	0	0	0	1	1
	199	147	76	52	345	186	168	169
12	0	1	2	1	2	0	3	2
	164	151	27	14	283	153	149	152
14	1	1	0	2	1	0	1	1
	133	42	25	14	243	124	127	127
15	0	1	1	0	3	1	5	1
	115	75	35	20	203	109	99	100
16	1	2	2	3	6	7	2	7
	205	66	61	304	287	193	100	110
17	0	4	5	6	8	9	3	1
	153	69	443	302	230	166	85	82
18	6	34	20	15	13	17	19	24
	555	2014	1102	550	411	382	213	211
24	20	164	128	98	118	118	76	126
	762	2109	1361	888	758	587	297	314
33+	17	135	72	42	30	37	22	9
	100	445	100	103	67	75	31	11

Source: Farmer *et al.* (1979).

Try to estimate the ED_{01} using your fitted model. Does your model produce a reasonable estimate? Next try deleting some of the data at the lowest doses and see how accurately your model fits the missing values.

What would happen if you consider doing a similar analysis, estimating the ED_{01} using the beetle data given in Table 8.1? It would be relatively easy for us to take the fitted logit or probit model and use the method in Section 8.6.1 to estimate the ED_{01}. This would provide a quick and inexpensive estimate.

What is wrong with following this procedure for the beetle data? A quick look at Figure 8.2 reveals that there is very little data anywhere near the ED_{01}. Most of the data is centered near the middle or ED_{50} of this figure. Advice worth repeating is

> Extrapolate at your peril.

Estimating properties about an event that occurs only 1% of the time will require a large and expensive experiment that will not provide the outcome 99% of the time. There is no shortcut for quality data in order to yield a reasonable estimate. Table 8.7 gives data on more than 20,000 mice. Obtaining this data took a great amount of time and planning.

Table 8.8. Summary of each drive in Super Bowl XXXVIII. Columns are: Team with the ball (N; New England Patriots; C; Carolina Panthers); Drive or possession number; Starting distance in yards to their goal line; Indication of a scoring drive (0 = no, 1 = yes).

Team	Drive	Dist	Score?	Team	Drive	Dist	Score?
N	1	48	0	N	2	62	0
N	3	49	0	N	4	68	0
N	5	76	0	N	6	20	1
N	7	77	1	N	8	75	0
N	9	90	0	N	10	71	1
N	11	73	0	N	12	68	1
N	13	60	1	← The game-winning drive			
C	1	78	0	C	2	79	0
C	3	89	0	C	4	92	0
C	5	62	0	C	6	72	0
C	7	95	1	C	8	52	1
C	9	59	0	C	10	90	0
C	11	81	1	C	12	90	1
C	13	80	1				

Reported by the *New York Times*, February 2, 2004.

8.6.4 Super Bowl XXXVIII

This football game was played in Houston on Sunday, February 1, 2004; between the New England Patriots and the Carolina Panthers. The Patriots won 32 to 29 on a play in the last 4 seconds of the game.

Notice that both teams were in possession of the ball the same number of times (13). Did one team begin significantly closer to their goal, on average? You might use a t-test to answer this question. Intuitively, the closer the team begins to their goal, the more likely it is that they will score. Is this the case with the present data? Here are some other questions you might use logistic regression to answer. Raise any other points you want to about this data:

- Do shorter distances to the goal increase the probability of a team scoring?
- Is there a trend for more scoring later in the game? The time of each play is not given here, but we can use the drive number as an indication of how early or late each event occurred. Why do you think there might be more scoring later in the game?
- Is there an interaction indicating that one team was increasingly likely to score later? What does this indicate?
- Is the effect of the distance to the goal smaller or greater than the later-in-the-game effect? What does this tell us?

Running a television ad during the game is very expensive. The price was approximately $2 million for a 30-second message during this game. If you were an advertiser,

Table 8.9. Outline of a SAS program for the Superbowl data.

```
title1 'Superbowl XXXVIII';
data Superbowl;
   input team $ drive dist score;
   label
      team = 'N=Patriots, C=Panthers'
      dist = 'distance to the goal line'
      drive= 'drive number'
      score= 'drive results in score or not'
      ;
   datalines;
      N  1 48 0
      N  2 62 0

        . . .

      C 12 90 1
      C 13 80 1
run;

proc print;   /* always do this */
run;

title2 'Logistic examination of drives';
proc logistic descending;
   class team;
   model score = drive team dist ;
run;
```

where would you want your ad to appear: early in the game when your audience is still alert; at half-time (where an elaborate on-field show included Janet Jackson's embarrassing "wardrobe malfunction"); or toward the end, when the earlier audience members may have changed channels? There was a joke that all sewers across the United States would overflow at halftime as millions of Americans simultaneously went to the bathroom. Comment on the element of uncertainty associated with these three different time points in the game.

An outline of a SAS program for this data is given in Table 8.9. We next describe some of the different options and statements used in `proc logistic`. Notice how all of the binomial n parameters are equal to 1 in this example. That is, one team has the ball, and they either score or they don't. Then the other team gets the ball under different conditions. There is no repetition of the binomial experiment. When all of the n parameters are equal to 1, there is no need to specify them in the model statement. We only need to include the `/ n` portion of the `model` statement when the *ns* are different from 1.

This leads to a certain ambiguity, however. When there is only a single binomial trial, it is not clear what value of the outcome variable is to be considered a "success." In this case, SAS considers a value of 0 to be the success. If we want to model the outcome value of 1 to be the success, we also need to use the `descending` option in `proc logistic`.

Another statement used in the `proc logistic` of Table 8.9 is the `class` statement. The team names are characters "C" and "N", and it doesn't make sense to talk about using these names in a regression equation. But we still want to distinguish between the two teams. One way to fix this is to create an indicator variable taking two different numerical values for the two teams. This is also called a dummy variable. An easier way is to let SAS do this for us. The `class` statement creates a numerical-valued surrogate variable that allows us to use the team names as an explanatory variable. In this case, SAS creates a new variable taking the value +1 for C and −1 for N. If this is not what you intended, then you should take the time to create the values you want. Sometimes an indicator variable taking the values 0 or 1 is easier to interpret.

9

Diagnostics for Logistic Regression

Let's review what was covered in the previous chapter. The logistic model is a useful method that allows us to examine the p parameter of binomial data. In order to keep our estimate of p between 0 and 1, we need to model functions of p. The log odds or $\log(p/(1-p))$ is called the *logit* and is modeled as a linear function of covariates. There are other variations on this idea. The *probit* models the cumulative normal distribution as a linear function of covariates. Both the logit and probit were designed to keep estimates of p between 0 and 1. The `link=probit` option in the model statement of `proc logistic` can be used to fit the probit model. There is little difference between the two fitted models, as we see when we look at Figure 8.2.

The SAS output in Table 8.3 provides a statistical significance of the regression slope, but it does not tell us anything about how well the model fits or even whether it is appropriate. In this chapter we want to discuss several diagnostic measures available that allow us to detect outliers and observations with high influence. Many of these have a parallel measure in linear regression, discussed in Chapter 5. There are options in `proc logistic` to print and plot these. Before we get to that, let's introduce another example.

The data in Table 9.1 is a list of men with prostate cancer.[1] If the cancer is localized, then the disease is still in an early stage. It is also easier to treat, and that treatment is more likely to be successful. Prostate cancer is more serious if it has already spread to the lymph nodes. Surgery is needed to determine if this spread has already happened. It would be better if we could find a less intrusive estimator of the risk of nodal involvement. Such a model would spare an unnecessary surgery for those men at lowest risk and also alert the physician to those patients at high risk.

The outcome (y) variable is nodal involvement and is binary valued. Binary-valued covariates (X-ray, stage, and grade) have been coded so that the "0" values are the less serious status. Age and serum acid phosphatase are continuous measures.

[1] Distributed as part of the R package: http://cran.r-project.org/.

Table 9.1. Nodal involvement in prostate cancer patients. The six columns are: x-ray status; stage of the cancer; grade of the tumor; age of the patient; serum acid phosphatase; and nodal involvement (1 = yes, 0 = no).

X-ray	Stage	Grade	Age	Acid	Nodes	X-ray	Stage	Grade	Age	Acid	Nodes
0	0	0	66	48	0	0	0	0	68	56	0
0	0	0	66	50	0	0	0	0	56	52	0
0	0	0	58	50	0	0	0	0	60	49	0
1	0	0	65	46	0	1	0	0	60	62	0
0	0	1	50	56	1	1	0	0	49	55	0
0	0	0	61	62	0	0	0	0	58	71	0
0	0	0	51	65	0	1	0	1	67	67	1
0	0	1	67	47	0	0	0	0	51	49	0
0	0	1	56	50	0	0	0	0	60	78	0
0	0	0	52	83	0	0	0	0	56	98	0
0	0	0	67	52	0	0	0	0	63	75	0
0	0	1	59	99	1	0	0	0	64	187	0
1	0	0	61	136	1	0	0	0	56	82	1
0	1	1	64	40	0	0	1	0	61	50	0
0	1	1	64	50	0	0	1	0	63	40	0
0	1	1	52	55	0	0	1	1	66	59	0
1	1	0	58	48	1	1	1	1	57	51	1
0	1	0	65	49	1	0	1	1	65	48	0
1	1	1	59	63	0	0	1	0	61	102	0
0	1	0	53	76	0	0	1	0	67	95	0
0	1	1	53	66	0	1	1	1	65	84	1
1	1	1	50	81	1	1	1	1	60	76	1
0	1	1	45	70	1	1	1	1	56	78	1
0	1	0	46	70	1	0	1	0	67	67	1
0	1	0	63	82	1	0	1	1	57	67	1
1	1	0	51	72	1	1	1	0	64	89	1
1	1	1	68	126	1						

Source: Brown (1980).

Questions to ask from this data: What are useful predictors of nodal status? Are the explanatory variables independent of each other, or are these correlated with each other? What does that say about their individual and collective use as diagnostic measures? Are there any outliers or highly influential observations that may unduly effect the fitted model?

9.1 Some Syntax for `proc logistic`

A SAS program to invoke the logistic procedure uses the code given in Table 9.2 for the nodal cancer example of the previous section. This program produces a number

Table 9.2. A logistic regression program that produces and captures values from `iplots`.

```
proc logistic descending;
   model node= xray acid stage grade age / lackfit iplots;
   output out=logout p=p h=h c=c cbar=cbar reschi=reschi
      resdev=resdev difchisq=difchisq difdev=difdev
      dfbetas= _ALL_;
run;

proc print data=logout;
run;
```

of informative plots that are described in this chapter, and it captures all of the diagnostic values in a new dataset called `logout`.

Part of the output from this program appears in Table 9.3. If $\widehat{p}$ is the estimated probability of nodal involvement, then the fitted model is

$$\begin{aligned}\text{logit}(\widehat{p}) &= 0.0618 + 2.0453\ \texttt{xray} + 0.0243\ \texttt{acid}\\ &\quad + 1.5641\ \texttt{stage} + 0.7614\ \texttt{grade} - 0.0693\ \texttt{age}.\end{aligned}$$

These values are called `p` and appear in the `logout` dataset. The `descending` option is used to model the probabilities of node=1. Notice also that there is no `/n` needed because all of the binomial n parameters are equal to 1. The `descending` option was described in the exercise of Section 8.6.4 and is useful when all $n = 1$ and we want to model response values of 1 as the success.

The `lackfit` option performs a test of the overall fit of the logistic regression. This test was proposed by Hosmer and Lemeshow (2000). The range of p is broken up into 10 intervals. Within each interval, we use the logistic model to provide the expected number of successes and failures. These expected values are compared with

Table 9.3. Part of the SAS output for the prostate cancer example.

Analysis of Maximum Likelihood Estimates

Parameter	DF	Estimate	Standard Error	Wald Chi-Square	Pr > ChiSq
Intercept	1	0.0618	3.4599	0.0003	0.9857
xray	1	2.0453	0.8072	6.4208	0.0113
acid	1	0.0243	0.0132	3.4230	0.0643
stage	1	1.5641	0.7740	4.0835	0.0433
grade	1	0.7614	0.7708	0.9759	0.3232
age	1	-0.0693	0.0579	1.4320	0.2314

the observed numbers of successes and failures using a chi-squared statistic with 9 df. This test is only available when all $n = 1$.

The new option we discuss in this chapter is the use of the `/iplots` option. The `iplots` option in `proc logistic` produces a large number of informative *index plots* that can be used to identify outliers and unusual observations. The aim of this chapter is to explain all of these plots. The index refers to the observation number. If you use a `proc print` after every `data` step, then you will be able to associate the index number with the rest of the data for that subject.

The `output` statement in Table 9.2 captures all of the numerical values of the `iplots` measures and puts these into a new dataset called `logout`. The program prints out the contents of this dataset. One important variable in this dataset is the fitted value $\widehat{p}$ of the binomial parameter for each observation.

9.2 Residuals for Logistic Regression

We have already seen the important use of examining residuals in identifying exceptional observations in the data. Despite their critical role in linear regression models, there is more than one definition of a residual in logistic regression. There is a simple explanation for this. In linear regression with normally distributed errors, one of the fundamental assumptions is that residuals have a constant variance. See Section 4.4 for a review of this. Similarly, we fit linear regression models using least squares of these residual values. So, in linear regression, we rely on residuals to both fit the model and then tell us how well it explains the data. In logistic regression there are several definitions of residuals, all interesting in their own way.

So, for example, we could simply use the definition of residuals from linear regression, namely, the difference between observed and expected. SAS calls these the *raw residuals*, which are defined as

$$\text{Raw residual} = \text{Observed} - \text{Expected} = y - n\widehat{p}$$

where $\widehat{p}$ is the value fitted by logistic regression.

What is wrong with looking at these raw residuals? A problem with logistic regression for binary-valued data is that the binomial distribution does not have a constant variance, unlike the assumption we make for linear regression with normally distributed errors. The formula for the binomial variance is $np(1 - p)$ and is given at (2.3). Specifically, when the p parameter is close to either 0 or 1 then all of the observations are likely to be failures or successes, respectively, with little variability.

A simple correction to the raw residual is to divide each of these by their estimated standard error. SAS calls these the *Pearson residuals* or the *chi-squared residuals*. These are defined as

$$\texttt{reschi} = \frac{y - n\widehat{p}}{\sqrt{n\widehat{p}(1 - \widehat{p})}}.$$

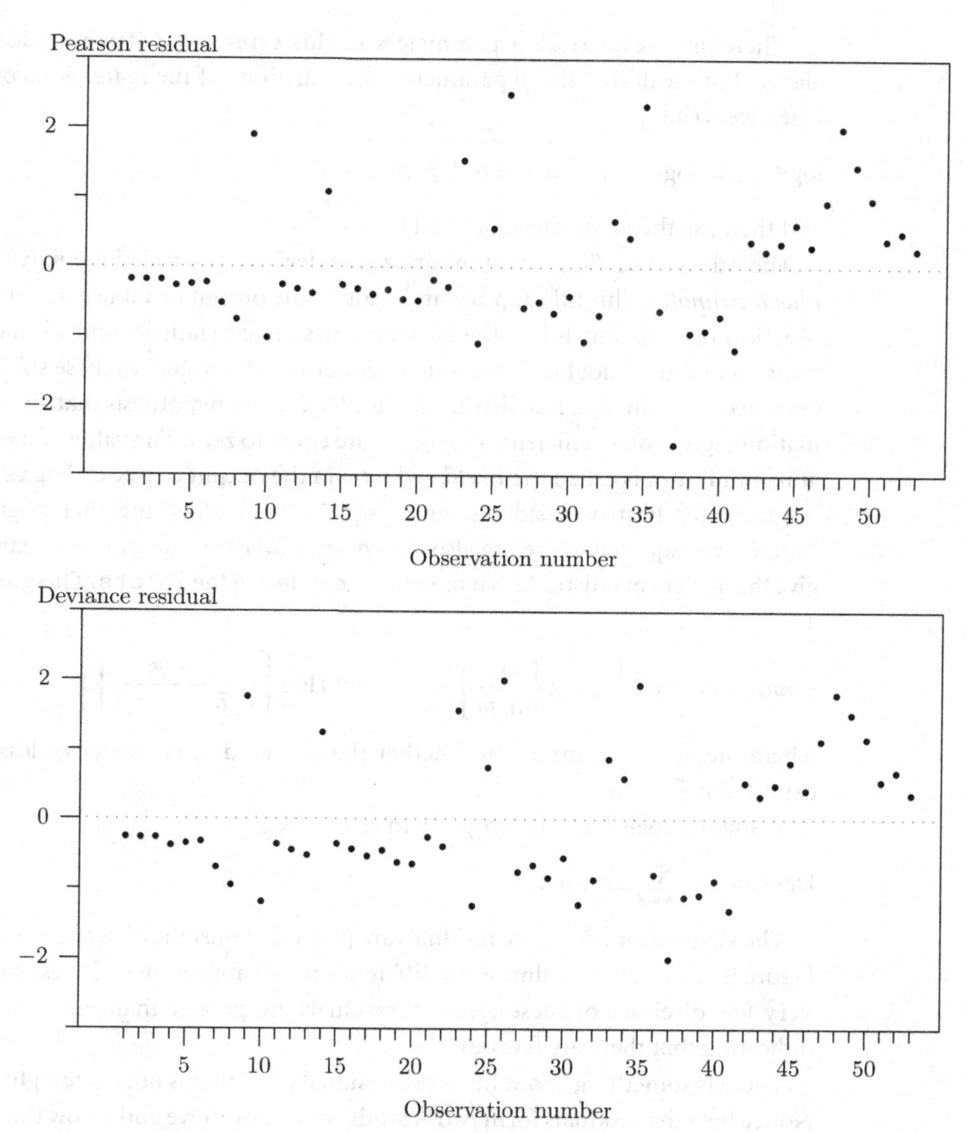

Figure 9.1 Pearson and deviance residuals for the prostate cancer data.

The Pearson residuals are plotted against the observation number when you use the `iplots` option. These appear in Figure 9.1.

This also leads us to raise the question: How does SAS fit the regression parameters in logistic regression? Unlike the residual sums of squares that are minimized in Section 3.2 on linear regression, estimates of the regression coefficients are obtained by minimizing the *deviance* function, which is defined as

$$\text{Deviance} = 2\sum_i \left[y_i \log\left\{\frac{y_i}{n_i\, p_i}\right\} + (n_i - y_i)\log\left\{\frac{n_i - y_i}{n_i(1-p_i)}\right\}\right]. \tag{9.1}$$

Where are the regression parameters in this expression? It is not clear at first glance, but recall that the p parameters are functions of the regression coefficients when we write

$$\text{logit}(p) = \log(p/(1-p)) = \alpha + \beta_1 x_1 + \cdots$$

and then use this in the deviance (9.1).

The values of α, $\beta_1, \ldots$ that minimize the deviance are called the *maximum likelihood estimates.* This title appears at the top of the output in Table 9.3. The deviance function behaves much like the Pearson chi-squared statistic, and in many situations there should not be a large difference between the values of these statistics. The deviance has a chi-squared distribution under the null hypothesis that all of the population regression coefficients $\beta_1, \beta_2, \ldots$ are equal to zero. The value of the deviance at its minimum is called the *likelihood ratio* in the output of `proc logistic`.

Just as the Pearson residuals can be squared and added together to give us the Pearson chi-squared, there are also *deviance residuals* whose sum of squared values give the deviance statistic. SAS names these `resdev` in the `iplots`. These are defined as

$$\texttt{resdev} = \pm\sqrt{2}\left[y_i \log\left\{\frac{y_i}{n_i \widehat{p}_i}\right\} + (n_i - y_i)\log\left\{\frac{n_i - y_i}{n_i \widehat{p}_i(1-\widehat{p}_i)}\right\}\right]^{1/2}$$

where the $\pm$ is determined by whether the observed y_i is greater or less than the expected $n_i \widehat{p}_i$.

These residuals have the property that

$$\text{Deviance} = \sum (\texttt{resdev})^2.$$

The Pearson and deviance residuals are plotted against the observation number in Figure 9.1, and there is almost no difference in the appearance of these two figures. Very few of either of these types of residuals are greater than ± 2 in magnitude, indicating that there are few outliers.

There is something about these two residual plots that is not quite right, however. Notice how the residuals form two "clouds" of values above and below the zero value line but do not actually touch it. This is even more striking in the plot of deviance residuals. Why does the residual plot take this peculiar shape?

Even though the residuals for this model have a mean of 0 and a standard deviation close to 1, there is no reason that they need to behave as though they were sampled from a normal, bell-shaped distribution. Specifically, in this example, recall that all of the binomial n parameters are equal to 1. The binomial response variables y will only take on the values 0 or 1, and the estimated $\widehat{p}$ parameter can take on any value between 0 and 1.

The raw residuals are defined as $y - \widehat{p}$. When $y = 1$ the estimated $\widehat{p}$ will always underestimate the response. Similarly, when $y = 0$, the estimate $\widehat{p}$ will always overestimate the response. In other words, the cloud of residuals above the zero line all

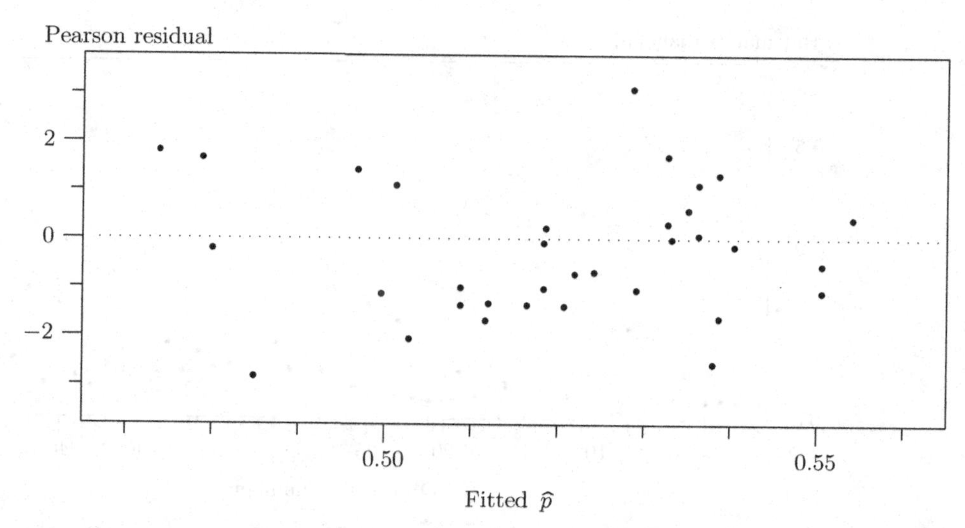

Figure 9.2 Pearson residuals and fitted $\widehat{p}$ for the toxoplasmosis data of Section 8.6.2.

correspond to values of $y = 1$, and the residuals below the zero line are all associated with $y = 0$ responses. The standardization of the raw residuals by their estimated standard error will change the scale of the residuals and actually pushes them further away from 0. See Exercise 9.2 for an explanation of this. You may have also noticed a trend in the residual plots of Figure 9.1 for these data. This is discussed in Exercise 9.3.

Does this mean that residuals are not useful in logistic regression? No, residuals are still useful, especially in identifying poorly fitting outliers in the data. The only problem is that when all of the binomial n parameters are equal to 1 or other small counts, then we cannot expect the responses to behave approximately as normally distributed. The residuals may not take values close to 0 even in a well-fitting model.

As another example of residuals, look back at the toxoplasmosis example of Section 8.6.2. In this example, a small number of villages had only $n = 1$ or 2 children tested, but most villages had much larger values. Let us fit a model in which the logit of the risk of infection in each village is expressible as a linear function of rainfall. The residuals are plotted against the fitted $\widehat{p}$ values in Figure 9.2. In this figure we see that the residuals appear to be reasonably distributed close to the zero line and that there are few large outliers to point out. The residuals on this figure behave more as we would expect them to, because most of the binomial n parameters are greater than 1.

9.3 Influence in Logistic Regression

Many of the diagnostic measures for logistic regression have a direct parallel and are borrowed from linear regression. For example, there is a hat diagonal for logistic

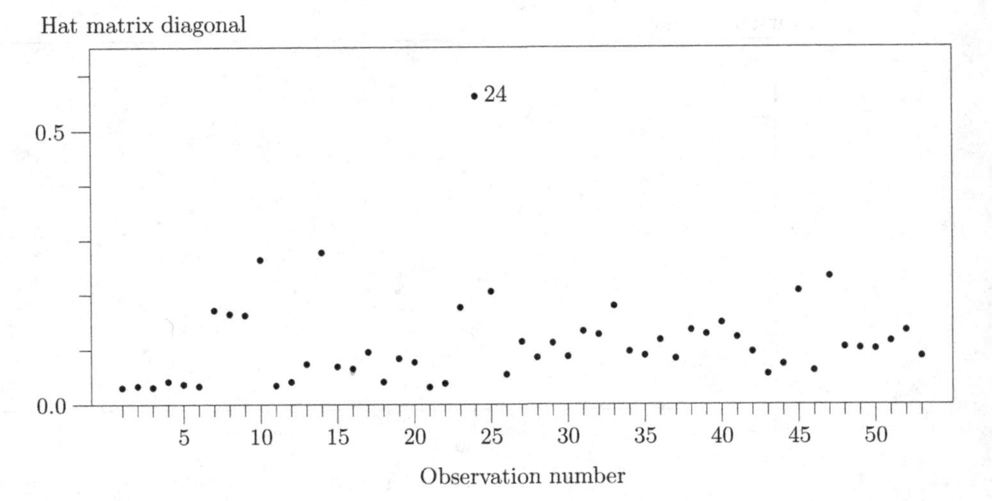

Figure 9.3 Hat matrix diagonal for the prostate cancer data.

regression that is similar to the influence measure we saw in Section 5.3. This measure is called `h` in the program in Table 9.2. The index plot of the hat diagonal appears in Figure 9.3.

This figure shows that most of the patients have reasonable influence in the logistic regression, but observation 24 really stands out from the rest. Recall that the hat diagonal only indicates outliers among the explanatory values, not the response. In Figure 9.1 we see that this observation has a negative residual that is not extreme. This observation appears to follow the form of the model, but something is not quite right. The hat matrix diagonal points this observation out to us, but it does not explain what the matter is. To find out, we need to examine the other diagnostics that are part of the `iplots`.

Two popular diagnostic measures are c and $\overline{c}$ (called `c` and `cbar` in SAS). Together, these two measures are referred to as the *confidence interval displacement.* These combine the Pearson residual (`reschi`) and the hat diagonal. They are calculated as

$$c = (\texttt{reschi})^2 \times \text{hat}/(1 - \text{hat})^2$$

and

$$\overline{c} = (\texttt{reschi})^2 \times \text{hat}/(1 - \text{hat}),$$

respectively.

Index plots of c and $\overline{c}$ for the prostate cancer data are given in Figure 9.4. These look much like that of the hat diagonal in Figure 9.3. As in that plot of the hat diagnostic, plots of c and $\overline{c}$ indicate that observation 24 is unusual but do not help to explain why this is the case.

The remaining diagnostics for logistic regression all derive from jackknife methods. Recall from Section 5.4 that the jackknife is a general technique that omits

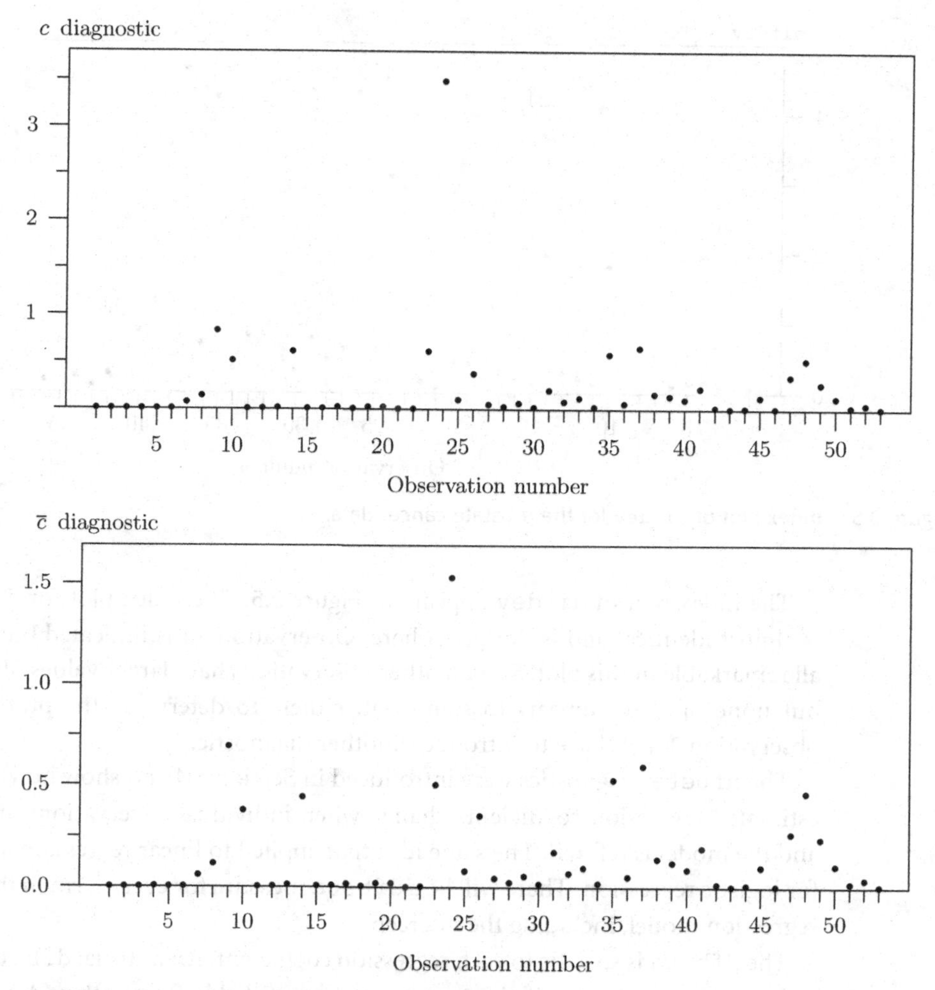

Figure 9.4 Confidence interval displacement from the logistic regression of the prostate cancer data.

an observation and then refits the model without that observation. The new fitted model is then compared to the original model fitted from all of the data.

Specifically, the `difchisq` and `difdev` are the change in Pearson chi-squared and the deviance functions when individual observations are deleted and then the model is refitted. These two measures are typically used to identify outliers because they indicate how much the overall fit is altered when observations are omitted. These statistics are calculated as

$$\texttt{difchisq} = \bar{c}\,/\,\text{hat} = (\texttt{reschi})^2\,/\,(1 - \text{hat})$$

and

$$\texttt{difdev} = (\texttt{resdev})^2 + \bar{c}\,,$$

respectively, for each observation.

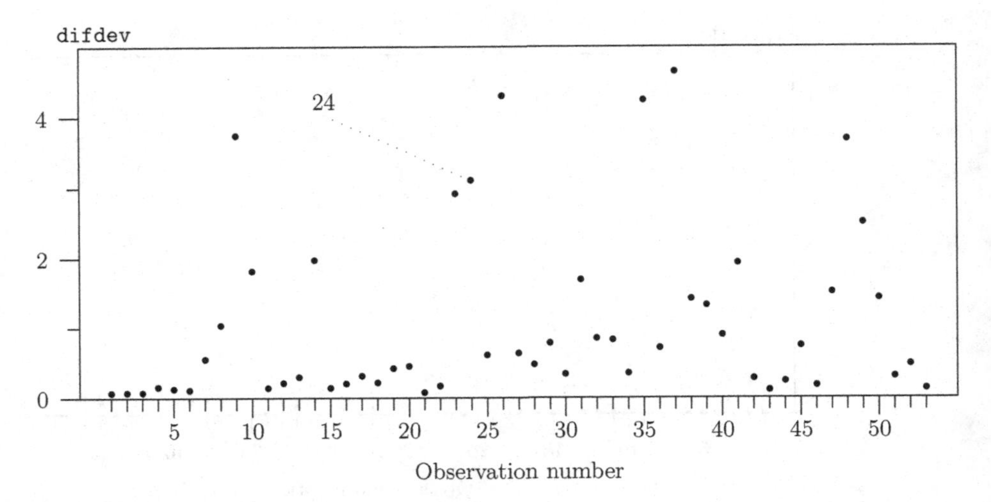

Figure 9.5 Index plot of `difdev` for the prostate cancer data.

The index plot of `difdev` appears in Figure 9.5. The index plot for `difchisq` is almost identical and is not given here. Observation 24 is indicated but is not at all remarkable in this plot. Several other observations have larger values of `difdev`, but none of these appears to stand out, either. To determine the problem with observation 24, we have to introduce another diagnostic.

The `dfbeta` diagnostics were introduced in Section 5.4 and show how much the estimated regression coefficients change when individual observations are deleted and the model is refitted. The same idea that applied to linear regression also works for logistic regression. There will be a `dfbeta` measure for every term in the logistic regression model, including the intercept.

The `dfbeta` is specific to each regression coefficient. An unusual `dfbeta` for one estimated regression coefficient may not be remarkable for another. A number of these `iplots` for the prostate cancer example are not remarkable, but one really stands out. The index plot for the serum acid phosphatase `dfbeta` is given in Figure 9.6.

In this diagnostic plot we can easily see how observation 24 is different from the others. Now we know something is unusual about the serum acid level for this subject. If we look back at the original data in Table 9.1, we see that his serum acid level is 187, much higher than any other individual. This extremely high acid level is the source of the influence of this cancer patient.

In this section we described a number of diagnostic measures that are produced in `proc logistic` using the `iplots` option. Not all of these will be useful all of the time, of course. Residuals are important and identify poorly fitting observations. The index plots are more concerned with unusual values among the explanatory variables. In the example of the prostate cancer patients, we saw that some measures, such as c and $\bar{c}$, are useful for identifying unusual observations. Other measures,

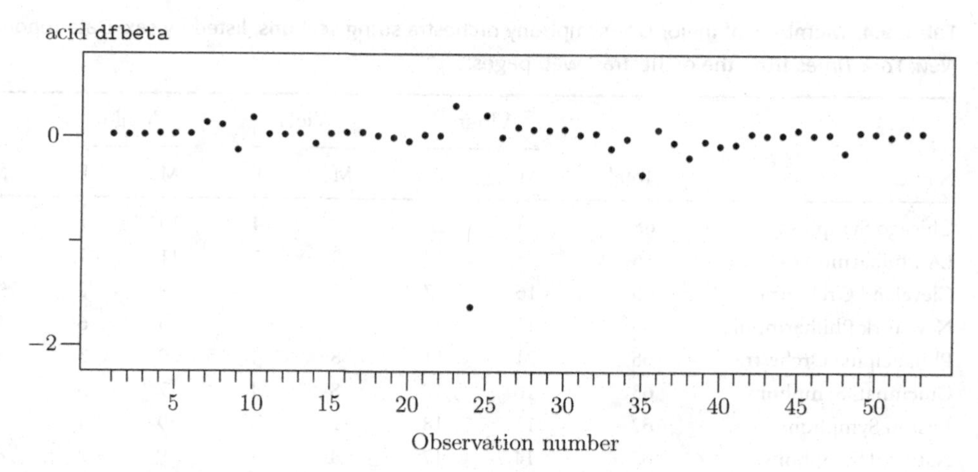

Figure 9.6 Index plot of the serum acid dfbeta for the prostate cancer data.

such as difdev and difchisq, may miss these influential observations if the model fits them well. Finally, the dfbetas are specific to each term in the model. Taken together, all of these diagnostics are helpful in identifying influential and unusual observations in our data.

9.4 Exercises

9.1 When all of the binomial n parameters are equal to 1, then we need to use the descending option in proc logistic. Otherwise we are modeling the binomial probability of "failure" $1 - p$ for $y = 0$ rather than the probability p of "success" for $y = 1$.

Suppose we forgot to do this and SAS treats $y = 0$ as the success event. Do we need to run the program again? What can be done to fix the problem? *Hint:* The log of a reciprocal is the negative of the log. That is, $\log(1/x) = -\log(x)$. What is the relationship between

$$\log\left\{\frac{p}{1-p}\right\}$$

and

$$\log\left\{\frac{1-p}{p}\right\},$$

and what should we do to the estimated regression coefficients in the logistic model?

9.2 When all of the n parameters are equal to 1 in a logistic regression, are the raw residuals closer to 0 or further away from 0 than the Pearson, reschi residuals? *Hint:* What can you say about the denominator of the Pearson residuals?

Table 9.4. Members of major U.S. symphony orchestra string sections, listed by sex. Data reported by the *New York Times* from the orchestras' web pages.

		Violin		Viola		'Cello		Bass	
Name	Total	M	F	M	F	M	F	M	F
Chicago Symphony	68	14	20	10	4	10	1	9	0
LA Philharmonic	66	15	17	8	5	11	1	9	0
Cleveland Orchestra	65	16	17	7	5	9	2	9	0
New York Philharmonic	65	13	20	5	7	5	6	7	2
Philadelphia Orchestra	65	21	11	8	4	9	3	9	0
Cincinnati Symphony	63	16	17	8	4	7	3	8	0
Boston Symphony	62	13	18	7	5	9	1	9	0
National Symphony	62	14	17	4	7	9	3	8	0
Baltimore Symphony	58	18	10	6	6	5	5	8	0

9.3 Notice the trend in the residual plots in Figure 9.1, especially among the negative residuals. Can you explain this? What does the horizontal axis in this plot represent? Could this be a risk factor for nodal involvement? Why do you think that might be the case? Run a logistic regression model and see if this is a useful and statistically significant measure of risk of nodal involvement.

9.4.1 Statistics in the News: Sex and Violins

In an article about a reverse sex-discrimination case, a male violinist was suing a major symphony orchestra claiming, among other things, that there were too many female violinists. The *New York Times* printed the data in Table 9.4 detailing the gender breakdown of the string sections of several major U.S. symphony orchestras. The data was obtained from the individual orchestras' web pages.

An opening for a position in a major symphony orchestra will bring hundreds of applicants from many countries. To ensure fairness to these performers, most modern symphony auditions are conducted anonymously. Orchestras will usually audition players for their positions behind screens so that they can be heard but not seen. The players' identities are usually not known by those doing the hiring until after a decision has been reached. The orchestras will often go so far as to provide thick carpeting so that even the performer's footsteps cannot be heard behind the screen.

Possible statistical analysis includes:

a. Show that female players appear more often in the higher pitched instruments. The order of deeper pitch is violin, viola, 'cello, bass. Notice, for example, there are almost no female bass players. Do you think that smaller or larger hands may be advantageous for some instruments?
b. Does the percentage of female membership change with size of the string section? Is the Total number of string players a useful covariate?
c. Which orchestras are more prone to males or females predominating?

Table 9.5. The start of a SAS program that reads and reformats the orchestra data.

```
title1 'Sex discrimination in major symphony string sections';
data raw;
   input name $ 1-18 size mviolin fviolin
       mviola fviola mcello fcello mbass fbass;
datalines;
   Chicago Symphony  68 14 20 10  4 10  1  9  0
   LA Philharmonic   66 15 17  8  5 11  1  9  0
   Cleveland Orch    65 16 17  7  5  9  2  9  0
   NY Philharmonic   65 13 20  5  7  5  6  7  2
   Philadelphia Orch 65 21 11  8  4  9  3  9  0
   Cincinnati Symph  63 16 17  8  4  7  3  8  0
   Boston Symphony   62 13 18  7  5  9  1  9  0
   National Symphony 62 14 17  4  7  9  3  8  0
   Baltimore Symph   58 18 10  6  6  5  5  8  0
run;
proc print;      /* Echo the raw data */
run;
title2 'Separate data lines for each instrument';
data string;    /* create a longer, more useful version */
   set raw;      /* begin with the raw data */
   keep name size total instrument m f; /* delete all other variables */
   instrument='violin';
   m=mviolin; f=fviolin; total= m+f; output;
   instrument='viola';
   m=mviola; f=fviola; total=m+f; output;
   instrument='cello';
   m=mcello; f=fcello; total=m+f; output;
   instrument='bass';
   m=mbass; f=fbass; total=m+f; output;
run;
proc print data=string; /* Print the reformatted data */
run;
title2 'A suggested analysis';
proc logistic data=string;
   class name instrument;
   model f / total = instrument size name / iplots ;
run;
```

The outline of a suggested SAS program is given in Table 9.5. The `data` step of this program creates another dataset called `string`, with each instrument within every orchestra listed on a different line. Run this program and see how the data is reformatted. Use this program as the basis of your examination of these data using logistic regression. As always, be on the lookout for outliers and points of high influence.

Table 9.6. Glove use among nurses for four observation periods. Missing values are indicated by blank spaces.

Years of experience	Period 1 obs	Period 1 gloved	Period 2 obs	Period 2 gloved	Period 3 obs	Period 3 gloved	Period 4 obs	Period 4 gloved
15	2	1	7	6	1	1		
2	2	1	6	5	11	10	9	9
3	5	5	13	13	8	7	15	14
10	2	0	2	2	2	2	5	4
20	12	0	2	2	3	3	3	0
8	3	0	8	8	3	2	4	2
9	4	4	4	4				
4	4	0	4	4	2	1		
15	2	0	3	2	1	1	2	1
8	6	1	1	1	2	2		
8	3	0	4	3	8	6	2	0
2	2	0	3	3	8	8	5	5
5	1	0						
15	1	0	3	3				
3	1	1	2	2	1	1	1	1
14	1	0					1	1
14			2	2	3	3	1	1
8			1	1	1	1	1	1
3			2	1				
6			1	1				
3			1	1				
1					2	2		
6							1	0

Source: Friedland, Joffe, Moore *et al.* (1992) and http://lib.stat.cmu.edu/DASL/Datafiles/Nurses.html.

9.4.2 Glove Use Among Nurses

In an effort to increase the use of gloves among pediatric nurses, a study was conducted in the emergency department of an inner-city pediatric hospital. Without their knowledge, the nurses were observed during a vascular procedure, and the observers recorded how often they used gloves. Observations were made at four time points: before a training period and at 1, 2, and 5 months following the training period. For each of the four periods, Table 9.6 gives the number of times the nurse was observed to perform the procedure (n) and how many of these times he or she wore gloves (y). The number of years of experience for each nurse is also given.

Notice the longitudinal nature of the data. The observations were collected over a period of time. It might help to review the discussion of methods for longitudinal data given in Section 6.5 and Exercise 6.7 for the approach in a specific example. In this present example, the outcomes (gloved or ungloved procedures) are binary valued, but most of the same principles remain.

Even though each nurse was observed at up to four different time periods, let us treat these as independent binomial experiments. Create a binary-valued indicator variable equal to 0 at the first period and 1 for all posttraining periods. Use this indicator in a logistic regression to see if there was a (marginal) difference in the use of gloves before and after the training period. Does the (marginal) rate of glove use increase or decrease with years of experience? Can you interpret this in simple terms? Look at the interaction between this pre/post indicator and period to see if there was a trend in the posttraining period. Is there evidence whether this posttraining trend is the same regardless of the experience of the nurse? Again, interpret this finding. Use the logistic regression diagnostics to identify outliers or influential observations.

Create an indicator variable for more or fewer than 5 years of experience. Is there a relationship between the number of observed procedures and this simple measure of experience? Interpret this finding. Does this mean that the procedure was performed more often by some nurses, or perhaps that some nurses were more likely to be observed and their data recorded?

In a transitional approach to this data, see if there is evidence that individual behavior was changed by the training. Specifically, did individuals with a low frequency of glove use before training change their behavior after training? To answer this question, we might classify every nurses's pretraining glove use as above or below 50%, and then classify their posttraining as above or below 50%. Tabulate the frequencies of these individuals in a 2×2 table. Look at the separate 2×2 tables for those whose experience is above and below 5 years. Is there a difference in these two frequency tables?

There are a large number of missing values in Table 9.6. These are indicated by blank spaces where data values should be. Missing values are common and play an important part in longitudinal data. Was the frequency of missing observations related to years of experience? Were the missing values more likely in pre- or posttraining for more or less experienced nurses? Can you explain this? In Section 6.5 we described a method called "last value carried forward" to fill in missing values. Does this technique change the conclusions for any of the other questions in this exercise?

9.4.3 Statistics in Sports: Pittsburgh Steelers Rushing Game

In Table 9.7 we are given a history of the Pittsburgh Steelers for 21 years, under the direction of three different coaches.[2] This includes a win/loss record for each year. "Rushing attempts" is the number of running plays. These are not listed as absolute numbers but instead given as ranks among all teams for each year. Similarly, the number of yards attained is given as the rank compared to all other teams. Of course,

[2] Available online at http://www.nytimes.com/2009/01/11/sports/football/11steelers.html.

Table 9.7. Pittsburgh Steelers rushing records. Reported by the *New York Times*, January 11, 2009.

	Games		Rank of		
Year	Won	Lost	Rushing attempts	Rushing yards	Coach
1988	5	11	13	6	Chuck Noll
1989	9	7	11	18	Chuck Noll
1990	9	7	14	13	Chuck Noll
1991	7	9	16	17	Chuck Noll
1992	11	5	2	4	Bill Cowher
1993	9	7	5	6	Bill Cowher
1994	12	4	2	1	Bill Cowher
1995	11	5	5	2	Bill Cowher
1996	10	6	2	2	Bill Cowher
1997	11	5	1	1	Bill Cowher
1998	7	9	8	7	Bill Cowher
1999	6	10	5	10	Bill Cowher
2000	9	7	2	4	Bill Cowher
2001	13	3	1	1	Bill Cowher
2002	10	5	3	9	Bill Cowher
2003	6	10	16	31	Bill Cowher
2004	15	1	1	2	Bill Cowher
2005	11	5	1	5	Bill Cowher
2006	8	8	14	10	Bill Cowher
2007	10	6	3	3	Mike Tomlin
2008	12	4	9	23	Mike Tomlin

each year's data represents the same team in name only, because most players' careers are relatively short. The coaches are working with different players from year to year. The number of teams has changed as well.

Some would argue that rushing, as opposed to passing, is a more conservative strategy. Passing, or throwing the ball, has a higher risk of failure, but more yards are gained when it succeeds. In some years there are changes in the rules that favor either passing or rushing, so the overall strategy of the game has changed over time. Similarly, the number of rushing plays is not as useful as the rank of plays attempted when compared to other teams. Let us use logistic regression to see how the rushing game affects the overall win/loss record for this team.

Is there an association of rushing and yards achieved with the win/loss record? Is there a difference between the three coaches? Do these coaches have a different emphasis on rushing? Are they more successful at it? Has the reliance of rushing plays changed over the years? is there an interaction between yards attempted and plays run? Are the running plays more successful in some years?

Look for influence and outliers. What was so unusual about the 2003 season? Notice that the years under coach Mike Tomlin are influential. The earliest years are influential as well. Why is that?

10

Poisson Regression

The Poisson distribution[1] is the approximation to the binomial model when the n parameter is large and the p parameter is small. This is the most important discrete distribution for public health. Many individuals are at risk for an event that is very unlikely to occur to any one of them. Shark attacks, lottery winners, and lightning strikes are all good examples. So is the incidence of cancer, industrial injuries, surgical complications, and the births of twins.

10.1 Statistics in the News: Lottery Winners

Let us consider the example of people winning the lottery in several different towns in the New Haven area. The data is given in Table 10.1. There are a large number of people playing, many tickets are sold, but the probability of winning remains very small. Yet, as the advertisements point out, some people do win. In a town with a population of a few thousand, how can we develop mathematical models to describe the numbers of winners? What about characteristics of different towns: Do rural or urban settings have more winners? Do towns with higher property taxes have a different number of winners? How do we take different population sizes of the various towns into account? We show how to answer some of these questions and leave the remainder for the reader to complete in the exercise of Section 10.6.4.

10.2 Poisson Distribution Basics

Recall the binomial experiment described in Section 2.1. A simple experiment is repeated N times, and each independent outcome occurs as "success" with probability p or "failure" with probability $1 - p$. The Poisson distribution is an approximation to the binomial model where N is large and p is small. In our lottery example,

[1] Siméon-Denis Poisson, French physicist and mathematician (1781–1840), published this statistical distribution in 1838. *Poisson* is the French word for fish.

Table 10.1. The number of lottery winners in towns near New Haven. Columns are town name; number of lottery winners; population (in thousands); area in square miles; mill rate; and number of library books per student.

Town	Winners	Pop.	Area	Mill	Books
Ansonia	6	17.9	6.2	28.9	16.4
Branford	11	28.0	27.9	22.6	18.0
Cheshire	6	26.2	33.0	27.1	21.0
Clinton	2	12.8	17.2	27.9	20.5
Derby	6	12.0	5.3	29.6	14.8
East Haven	9	26.5	12.6	37.1	13.5
Guilford	6	20.3	47.7	28.6	30.9
Hamden	9	52.0	33.0	34.1	17.4
Madison	5	16.0	36.3	22.3	24.2
Milford	10	49.5	23.5	30.8	19.7
N. Branford	2	13.1	26.8	26.9	14.0
North Haven	12	21.6	21.0	23.4	23.2
Old Saybrook	1	9.3	18.3	15.3	23.4
Orange	9	12.5	17.6	23.8	29.7
Oxford	3	9.1	33.0	29.0	15.3
Seymour	1	14.5	14.7	40.5	18.7
Shelton	7	36.0	31.4	21.6	17.3
Trumbull	14	33.0	23.5	24.1	21.6
West Haven	12	54.0	10.6	41.4	17.2

Source: New Haven Register, August 17, 1995, and U.S. Census data.

there are many lottery players and many tickets are sold, but the chance that any one ticket wins a major prize is very small.

> The Poisson distribution is the approximation to the binomial for large N and small p.

It is hard to say exactly where this approximation takes over. Larger N and smaller p make it better, but there are no quick rules about when the Poisson is to be preferred to the binomial model. If it were really critical that we get the right value, then we should not cut any corners in getting it correct and use the binomial distribution. On the other hand, finding factorials of really large numbers in order to calculate the binomial probability may quickly dissuade us from using it. Exercise 10.1 asks the reader to calculate some probabilities and note how well the approximation works for a simple example.

The Poisson model assumes that the binomial mean Np is fixed and moderate. We don't want to talk about a setting where Np is small so that there are too few rare events expected. Similarly, if Np is large, then we would do better to use the normal approximation to the binomial model.

Recall from (2.3) that the variance of the binomial distribution is equal to $Np(1-p)$. When p is very close to zero, then $1-p$ is very close to 1 and can be ignored in the variance. This makes the variance very close to the value Np, or the same as the mean. So, when N is large and p is small, we see that the mean and the variance are very close in value.

In the Poisson distribution, the mean and variance are equal in value.

In the Poisson distribution we do not talk about the N and p parts separately. Instead we refer to the distribution by its mean, which we denote using the Greek letter lambda, λ. The value of λ can be any positive number, and it does not need to be an integer. The value of λ is both the mean and the variance, as we just pointed out.

As with the binomial distribution, the outcome must be a nonnegative integer number of events. The range of the Poisson distribution is also infinite because the N part of the binomial is considered to be infinite.

In a Poisson distribution with mean λ, the probability of j events (for any value of $j = 0, 1, 2, \ldots$) is equal to

$$\Pr[j \text{ events}] = e^{-\lambda}\lambda^j / j!. \tag{10.1}$$

We do not need to know this formula in order to use the Poisson distribution or fit models to it in SAS. The formula is useful to illustrate the shape of the distribution. Examples of the Poisson distribution are given in Figure 10.1 for values of λ equal to 0.5, 2, and 8.

When the Poisson mean λ is equal to 0.5, we see in Figure 10.1 that most of the probability is concentrated at 0 and 1 events, and larger values are unlikely to occur. Even though the distribution continues on to the right forever, these probabilities quickly become very small. When λ is increased to 2, Figure 10.1 shows that the variance as well as the mean have increased. The range of likely values has increased to between 0 and 5, and values larger than 7 should rarely appear. When $\lambda = 8$, this figure shows that the Poisson is starting to look much like a normal distribution.

The Poisson distribution with a large mean is approximately normal.

10.3 Regression Models for Poisson Data

In Poisson regression, we model the mean λ of the number of events. The aim is to see how λ varies with additional covariate information available in the data. Are there more lottery winners, for example, in towns with larger areas?

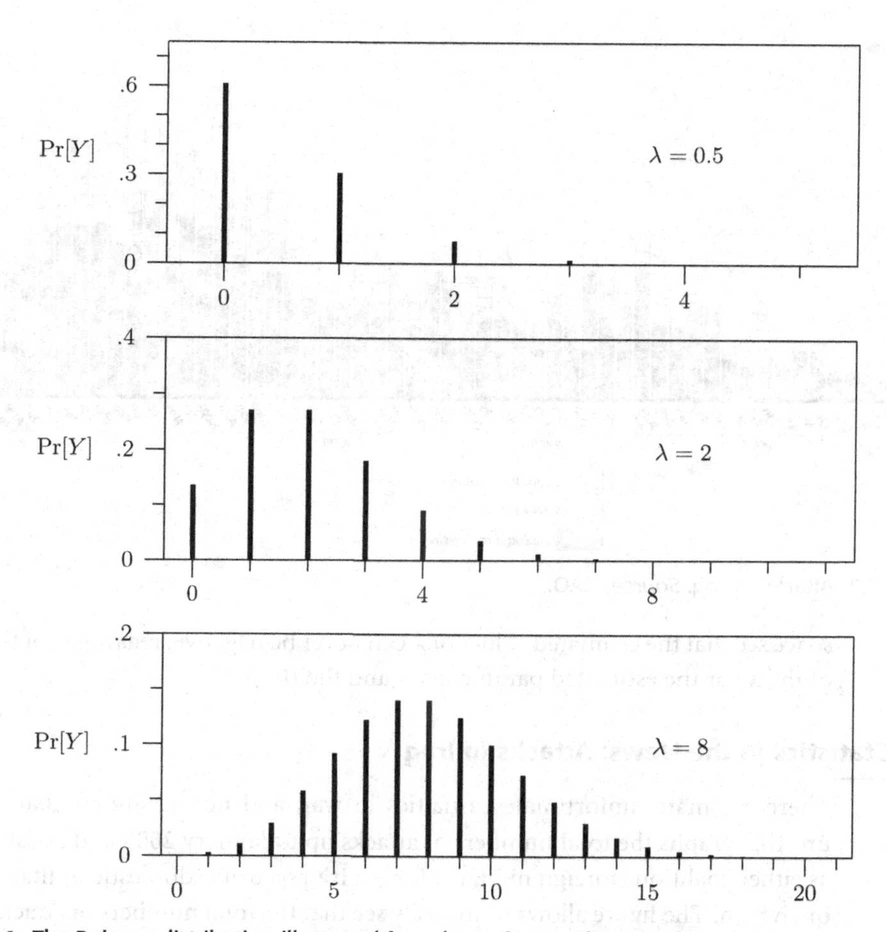

Figure 10.1 The Poisson distribution illustrated for values of λ equal to 0.5, 2, and 8.

We should not simply try to fit a model of the form

$$\lambda = \alpha + \beta_1 \text{ Area} + \beta_2 \text{ Population} .$$

For some values of the area and population, this might result in a negative number and we must always have $\lambda > 0$.

Instead, we need to use a link function, just as we used in Chapter 8 for logistic regression. The specific link used in Poisson regression is the log function. (The logarithm, as elsewhere in this book, is to the base e = 2.718). In Poisson regression, we fit models of the form

$$\log(\lambda) = \alpha + \beta_1 x_1 + \beta_2 x_2 + \cdots$$

for explanatory variables $x_1, x_2, \ldots$.

Equivalently,

$$\lambda = \exp(\alpha + \beta_1 x_1 + \beta_2 x_2 + \cdots),$$

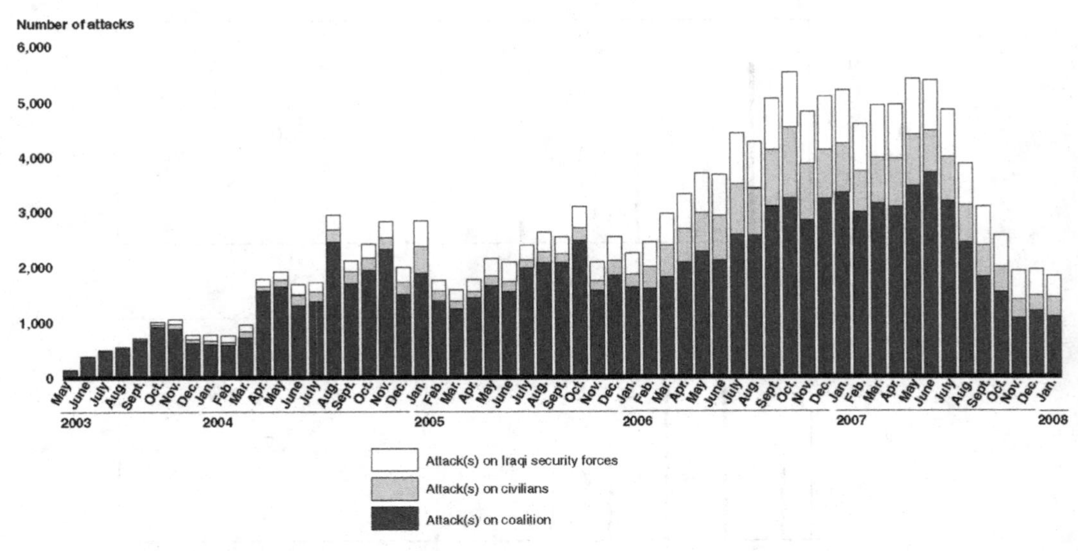

Figure 10.2 Attacks in Iraq. *Source:* GAO.

so we see that the estimated values of λ can never be negative, regardless of the values of the xs or the estimated parameters α and the βs.

10.4 Statistics in the News: Attacks in Iraq

There are many unfortunate casualties in war, and not all are combatants. Figure 10.2 graphs the total numbers of attacks up to January 2008 and classifies these as either coalition (foreign military) forces; Iraq security (domestic military) forces; or civilian. The figure allows us to easily see that the total numbers of attacks greatly increased from 2003 to 2007 but had decreased in the last few months of this graph.

Many people are involved in the conflict. The chance of an attack on any one person in a given month is small, so the Poisson assumptions appear to be met. As the mean number of attacks gets larger, the values of these counts also tend to vary by larger amounts. That is, the variances increase with the means, as we would expect for Poisson distributed data.

Are all persons in Iraq equally likely to be the target of an attack? Clearly not. There are many more civilians than military forces at risk in the country, but most attacks are directed at the military. It appears from this figure that the proportion of civilian attacks has remained the same over time and has only increased along with the total numbers of attacks.

Are the counts independent from one month to the next? Probably not, because these depend on troop movements into different areas and other coordinated activities by combatant forces. Notice that the overall trend in Figure 10.2 is increasing, but this appears as waves: a few months of high levels of attacks are followed by several months of lower levels. Perhaps this is due to the changing seasons. The trend within each year seems to increase into the summer and autumn months, and then a drop of the numbers of attacks appears every January.

Whatever the reason, counts in adjacent months of a *time series* such as this should be more highly correlated than those more distant in time. Such data is often said to be *autocorrelated*, meaning that the correlation between observations at two points falls off with the time difference between them. Autocorrelated time series data, usually with calendar effects, often appears in studies of economic activity in which events in one time period have bearing on the next but little effect years later.

10.5 Poisson Regression in SAS

A SAS program to fit a Poisson regression model to the lottery data is given in Table 10.2. The `data` step reads the variables and provides a `label` for each. The town names have character values. This needs to be specified in SAS using `input name $ 1-14`. The dollar sign indicates that character data is to be read, and the numbers indicate that columns 1–14 contain these values. The `proc print` following the `data` step is an important check that everything was read correctly.

The `genmod` procedure in Table 10.2 fits models for `winners` as a Poisson count. The `dist=Poisson` option specifies that the response variable (`winners`) has a Poisson distribution. The log of the mean number of winners is linear in the covariates area and population. The `model` statement specifies the model

$$\log(\lambda_i) = \alpha + \beta_1\, \texttt{area}_i + \beta_2\, \texttt{population}_i, \tag{10.2}$$

where λ_i is the mean number of lottery winners we would expect in the ith town.

10.5.1 Basic Output for Poisson Regression

A portion of the output is given in Table 10.3. This output contains the fitted parameters for α, and the two βs. Each of these estimated parameters is accompanied by its estimated standard error and a 95% confidence interval. The `Chi-square` statistic is the square of the ratio of the parameter estimate divided by its estimated standard error. This statistic tests the null hypothesis that the underlying (population) parameter value is 0. The p-value for the chi-squared test is given in the last column of the table. In this output we can see that the town population is very important in explaining the mean number of lottery winners in the various towns, but the town's area has little explanatory value in this model.

The top of Table 10.3 provides a rough guide to the fit of the model using the chi-squared statistic

$$\chi^2 = \sum_i\, (\texttt{winners}_i - \widehat{\lambda})^2 / \widehat{\lambda}_i$$

summed over all of the towns in the dataset.

Table 10.2. A SAS program to fit a Poisson regression model to the lottery data.

```
title1 'Lottery winners in towns near New Haven';

data lottery;
   input name $ 1-14 winners pop area mill books;
   label
      winners = '# of major lottery winners'
      pop     = 'population in thousands'
        area    = 'area in sq miles'
        mill    = 'mill rate for property taxes'
        books   = 'number of books per student' ;
   datalines;
Ansonia          6   17.9    6.2   28.9   16.4
Branford        11   28.0   27.9   22.6   18.0
Cheshire         6   26.2   33.0   27.1   21.0
Clinton          2   12.8   17.2   27.9   20.5
          .  .  .  .  .  .  .  .
Trumbull        14   33.0   23.5   24.1   21.6
West Haven      12   54.0   10.6   41.4   17.2
run;

proc print;     /* Always check to see if data step is OK */
run;

proc genmod data=lottery;
   model winners = area pop / dist=Poisson obstats;
   ods output obstats=fitted;
run;

title2 'Fitted information from proc genmod';
proc print data=fitted;
run;
```

The $\widehat{\lambda}_i$ are the estimated mean number of winners for each of the towns and winners; denotes the observed numbers. This chi-squared statistic (given in the top half of Table 10.3) is a reliable measure of model fit provided all of the λs are large. SAS recognizes that having large λs is not always the case, and so it provides another rough measure of fit in terms of this chi-squared divided by its degrees of freedom. Values of this ratio near 1 are indicative of a good fit.

The *deviance* is another statistic that behaves similarly to the chi-squared statistic. In Poisson regression, the estimated values of the βs are found by minimizing the

Table 10.3. A portion of the fitted Poisson regression for the lottery data.

Criteria For Assessing Goodness Of Fit

Criterion	DF	Value	Value/DF
Deviance	16	29.4934	1.8433
Scaled Deviance	16	29.4934	1.8433
Pearson Chi-Square	16	28.2003	1.7625
Scaled Pearson X2	16	28.2003	1.7625
Log Likelihood		130.3048	

Algorithm converged.

Analysis Of Parameter Estimates

Parameter	DF	Estimate	Standard Error	Wald 95% Confidence Limits		Chi-Square	Pr > ChiSq
Intercept	1	1.4076	0.2630	0.8922	1.9230	28.65	<.0001
area	1	-0.0045	0.0084	-0.0210	0.0119	0.29	0.5882
pop	1	0.0233	0.0055	0.0125	0.0341	17.76	<.0001
Scale	0	1.0000	0.0000	1.0000	1.0000		

deviance, rather than through least squares as is the case in linear regression. The deviance statistic for Poisson regression is

$$\text{Deviance} = 2 \sum_i (y_i - \lambda_i) + y_i \log(\lambda_i / y_i),$$

where y_i is the observed Poisson count.

In this example, as with the Poisson distribution more generally, the mean and variance are equal in value. The `scale` in the last row of Table 10.3 provides an option to fit a Poisson model with a variance that is greater than or less than the mean. The `scale` is specified by the programmer and is not estimated by SAS. Specifying a scale different from 1 will also rescale the chi-squared and deviance statistics as well as all of the standard errors of the estimated parameter values. Suggested values for the scale are given by the `Value/df` section of the output in Table 10.3.

10.5.2 The `obstats` Output

Specifying the `obstats` (for *observed statistics*) option in the `model` statement produces a collection of useful values including residuals, fitted values, and other measures. These are given in Table 10.4 for the first four towns in the lottery data.

Table 10.4. Part of the `obstats` output from the program in Table 10.2.

```
                         Lottery winners in towns near New Haven
                          Fitted information from proc genmod

Obs   winners    area     pop     Pred    Xbeta     Std  Hesswgt    Lower

  1         6     6.2    17.9   6.0282   1.7964  0.1753   6.0282  4.27507
  2        11    27.9      28   6.9120   1.9332  0.0976   6.9120  5.70806
  3         6      33    26.2   6.4764   1.8681  0.1238   6.4764  5.08033
  4         2    17.2    12.8   5.0921   1.6277  0.1351   5.0921  3.90706

   . . . . .

Obs     Upper   Resraw    Reschi     Resdev  Stresdev  Streschi    Reslik

  1   8.50052  -0.0282  -0.01152   -0.01153  -0.01278  -0.01277 -0.012778
  2   8.36995   4.0879   1.55490    1.43036   1.47996   1.60882  1.488804
  3   8.25625  -0.4764  -0.18722   -0.18959  -0.19977  -0.19728 -0.199532
  4   6.63675  -3.0921  -1.37029   -1.56400  -1.64226  -1.43885 -1.624414
   . . . . .
```

This information was obtained using the `output` statement or through the *output delivery system* (`ods`). The `output` statement is one way to capture the `obstats` information. The `ods` is more flexible and can be used to manage output from SAS procedures, including turning on and off various segments of the output as well as saving it for use in a later step. The `ods` statement in the program of Table 10.2 captures this information and creates a new data set called `fitted` that contains these statistics for use in a later step of the program.

The output in Table 10.4 includes the dependent variable (`winners`) and each of the explanatory variables (`area` and `pop`) that were included in the `model` statement of `proc genmod`. The estimated mean $\widehat{\lambda}_i$ for each town is called `Pred`. The estimated log of the mean given in (10.2) is called `Xbeta` in this output. The variable `Xbeta` is often called the *linear predictor*. The estimated standard error of `Xbeta` is listed under the `Std` column.

The `Xbeta` and `Std` can be combined to create a 95% confidence interval for each of the estimated means. The endpoints of these intervals are called `Lower` and `Upper` in this output. This confidence interval is calculated as

$$\exp(\texttt{Xbeta} \pm 1.96\,\texttt{Std}).$$

The raw residual (`Resraw`) is the difference between observed and expected:

$$\texttt{Resraw}_i = y_i - \widehat{\lambda}_i$$

where y_i is the response variable or `winners` in the ith town for the present example.

The raw residual is intuitive, but not the most appropriate way to look for outliers. This is because the mean and variance are equal in the Poisson distribution, so different raw residuals will have different variances. (Recall that an important assumption made in Section 4.4 for linear regression is the equality of the variances of all observations.) A better residual for Poisson regression standardizes each by its standard deviation. These are called `Reschi` and defined by

$$\texttt{Reschi}_i = (y_i - \widehat{\lambda}_i) \Big/ \sqrt{\widehat{\lambda}_i}\,.$$

These residuals are more comparable because they all have approximately the same variances. They are called the *chi-squared residuals* because they each represent the individual contribution to the familiar chi-squared statistic

$$\chi^2 = \sum_i (\texttt{Reschi}_i)^2 = \sum_i (y_i - \widehat{\lambda}_i)^2 \big/ \widehat{\lambda}_i\,.$$

The remaining statistics (`Resdev`, `Stresdev`, `Streschi`, `Reslik`) given in Table 10.4 are other definitions of residuals. These should all be similar in value to each other and to the `Reschi` residual. The Hessian weight (`Hesswgt`) is the estimated variance of each observation and is equal to the estimated mean.

10.5.3 The `offset` Option

Suppose we want to model the mean number of lottery winners as proportional to the town's population. In a town with twice the population, we should expect to see twice the number of lottery winners, all other things remaining equal. In vital rates, for another example, we want to talk about the rates of mortality and morbidity relative to the population at risk. How do we do this in SAS? Before we can answer that question, we need to describe what it means to be "proportional to."

If population was the only thing that mattered in describing the expected number of lottery winners λ_i in the ith town, then we would have the model

$$\lambda_i = C \times \text{Population}_i$$

where C has the same value for all towns, like a regression coefficient.

Then the log-link gives the model

$$\log(\lambda_i) = \log(C) + \log(\text{Population}_i).$$

This last equation illustrates the problem in fitting a "proportional to" model. We need to estimate C, but there is no regression coefficient to be estimated for the $\log(\text{Population}_i)$ term. More accurately, the regression coefficient in front of

$$\log(\text{Population}_i)$$

is always equal to 1.

Table 10.5. SAS program that uses an `offset` in Poisson regression.

```
title2 'Fit an offset for mean proportional to population';
data propto;                /* build a new dataset */
   set lottery;             /* start with the data of lottery dataset */
   logpop = log(pop);       /* add the new variable: log population */
run;

proc genmod data=propto;
   model winners = area  mill / dist=Poisson  obstats  offset=logpop;
run;
```

If we want to include covariates $\boldsymbol{x}$ (such as area and mill rate) in our model but still keep the mean number of lottery winners proportional to the population, then we might fit a model of the form

$$\lambda_i = C(\boldsymbol{x}) \times \text{Population}_i$$

so that

$$\log(\lambda_i) = \log\{C(\boldsymbol{x})\} + \log(\text{Population}_i)\,.$$

Again we see that the term $\log(\text{Population}_i)$ is not associated with an estimated regression coefficient.

In this last model, in order to include the effects of area and mill rate in our model, it is convenient to write

$$\log\{C(\boldsymbol{x})\} = \beta_0 + \beta_1\,\texttt{area} + \beta_2\,\texttt{mill}$$

for regression coefficients β_0, β_1, β_2 that can be estimated using the Poisson regression methods we have already described.

Together these give us a model

$$\log(\lambda_i) = \log(\text{Population}_i) + \beta_0 + \beta_1\,\texttt{area} + \beta_2\,\texttt{mill} \qquad (10.3)$$

that adjusts for the effects of the covariates area and mill rate but also estimates the mean number of lottery winners proportional to the population size.

We have just illustrated the models that we need to fit in order to produce estimates based on a "proportional to" model. In these cases we have to fit a model that looks like Poisson regression, but the log(Population) term in model (10.3) doesn't have a regression coefficient. Or, more correctly, it has a regression coefficient that is identically 1. Such a term can be added to the model using the `offset` in SAS `genmod` procedure.

An example of the use of an `offset` is given in the program in Table 10.5. The `data` step creates a new data set called `propto` based on the earlier `lottery` data using a `set` statement. No data has to be read. Instead, the older dataset is used as the basis of a new dataset. This new dataset creates a new variable called `logpop` that is defined as the log (base e) of the population variable.

The `model` statement in `proc genmod` lists the dependent variable (`winners`), the explanatory variables (`area, mill`), specifies a Poisson distribution (`dist= Poisson`), requests the observational statistics (`obstats`), and specifies that the logarithm of the population is the offset variable. The regression coefficient associated with the offset variable is identically 1, so there is no coefficient to estimate in this model. Similarly, SAS does not perform a test of statistical significance for this variable. For more information on the `offset`, see Exercise 10.3.

10.6 Exercises

10.1 In a Poisson distribution with a mean of 1, find the probability of 2 or fewer events. In a binomial experiment with $N = 4$ and $p = 1/4$, what is the probability of 2 or fewer events? In a binomial experiment with $N = 8$ and $p = 1/8$, what is the probability of 2 or fewer events? What is the mean for both of these binomial experiments? What are the variances? Do the variances in these two binomial models become closer to the means as N gets larger and p becomes smaller? Do the probabilities of 2 or fewer events get closer to the Poisson approximation?

10.2 In an example described as part of the newspaper article in Section 10.6.3 on airlines bumping passengers from overbooked flights, a specific flight is described. The airline routinely reserves up to 194 seats for this flight on an airplane that has only 185 physical seats. From experience the airline expects 5% of those passengers to fail to show up at the time of the flight. Is the Poisson distribution an appropriate model for this data? Explain why or why not. Estimate the Poisson parameter λ for the number of "no-shows" out of 194 potential passengers on this flight. How many reservations can the airline accept for this flight and still remain 99% confident that there will be no need to bump any passengers?

10.3 In the example program in Table 10.5, we used log population as an offset where the population is measured as thousands of persons. What happens if we measure population in counts of individual people? Does it matter which definition we use? Run the program in Table 10.5 using both definitions and note the differences in the output. Can you explain the differences in the outputs?

10.6.1 Coronary Bypass Mortality, Revisited

Reexamine the mortality data in Section 5.7.3 using Poisson regression. Specifically, consider the number of in-hospital deaths as a Poisson-distributed outcome. Why is this a reasonable assumption? Do the residuals of the fitted regression model

Table 10.6. Number of cases of mental illness in Massachusetts by county in 1854.

County	Cases	Distance to mental health center	Population in 1000s	Population density	Percent cared for at home
Berkshire	119	97	26.656	56	77
Franklin	84	62	22.260	45	81
Hampshire	94	54	23.312	72	75
Hampden	105	52	18.9	94	69
Worcester	351	20	82.836	98	64
Middlesex	357	14	66.759	231	47
Essex	377	10	95.004	3252	47
Suffolk	458	4	123.202	3042	6
Norfolk	241	14	62.901	235	49
Bristol	158	14	29.704	151	60
Plymouth	139	16	32.526	91	68
Barnstable	78	44	16.692	93	76
Nantucket	12	77	1.740	179	25
Dukes	19	52	7.524	46	79

Source: http://lib.stat.cmu.edu/DASL/Datafiles/lunaticsdat.html.

correspond to the indications of higher and lower death rates given by the last column of Table 5.9?

10.6.2 Cases of Mental Illness

A historical survey of cases of mental illness (people who were then called "lunatics") in Massachusetts in the 1850s is presented in Table 10.6. For each of the 14 counties, we have the number of lunatics, the distance to the nearest mental health center, the population (in thousands), the population density (per square mile), and the percent of lunatics cared for at home.

The counties have very different characteristics: Suffolk County includes Boston; Duke County (Martha's Vineyard) and Nantucket are islands; and Berkshire County is farthest from Boston, in the western part of the state. The great differences in population argue for using the logarithm of population rather than the original population values.

Show that the number of cases varies with population, or log population, as we would expect. Why is the population density such a good explanatory variable in this dataset? Does the distance to a mental health center explain the number of cases, or does it explain the number of diagnosed cases? In other words, is there evidence of undiagnosed or missing cases? Does the reciprocal distance provide a better interpretation or offer better explanatory value? In a separate analysis using regression methods, does the rate of home treatment vary with population density or distance to a center? Why is this the case?

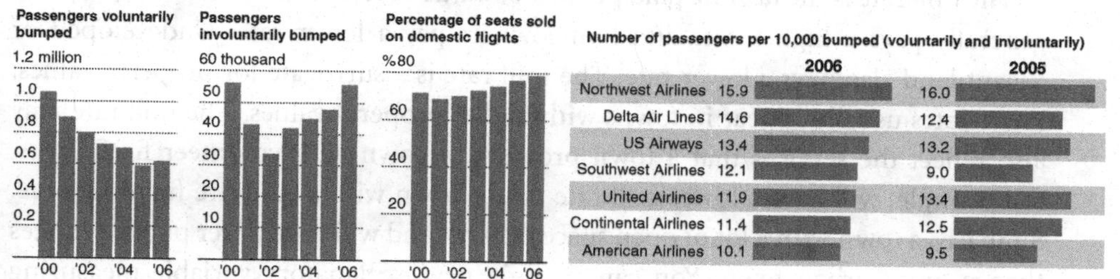
Bumping on the Rise
The number of domestic airline passengers voluntarily bumped – those who agree to take a flight voucher or other inducement to miss their original flight because it was overbooked – has declined since 2000. But those bumped involuntarily last year were at the highest level since 2000, in part because passengers know that all flights are so crowded these days that the "next available flight" can involve a much longer wait.
Passengers voluntarily bumped
1.2 million
1.0
0.8
0.6
0.4
0.2
'00 '02 '04 '06
Passengers involuntarily bumped
60 thousand
50
40
30
20
10
'00 '02 '04 '06
Percentage of seats sold on domestic flights
%80
60
40
20
'00 '02 '04 '06
Number of passengers per 10,000 bumped (voluntarily and involuntarily)
2006
2005
Northwest Airlines 15.9 16.0
Delta Air Lines 14.6 12.4
US Airways 13.4 13.2
Southwest Airlines 12.1 9.0
United Airlines 11.9 13.4
Continental Airlines 11.4 12.5
American Airlines 10.1 9.5

Figure 10.3 Statistics on airline bumping of passengers. *Source: New York Times*, May 30, 2007, p. C4.

10.6.3 Statistics in the News: Airlines Bump Passengers

An article about airline "bumping" included the graphic in Figure 10.3.[2] Running an airline is an expensive business, and unsold seats cut into profits. Airlines have long known that each flight will have a small number of passengers with reservations who do not show up. To decrease the chances of lost revenue, the airlines will usually sell more seats than exist. If too many passengers show up, the airlines will need to bump passengers to a later flight, first asking for volunteers by offering successively higher incentives (such as cash or vouchers for future flights and hotels) and finally involuntary measures. This, of course, creates a lot of bad feelings and publicity. Anxious passengers have taken to making several reservations under fictitious names (Mickey Mouse is reported to be a popular name) in order to ensure that the real passengers are unlikely to be bumped.

Why do you think that a Poisson distribution would be appropriate to model the number of "no-shows" on a flight? What assumptions do you consider? Each airline has its own formula, and the rates of bumping vary by as much as 50% according to Figure 10.3. What information would you need to estimate the number of "no-shows" on future flights? Would flights with a large percent of business travelers have a different rate than flights to vacation destinations? Would the rate for large planes to big cities differ from smaller regional flights with fewer seats? Explain why or why not you think this may be the case.

Compare the graphics of the number of passengers who were voluntarily bumped with those who were involuntarily bumped. One rate is decreasing and the other is increasing in recent years. Comment on the use of two different scales. One scale is 20 times larger than the other.

10.6.4 Lottery Winners

Table 10.1 lists the number of lottery winners in several towns near New Haven. The columns in this table are town name; the number of lottery winners (the response

[2] Available online at http://www.nytimes.com/2007/05/30/business/30bump.html.

or Y variable); the town's area in square miles; mill rate; and the number of library books per student.

The mill rate is the tax rate paid per $1,000 value of real estate. Industrial property generally pays a higher rate and homeowners pay a lower rate. Undeveloped or vacant land also pays a lower rate. The mill rate is a surrogate for property values: lower rates usually appear in towns with higher property values. The mill rate may also reflect the services that a town provides. A town with volunteer firefighters, for example, will have a lower mill rate than a town with a paid fire fighting force. Similarly, a town with a lot of open space or farmland will have fewer public services than a more urban town. You can create a new explanatory variable measuring population density (population divided by area). Density is a measure of urban or rural character of a town.

Use your final model to estimate the number of lottery winners expected in the city of New Haven with a population of 126,000; an area of 21.1 square miles; and a mill rate of 37.0. What about the town of Durham with 6,000 people; 23.3 square miles; and a mill rate of 26.4? Are these appropriate uses of your model? Explain.

Are some towns luckier than others? Is the number of winners proportional to the population? Should it be? What can you say about the intercept, on a log scale? What other covariate values might be useful to you? Is the Poisson distribution appropriate for this example? Why?

10.6.5 Species on the Galápagos Islands

Follow Charles Darwin to the Galápagos Islands! These islands are hundreds of miles from the nearest continent, and their flora and fauna are the study of many scientific studies. The summary of one such survey is given in Table 10.7. The data variables are island name; the number of species (the Y variable); area in square kilometers; distance to nearest neighboring island; distance to Santa Cruz (the second largest island, near the center of the archipelago); and the number of species on the nearest neighboring island.

Use the Poisson distribution to model the number of species on each of these islands. Larger islands support a larger diversity of life forms. Isabela is so much larger than all of the other islands that it exerts a high amount of leverage. You might want to create an indicator for Isabela. Create new variables such as products (interactions) and ratios of variables that you can interpret. Are there outliers in the data? Are small islands similar to each other or very different from each other? What about the larger islands?

Is the Poisson model appropriate for this data? You can sometimes use the Poisson distribution for settings where there is no underlying binomial model to be approximated: that is, where there is no N or p. Another unusual use of the Poisson model without an underlying binomial model appears in Exercise 10.6.6.

Is there an evolutionary advantage to species on an island with a larger diversity of lifeforms? We might see this if the islands with large estimated numbers of species

Table 10.7. Diversity of Species on Each of the Galápagos Islands.

Island	Species observed	Area in km^2	Distance (km) To nearest neighbor	Distance (km) To Santa Cruz	Species on adjacent island
Baltra	58	25.09	.6	.6	44
Bartolomé	31	1.24	.6	26.3	237
Caldwell	3	.21	2.8	58.7	5
Champion	25	.10	1.9	47.4	2
Coamaño	2	.05	1.9	1.9	444
Daphne Major	18	.34	8.0	8.0	44
Daphne Minor	24	.08	6.0	12.0	18
Darwin	10	2.33	34.1	290.2	21
Eden	8	.03	.4	.4	108
Enderby	2	.18	2.6	50.2	25
Española	97	58.27	1.1	88.3	58
Fernandina	93	634.49	4.3	95.3	347
Gardner A	58	.57	1.1	93.1	97
Gardner B	5	.78	4.6	62.2	3
Genovesa	40	17.35	47.4	92.2	51
Isabela	347	4669.32	.7	28.1	91
Marchena	51	129.49	29.1	85.9	104
Onslow	2	.01	3.3	45.9	25
Pinta	104	59.56	29.1	119.6	51
Pinzón	108	17.95	10.7	10.7	8
Las Plazas	12	.23	.5	.6	58
Rábida	70	4.89	4.4	24.4	237
San Cristóbal	280	551.62	45.2	66.6	58
San Salvador	237	572.33	.2	19.8	70
Santa Cruz	444	903.82	.6	.0	8
Santa Fé	62	24.08	16.5	16.5	444
Santa María	285	170.92	2.6	49.2	25
Seymour	44	1.84	.6	9.6	58
Tortuga	16	1.24	6.8	50.9	108
Wolf	21	2.85	34.1	254.7	10

Source: Johnson and Raven (1973), and Andrews and Herzberg (1985, pp. 291–3).

appear to have too many species, and similarly, if those with small estimated numbers would tend to have fewer than expected. The result would be that both the upper and lower tails of the Poisson distribution extend out further than we would expect. Does this help explain some of the outliers in the data? Are there other explanations for these outliers? Should all species be treated equally, for example?

Table 10.8. Pro Bowl appearances by running backs.

		Career	
Name	Active?	Yards	Pro Bowls
Emmit Smith		18,355	8
Walter Payton		16,726	9
Barry Sanders		15,269	10
Curtis Martin		14,101	5
Jerome Bettis		13,662	6
Eric Dickerson		13,259	5
Tony Dorsett		12,739	4
Jim Brown		12,312	9
Marshall Faulk		12,279	7
Marcus Allen		12,243	6
Franco Harris		12,120	8
Thurman Harris		12,074	5
John Riggins		11,352	1
Corey Dillon		11,241	4
O. J. Simpson		11,236	5
Edgerrin James	Y	10,988	3
Ricky Watters		10,643	5
Tiki Barber		10,449	3
Eddie George		10,441	4
Ottis Anderson		10,273	2
Fred Taylor	Y	9,933	0
LaDainian Tomlinson	Y	9,793	4
Warrick Dunn	Y	9,753	3
Earl Campbell	Y	9,407	5
Shaun Alexander	Y	9,173	3

Reported by the *New York Times*, November 2, 2007.

10.6.6 Statistics in the News: Pro Bowl Appearances

Football is a game of strength and speed. Running with the ball is appropriately called *rushing*, and the total career distances covered by the most accomplished players at the time of the source publication[3] are listed in Table 10.8. Most of the players listed had retired, and the men whose names are listed as active were still playing. The article that accompanied this table concentrated on Fred Taylor, who was close to having rushed 10,000 career yards but had not yet appeared in a Pro Bowl.

The Pro Bowl is played at the end of the regular season by players who are judged to be the best individual players, regardless of their regular team. The game itself is

[3] Available online at http://www.nytimes.com/2007/11/02/sports/football/02taylor.html.

not taken very seriously, because these are players who have never practiced together. There is a lot of friendly comradeship, and the play is not competitive. Instead, it is considered a great honor to be chosen to play. Table 10.8 lists the players with the top 25 rushing records and includes the number of Pro Bowl appearances of each.

Use Poisson regression to show that larger numbers of rushing yards are associated with a larger number of career Pro Bowl appearances. Create an indicator variable for active versus retired status and include this in your model. Is there a significant interaction between this indicator and total rushing yards? How do you interpret this finding? Does Fred Taylor appear to be an outlier, never having been chosen to play in the Pro Bowl? Compare his residual with that of John Riggins, for example, who had only one Pro Bowl appearance. Are there other outliers in these data worth noting? Can you identify players whose records were overrated, resulting in too many Pro Bowl appearances?

A small number of players appear to have much stronger rushing records than the rest. Try transforming the rushing yards variable by log or square root to remove the influence these players have on the fitted model. Does this model result in a better fit?

Say something about the overall fit of the model. Does this appear to be a valid use of the Poisson model? Can you justify the use of the model in this case? Is the use of the Poisson model any less valid than its use in the species data of Exercise 10.6.5?

10.6.7 Cancer Rates in Japan

Vital rates are important for many reasons and are collected by government agencies. We saw an example of this in Section 3.5.5. This exercise represents another example of official mortality data. The data of Table 10.9 summarizes the number of men in Japan who died of cancer of the testis in 1946–70 by 5-year intervals. The populations are given in thousands. The rows are the ages given in 5-year groups. Missing data are indicated by asterisks; and these should be omitted in any examination of these data.

A SAS program that reads and reformats these data appears in Table 10.10. The ages are converted to categories with values 1, 2, ..., 18, and the five time periods are similarly converted. The `class` statement in `proc genmod` allows us to list all ages and periods as a single entry in the `model` statement. The `array` statement allows us to refer to the five population and death rates on each line of input either as `p1` through `p5` or as `p(i)` where `i` ranges between 1 and 5. See Exercise 6.6.8 for another example of the `array` statement.

Is the Poisson distribution appropriate for this data? Why? Fit a model with effects for years and ages. Look at the residuals. Are there any trends over the years? Notice that the risk of cancer increases after age 40 but then appears to decrease after age 80. Can you explain this decreased rate among the oldest men? Read about the `offset` option in Section 10.5.3 if you want to fit a model in which cancer rates are proportional to the population.

Table 10.9. Deaths in Japan due to cancer of the testis by age, year, and population (in thousands). The values indicated by '*' are missing.

	1947–49		1951–55		1956–60		1961–65		1966–70	
Age	Pop.	Deaths	Pop.	Deaths	Pop.	Deaths	Pop.	Deaths	Pop.	Deaths
0	15501	17	26914	51	21027	65	20246	69	21596	74
5	14236	*	25380	6	26613	7	20885	8	20051	7
10	13270	*	23492	3	25324	3	26540	7	20718	11
15	12658	2	21881	6	23211	15	24931	25	26182	39
20	10696	5	20402	27	21263	39	22228	56	24033	83
25	7563	5	17242	40	19994	58	20606	97	21805	125
30	7074	7	12609	18	17128	54	19864	77	20750	129
35	7038	10	11712	13	12476	36	17001	70	19890	101
40	6418	9	11478	26	11450	32	12275	29	16794	67
45	5981	7	10274	16	11157	26	11147	34	11962	37
50	4944	7	9325	16	9828	27	10705	27	10741	29
55	3994	7	7562	17	8718	19	9206	32	10086	39
60	3098	6	5902	13	6796	21	7869	21	8399	31
65	2317	4	4244	12	4911	26	5728	29	6715	34
70	1513	7	2845	17	3197	22	3737	25	4448	33
75	688	5	1587	9	1812	10	2061	25	2482	31
80	264	2	583	6	787	6	904	14	1068	9
85	73	2	179	2	246	3	335	3	419	3

Public domain: *Journal of the National Cancer Institute*, Oxford University Press. See also Lee *et al.* (1973), Andrews and Herzberg (1985, pp. 233–5).

A *cohort* is the same group of men appearing several times in this table. Five years later, the men from one age/year group are 5 years older and will appear again in the next age/year group. The cohort runs diagonally from upper left to lower right. The SAS program creates a cohort number in the line

```
cohort=age-i;
```

where `i` is the period number.

Try to fit a model that includes the three separate effects of age, period, and cohort. What happens? Can you explain the problem that occurs? Reread the discussion of multicolinearity in Section 6.1 and describe the difficulty with the *age, period, cohort model.*

10.6.8 Tourette's Syndrome

In an experiment conducted at the Yale Child Study Center, van Wattum *et al.* (2000) studied the effects of naloxone on patients diagnosed with Tourette's syndrome. Patients with Tourette's syndrome suffer from frequent involuntary twitches (motor)

Table 10.10. SAS program to read and format the Japanese cancer data.

```
title1 'Death rates for testicular cancer in Japan';
data cancer;
   array p(5) p1-p5;
   array d(5) d1-d5;
   input age  p1 d1  p2 d2  p3 d3  p4 d4  p5 d5;
   age=1+age/5;   /* make age categories 1,..,18 */
   do i=1 to 5;
      keep pop death age period cohort;
      cohort=age-i;
      period=i;
      pop=p(i);
      death=d(i);
      output; /* one input line equals five on output */
   end;
   datalines;
 0  15501  17  26914  51  21027  65  20246  69  21596   74
 5  14236   .  25380   6  26613   7  20885   8  20051    7
10  13270   .  23492   3  25324   3  26540   7  20718   11
15  12658   2  21881   6  23211  15  24931  25  26182   39

                         . . .

75    688   5   1587   9   1812  10   2061  25   2482   31
80    264   2    583   6    787   6    904  14   1068    9
85     73   2    179   2    246   3    335   3    419    3
run;

proc print;   /* examine the reformatted data */
run;

proc genmod;
   class age period cohort;
   model death = pop age period / dist=Poisson obstats;
run;
quit;
```

or verbal (phonic) outbursts. Naloxone is usually administered to counteract the effects of narcotic drug overdoses. It was thought that naloxone inhibits certain receptors in the brain and perhaps that small amounts could reduce the symptoms of Tourette's.

Fourteen patients were each given one of three different doses of naloxone, and their behaviors were recorded during three 1-hour periods of observation. Motor

Table 10.11. Motor and phonic tics in Tourette's patients treated with naloxone during three 1-hour time periods.

Patient number	Naloxone dose (mcg)	Period I		Period II		Period III	
		Motor	Phonic	Motor	Phonic	Motor	Phonic
1	300	90	45	86	51	106	57
2	30	75	0	243	0	152	0
3	30	58	0	9	0	22	0
4	30	13	0	6	0	12	0
5	30	13	0	16	0	29	0
6	300	150	0	161	0	121	0
7	30	49	1	16	0	29	1
8	30	27	0	28	0	24	0
9	0	25	7	9	0	4	4
10	0	13	2	14	17	14	18
11	300	51	0	42	0	43	0
12	300	35	16	28	33	49	20
13	300	19	9	8	15	12	30
14	30	8	6	18	13	8	22

Source: van Wattum *et al.* (2000).

and phonic tics were counted separately for each of the three time periods. The data for the patients, naloxone dose, and tics for each of the three time periods is given in Table 10.11.

It is not clear whether we should be separately modeling the motor and phonic tics. Perhaps the sum of these two measures is more appropriate. As with the species example in Section 10.6.5, there is no underlying binomial experiment that we can refer to, so there are no N or p parameters. Instead, we might think of a subject's brain sending and receiving a great many signals, and that a small fraction of these are either misinterpreted or sent incorrectly.

The three separate periods were part of the experiment to see if the number of tics would change as the subject became acclimatized to the investigators and the settings. The investigators thought that a subject in unfamiliar surroundings would be more self-conscious and the number of tics would decrease. Similarly, after the subjects relaxed on their second or third visits, perhaps their tics might resume. Do you see evidence of a "period effect" in the numbers of either the motor or verbal tics? How can you justify modeling the log mean for this data?

Naloxone is used for other medical treatments, so the appropriate dose in this setting was not obvious to the investigators. Examine the two separate doses and compare the tic rates with those of the control. Is there any difference in these rates? Include a period effect in your model. Is the naloxone effect larger or smaller than the period effect?

11 Survival Analysis

Survival data, despite its name, is concerned with the time to an event, not just the death of the subject. The event could be a child learning how to tie her shoes, for example, and the survival time would be the age at which she masters this task. Survival data is different from any of the topics we have described so far, because at the time of the analysis not all of the subjects' data has been completely observed for the event of interest. This is called *censoring*. We describe a number of examples of time to event data and different types of censoring in this chapter. Survival curves graphically depict the time-to-event data for a data sample, much as a histogram does in elementary statistics. There are some simple statistical comparisons we can make of survival curves. In Chapter 12 we describe a regression model that is useful for modeling survival curves with several explanatory variables in a regression setting.

11.1 Censoring

Survival analysis is a collection of statistical methods to model the time it takes for an individual to achieve a specified event. The event could be death, as the name implies, or something less dramatic, such as how long it takes to complete a master's degree, or how long it takes a legislature to pass a bill into law. We provide a number of other examples in this section.

The study of survival data stands apart from other statistical topics because of *censoring*. Specifically, the exact time of the event for every individual under study may not be available to us at the time of the analysis. There are different types of censoring, as the following examples illustrate.

It is often useful to think of the time line traveling from left to right. The most common type of censoring is called *right censoring*: the left end point, the start of the time line, is known, but the right end point may not have yet occurred at the time we examine the data. The amount of time that students spend in a degree program is one example. We know the date when they were admitted to the degree program. Some students will breeze through and complete all of their requirements early. Others take longer. Some will either drop out or continue working at a slower pace. When it comes time to study the data on time to degree completion, many will (we hope) already have graduated, but there will also be some who have not yet completed their degrees. We can't tell if and when they ever will. Those who have not yet completed the program at the time of the examination of their data are said to be right censored: we know when they began, but the graduation event may not yet have occurred.

> In right censoring, we know the starting time, but the end point may not yet have been reached by all subjects.

The study of HIV involves another type of censoring. Sometimes we can trace a patient's initial infection to a single blood transfusion or sexual contact. In this case we know the start of the infection. Sometimes we do not. For some we may only know that the infection occurred before some date when the infection was first detected. In this case, the left end point of disease progression time line is said to be *left censored* because we do not know the starting date, we know only that it occurred before the date of the HIV diagnosis.

Perhaps we can trace the patient's initial HIV infection to one of a series of transfusions or sexual contacts that occurred over a period of time. In this case we might say that the left end point is *interval censored* because it could have occurred at any point within that time interval.

The time of progression from HIV infection to AIDS often involves another interval censoring. Some AIDS-defining events can only be determined by a blood test, such as when the patient's count of CD4+ cells falls below the threshold value of 200. The CD4+ counts are not monitored continuously, and these values are known only at discrete testing times. If one lab value is above the threshold and the subsequent value is below 200, then we do not know exactly when the threshold was reached. The threshold of 200 could have been passed at any time in between the two adjacent lab dates. In other words, in this examination of the progression from HIV infection to AIDS, both the starting and ending time points may be interval censored.

Here is another example that combines different types of censoring. Let us consider the age at which children learn to tie their shoes. A psychologist decides to sit in at a day-care facility for a period of six months to watch the children. During the six-month observation period, some children will learn to tie their shoes, and their exact ages of acquiring the skill will then be known. Some children will already know how to tie their shoes when the psychologist arrives, and their ages will be censored to the left. Similarly, some children will still not have this skill when the psychologist's observation period ends, and these children will be right censored.

These are examples of the most common types of censoring. An important assumption we make about censoring is that it is unrelated to the actual, unobserved event time. That is,

> We assume that whether or not a subject is censored is independent of the actual time to the event.

We need to get at the root cause of censoring in the first place. In a clinical trial of a new medical treatment, suppose patients were censored because they dropped out and their event times were not recorded. The data would be more difficult to analyze if those patients most likely to drop out were also the ones who were doing very well (or perhaps very poorly). In either of these cases, we would say that the study has *informative censoring*. That is, having a censored observation tells us something about the unobserved outcome. Instead, in the analysis of survival data, we assume that censoring is noninformative and contains no useful information concerning the event times. Noninformative censoring might occur if the reason for observations being censored had nothing to do with the actual event time. For example, censored patients might have moved to another city, or perhaps the statisticians had to meet a deadline and the patients still under study were censored at the time of the data analysis.

Although we have described most different types of censoring, but by far the most common is right censoring with a known (left), starting end point. Right-censored data has received the largest amount of statistical theoretical development and also has the largest amount of software available to analyze the data. Before we talk about software, we need to describe the survival curve.

11.2 The Survival Curve and Its Estimate

The *survival curve* estimates the proportion of subjects who have already experienced their event by a given time. Just as we would draw a histogram to graphically examine a new set of data, the plotting of a survival curve is usually the first step we take when we examine right-censored survival data. A survival curve begins at 1 (or 100%) at time zero and continues to drop in a series of steps. A survival curve can be flat in places, but it can never rise. The estimate of the survival curve is sometimes called the *product limit* or *Kaplan-Meier curve* and is attributed to E. L. Kaplan and Paul Meier, who published this method in 1958.

A typical example of a pair of survival curves is given in Figure 11.1. The data given in Table 11.1 presents the remission times for patients with acute myelogenous leukemia (AML). The outcome is not survival, but the length of time (in weeks) before their symptoms return. Notice, that we are not measuring time to death of these patients, but rather the time it takes for their leukemia symptoms to return

Table 11.1. Length of remission time, in weeks, for AML patients who were either on maintained treatment or not. Every patient has an indicator of whether their observed time was censored and they were still in remission (0), or whether they had relapsed and the time of their disease recurrence was known (1).

Treatment maintained											
9	1	13	1	13	0	18	1	23	1	28	0
31	1	34	1	45	0	48	1	161	0		
Treatment not maintained											
5	1	5	1	8	1	8	1	12	1	16	0
23	1	27	1	30	1	33	1	43	1	45	1

Source: Embury *et al.* (1977).

following treatment. The patients received one of two different treatments for their AML: either maintenance of their treatment or no additional treatments.

Initially, at time zero, all patients are in remission. As time progresses, most of these patients relapse. This figure estimates the proportion of patients in remission at each time point. The upper curve is for the treatment-maintained group of patients, so we can conclude that these patients will generally have longer remission times. At any time point, we see that a greater proportion treatment-maintained patients remain relapse-free. In Section 11.3 we examine these data again and perform tests of statistical significance comparing the two curves. For the moment, we can see that treatment maintenance is better and results in longer remission times. At

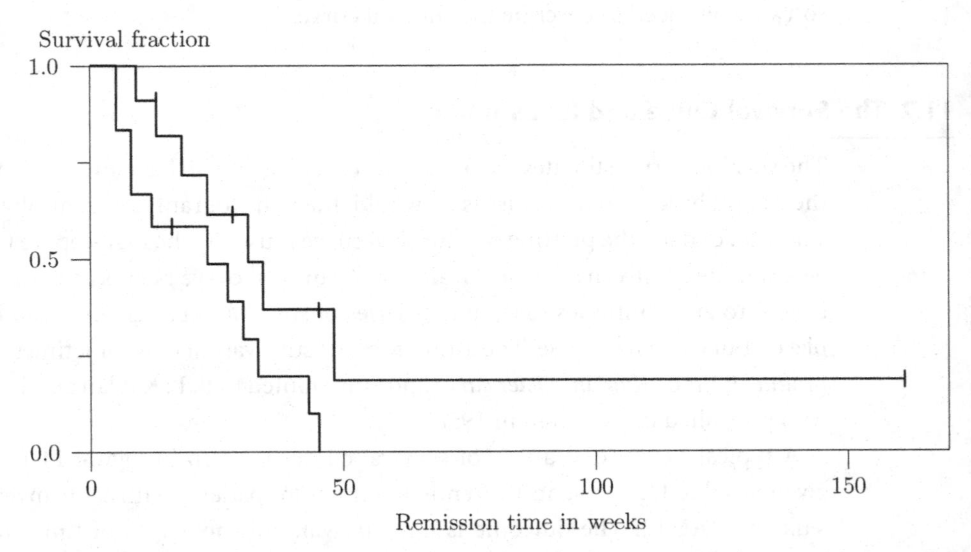

Figure 11.1 Kaplan-Meier survival curves for the AML data in Table 11.1. The upper line is for the treatment-maintained group.

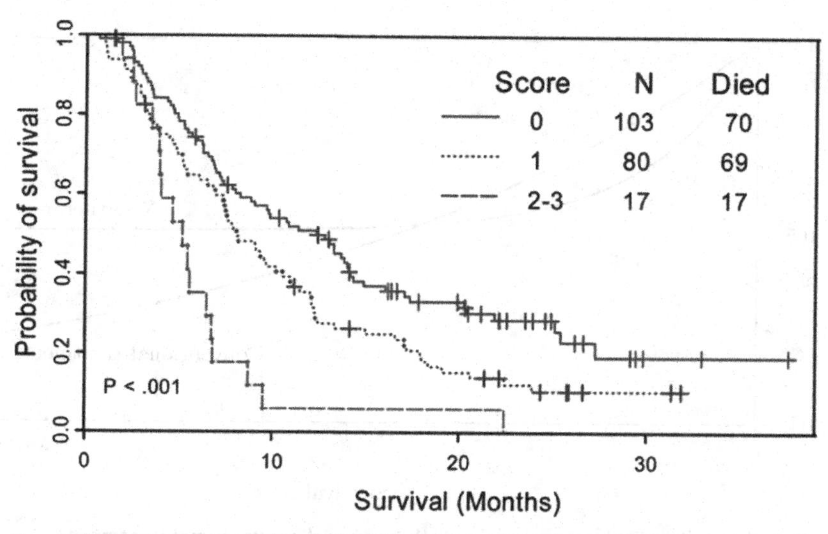

Figure 11.2 Survival of three groups of cancer patients. *Source:* Wheler *et al.* (2009).

any remission time, shortly after the start of this study, there are always a greater proportion of treatment maintained patients.

There are two additional features worth mentioning in Figure 11.1. One of these is the small vertical marks. These indicate the locations of the censored observations. This is an optional feature and is not always performed in practice. The inclusion of these small marks allows the reader to see the distribution of censored observations. If there are many censored observations and these occur very early in the study, this shows inadequate follow-up time. Similarly, if there are many more censored observations in one treatment group, this indicates that censoring may not be independent of outcome, a key assumption we stated in the previous section. In the present study, neither of these appears to be a problem.

A second feature of survival curves is the tendency for our eyes to concentrate on the long upper tail extending to the right of this figure. The nonmaintained group has a survival curve that drops to zero, but the maintained group does not. Does this indicate a long-term cure? No, because the long tail to the right is only indicative that the longest remission time was censored. That is, the long tail to the right is based on only one observation. If the longest observation is censored, then the survival curve does not go all the way to zero. The message from this remark is that we need to pay more attention to the portion of the survival curve in the upper left corner where most of the data is concentrated. As the curve extends to the right, there will be fewer observations.

Figure 11.2 presents a published set of survival curves for three groups of cancer patients enrolled in a Phase I clinical trial. A Phase I trial studies a new drug in its first use in humans. Because of the experimental nature of such studies, these trials typically enroll patients who have failed other conventional treatments. Indeed, we see in Figure 11.2 that few of these patients survived two years.

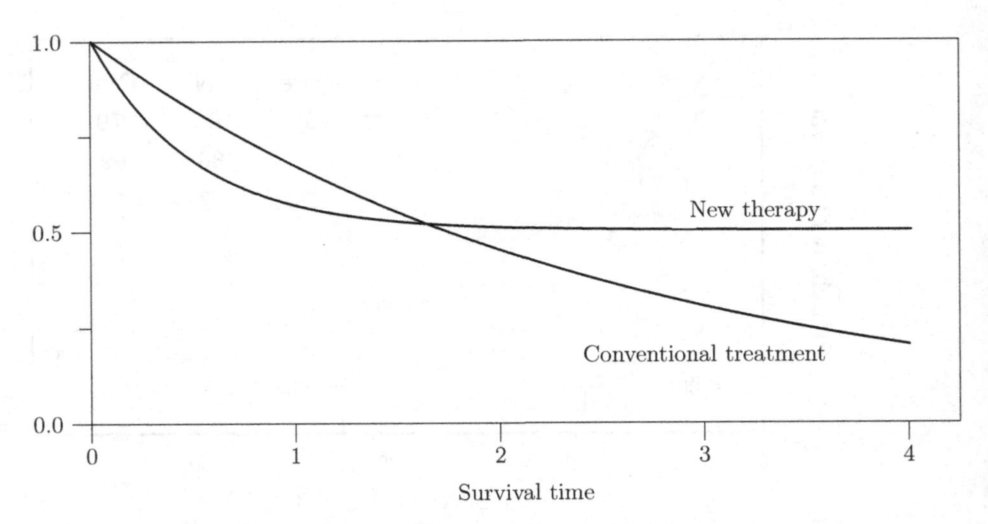

Figure 11.3 Hypothetical survival curves for a new therapy and conventional treatment.

The authors of the article presenting these data divided their patients into different groups by assigning a score based on their disease severity. We can clearly see that those patients who had lower scores survived longer. Most of the censoring occurred in the longest surviving group. The figure contains details on how many patients were in each of the three groups and how many died. The p-value in this figure tests the null hypothesis that the patients were sampled from populations with identical survival characteristics. In Section 11.3 we describe how this statistical test was performed.

Consider next a hypothetical situation in which a new therapy is being compared to a conventional treatment with survival times plotted in Figure 11.3. The new method (such as a heart transplant) has considerable risk, and there is a high rate of mortality associated with it. But once patients survive the initial stress, they appear to do much better than those receiving the conventional therapy. Which procedure would you prefer? This figure presents a difficult situation in which it is not at all clear which is the better group to be in. Compare Figure 11.2 with Figure 11.3. Sometimes survival curves may be different, but when they cross as in Figure 11.3, neither population has a higher survival fraction at all times. A test of statistical significance for comparing survival curves is described in the following section, but this method only tests whether curves are different.

Let us end this section with a description of the method of Kaplan and Meier to illustrate exactly how to construct a survival curve with censored data. Let us consider a small dataset with the following survival times observed for eight subjects:

$$1 \quad 2.5+ \quad 3 \quad 3 \quad 3+ \quad 4 \quad 4.5+ \quad 6$$

where a plus + sign indicates a right-censored value.

Table 11.2. Construction of the Kaplan-Meier estimate of the survival curve.

	Event times							
	1	2.5+	3	3	3+	4	4.5+	6
Number at risk	8	—	6		—	3	—	1
Number of events	1	—	2		—	1	—	1
Est'd. Pr[event]	1/8	—	1/3		—	1/3	—	1
Est'd. Pr[no event]	7/8	—	2/3		—	2/3	—	0
K-M estimate	7/8	—	7/8 × 2/3 =7/12		—	7/8 × 2/3 × 2/3 =7/18	—	0

Table 11.2 shows how to construct a Kaplan-Meier estimate of the survival curve for these data. The number of subjects at risk at any specified time is the number of individuals who are known to have their event times at this time or later. So, at time 1, all eight subjects were considered to be at risk for their events. At time 2.5, there was a censored observation. Censored observations are part of the risk set and denominator, but are not event times, so notice that no computation is done at this time value. At time 3 there were six individuals at risk. It is not known whether the "2.5+" person had his or her event at time 3 or later, so this subject is not considered to be at risk at time 3.

The two individuals with events at time 3 are combined. The "number of events" entry in this table shows these as two events at a single time. All other survival times indicate a single event. The censored 3+ time is considered to have occurred after the two events that occurred at time 3.

The estimated probability of an event is

$$\text{Pr[event]} = \frac{\text{Number of events}}{\text{Number at risk}}$$

at every event time. This probability is zero where there are no events, such as at censored time.

Similarly, the probability of no event is

$$\text{Pr[no event]} = 1 - \text{Pr[event]}.$$

Finally, the probability of surviving up to any given time is the product of all the survival probabilities up to this point. This is the product-limit (Kaplan-Meier) estimate of the survival curve. The actual survival curve is plotted in Figure 11.4.

The key point to remember about plotting survival curves is that the curve drops at event times but is flat at censored times and other nonevent times. Whether the longest survival time is censored determines whether the survival curve falls to zero or not. This point was also made in the discussion of Figure 11.1. We next show how to statistically compare two survival curves in SAS.

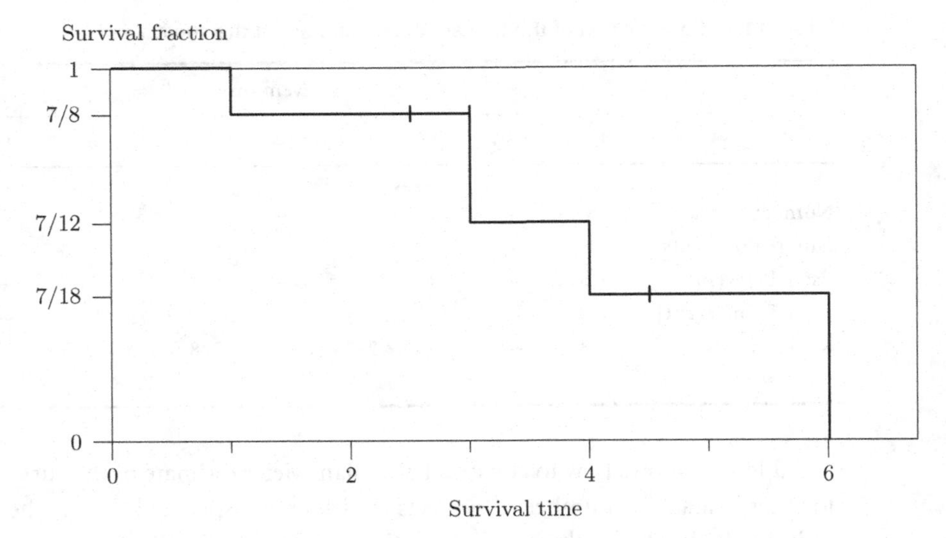

Figure 11.4 The Kaplan-Meier survival curve for the example data in Table 11.2.

11.3 The Log-Rank Test and SAS Program

The log-rank test is one of the oldest and most popular methods for comparing two survival curves. The approach is nonparametric. The null hypothesis is that groups of subjects are sampled from the same population. The alternative hypothesis is that the population survival curves are different. Let us illustrate the SAS program comparing the two groups in the AML data given in Table 11.1.

Table 11.3 contains a program to run `proc lifetest` in SAS. In this program, `surv` is the survival time, `cens` is the censoring variable, and 0 is the indicator of censored observations. Observations with `cens`=1 indicate an event was observed by the time these data were recorded. The `group` variable indicates which group (control or continued treatment) the patients belong to. The program computes a p-value comparing the two different groups. The `plots=(s)` option in the program produces the product-limit or Kaplan-Meier estimate of the survival curve we saw in Figure 11.1.

The log-rank test is a comparison of the observed and expected counts in a series of 2×2 tables. Every time an event occurs in either of the two patient groups, we construct a 2×2 table. So for example, at 23 weeks there was one event in both groups. At this time there were also six patients at risk in the treatment-maintained group and seven patients at risk in the nonmaintained group.

We summarize this information in a 2×2 table:

	Treatment maintained	Nonmaintained control
Events	1	1
No events	5	6
Patients at risk	6	7

Table 11.3. SAS program to compare remission times in the AML data.

```
data;
    input surv cens group;
    datalines;
      5 1 0
      5 1 0
      . . .
     45 1 0
      9 1 1
     13 1 1
     13 0 1
      . . .
    161 0 1
run;
proc print;    /* We are in this habit by now */
run;
proc lifetest plots =(s); /* plots=(s) draws the survival curve */
   time surv * cens(0);
   strata group; /* Compare the survival curves of two groups */
run;
```

We can also calculate the expected counts in this table just as we do when we compute the Pearson chi-squared test. Under the null hypothesis that events occur independently of group membership, the observed counts and expected values should be close.

There will be one such 2×2 table for every event time in the data. We only need a way to combine these tables. Let o_i be the observed number of events in the upper left corner of each 2×2 table, and let e_i denote the corresponding expected count under the null hypothesis of independence. The log-rank test is based on the statistic

$$\text{Log-rank statistic} = \sum_i (o_i - e_i),$$

which simply adds up all of these differences.

> The log-rank test compares the difference of observed and expected numbers of events at every event time.

Under the null hypothesis of identical population survival curves, events will occur independently in the two groups. More precisely, events are more likely to occur in proportion to the number of subjects at risk in the two groups. This corresponds to subjects in both groups being sampled from the same population survival curve.

Under this null hypothesis, the log-rank statistic should have a value near zero. Values far from zero indicate that one group has too many events when few are

Table 11.4. Survival times, in days, of patients treated for bile duct cancer. Censoring is indicated by Cens = 0, and the death of the patient by Cens = 1. Patients were treated with either placebo (Trt = 1) or radiation and 5-FU (Trt = 0).

Surv	Cens	Trt	Surv	Cens	Trt	Surv	Cens	Trt	Surv	Cens	Trt
57	1	0	58	1	0	74	1	0	79	1	0
89	1	0	98	1	0	101	1	0	104	1	0
110	1	0	118	1	0	125	1	0	132	1	0
154	1	0	159	1	0	188	1	0	203	1	0
257	1	0	257	1	0	431	1	0	461	1	0
497	1	0	723	1	0	747	1	0	1313	1	0
2636	1	0									
30	1	1	67	1	1	79	0	1	82	0	1
95	0	1	148	1	1	170	1	1	171	1	1
176	1	1	193	1	1	200	1	1	221	1	1
243	1	1	261	1	1	262	1	1	263	1	1
399	1	1	414	1	1	446	1	1	446	0	1
464	1	1	777	1	1						

Source: Fleming *et al.* (1980).

expected under the model of independence. Similarly, the opposite could occur, so this is a two-tailed test.

The log-rank statistic also needs to be normalized by its standard deviation. This is done for us in `proc lifetest` and gives a p-value of .0653, indicating a moderate amount of statistical evidence for a difference in the two survival curves.

There are other popular variants on the log-rank test. Notice that every observed event time is given equal weight in the definition of the log-rank statistic. Some might argue that we should give more weight to events that occur when there is more data available to us. Similarly, the Wilcoxon test gives more weight in this sum to earlier event times when more subjects are still at risk. The Wilcoxon test has the p-value .0989, providing about the same amount of evidence as the log-rank test for a difference in the survival curves. There are a variety of other ways of weighting the observed and expected numbers of events. These are described in the SAS help file for `lifetest`.

Did you notice how the log-rank and Wilcoxon tests are nonparametric? Nowhere did we need to know the actual times at which the events occurred. In the computation of these statistics, we only need to know the number of subjects at risk when an event occurs in either of the two groups. More specifically, we only need the ranked order in which these events happened. Similarly, the p-values for these tests will remain unchanged if we take logs of survival times or otherwise transform these in a way that maintains the order of the events.

A hard question to answer is whether the censored patients dropped out of the study for reasons related to their outcome. Did they improve and move away, or did they leave their treatment because it wasn't working for them? More generally, is there information in the censoring? Sometimes we can't know the answer to this, but an important assumption is that censoring is independent of the ultimate survival time.

Another difficult question is the resolution of the comparison of survival curves in Figure 11.3. These curves cross and may be statistically different using the log-rank test. The log-rank test tells us only whether these curves are different; it does not indicate which, if any, is better. That difficult decision is one we need to make.

In the following chapter we describe a regression method for modeling survival times using the effects of covariate information.

11.4 Exercises

11.1 Why can't we compare right-censored survival times using a t-test?

11.2 Suppose you transformed the survival times using log(time) or time squared. Would this affect the comparison of survival data using the log-rank test? Why?

11.3 In Figure 11.3, which group would you prefer to be in?

11.4.1 Cancer of the Bile Duct

Cancer of the bile duct is a terrible disease, and most patients die within a year of their diagnosis. A group of patients with this disease were randomized to two treatment groups. One group was treated with radiation and 5-fluorouracil (5-FU). This is a common treatment regime for many types of cancers. The second group was left as untreated with a placebo.

What do you see when you compare the two different treatment groups? Is there a difference between the shapes of the survival curves? Can you see a survival advantage to one group or the other? That is, is there one group that you or a loved one would prefer to belong to?

What can you say about this disease if the active treatment is not much better than doing nothing at all? Is the lack of an active treatment ethical for the patients in the control group? Is it ever ethical to assign a placebo to patients? These are hard questions that we should consider when performing medical research. We cannot ethically randomize patients to one of several different treatments unless we honestly do not know whether one is better than the others. This principle of equally valid treatments is called *equipoise.*

11.4.2 Survival of Centenarians

What are the limits of human longevity? Are there any limits? These are important questions to demographers, who debate the existence of such limits and what they

Table 11.5. Survival of centenarians.

Age at last birthday	Number at risk	Deaths	Number censored
100	52,947	20,845	2256
101	29,846	12,213	1317
102	16,316	6799	716
103	8801	3852	392
104	4557	2030	193
105	2334	1169	103
106	1062	500	63
107	499	271	9
108	219	129	16
109	·74	46	1
110	27	24	
111	3	2	
112	1	1	

Source: Kannisto (1988); Zelterman (1992).

might be. Part of the answer may lie in a study of survival of very old people. An example of such data appears in Table 11.5.

A *centenarian* is a person who is 100 years old. The data represents the survival of female centenarians from 13 countries in northern Europe and Scandinavia. This data was carefully collected by Kannisto (1988), who was concerned that individuals did not intentionally overstate their age in order to claim to be centenarians.

Construct a survival curve for these data. Is this the right way to display this data? The ages begin at 100, so it is best to use this as the starting value for the time axis. The survival curve falls very quickly. Why is that? Perhaps the vertical survival axis should on the log of the survival proportion. If we do that, the survival curve is always negative. Why is that?

Construct the survival curve following the example of Table 11.2. Plot values of Pr[event] in this table against age at last birthday. Do these probabilities generally increase or decrease over time? Why do you think that may be the case? These probabilities estimate the *hazard function* that is important to the model described in the following chapter.

Does there appear to be a limit of longevity? Can it be estimated from these data? Can this be done without extrapolating from the observed data?

12

Proportional Hazards Regression

Much of the language of survival analysis dates back to the 1600s with the early Dutch traders. Ships would leave Europe on a long and dangerous journey to India and China. When they returned with spices and silk, they brought great wealth and fortune to sailors who risked their lives and bankers who invested in the ship and its crew. Along the way there were storms, pirates, even sea monsters to contend with. Sometimes traders failed to return and were never heard from again, leaving behind widows and orphans, and financial ruin for their backers. The need to spread the risks involved in these journeys gave rise to an insurance industry.

Survival analysis uses a lot of the language of life insurance. If we think of life insurance as a bet, then we also need to think of the company that is taking the other side of this bet. *Actuaries* are special types of statisticians who assess these risks and then set the rates for the insurance company. If an actuary overestimates the risk, the company will charge high rates and will lose customers to their competitors. If the actuary underestimates the risks, the company risks financial disaster. Many of the terms used in this chapter will be familiar to actuaries and were originally developed by them. The hazard function is a natural way to describe the risk. It leads us to a popular and effective regression method for modeling survival data.

12.1 The Hazard Function

The *hazard function* (also called the *failure rate*) is a conditional probability. The hazard is the probability of having an event occur at the next instant of time for a subject who has not yet had the event occur. The people who sell life insurance want to know the probability that somebody will die within the next year given that they are alive at the beginning of the year. In our use we define the hazard to be the probability of the event occurring during the next small instant of time for an individual, provided that it has not yet happened for that person.

> The hazard at a given time is the probability that an event will occur in the next instant for a person who has not already experienced the event.

Intuitively, large values of the hazard mean that the event is likely to occur soon. Larger values of the hazard function also mean that the survival curve is falling faster. Similarly, if the survival curve is falling slowly, then the hazard is low.

The mathematical definition of the hazard function at time t is

$$\text{hazard}(t) = \Delta^{-1} \frac{\Pr[\text{event happens between } t \text{ and } t + \Delta]}{\Pr[\text{event has not happened by time } t]}$$

for values of Δ close to zero.

We won't be needing this formula, but here is some intuition about what it measures. The probability in the denominator restricts our attention to only those individuals who have not experienced their event by time t. This is the proportion of people at risk, also described in Table 11.2. When Δ is very small, then the probability in the numerator is also very small. We divide the ratio by Δ to magnify this very small probability.

The hazard function is not the probability that we will live to be a certain age. Instead, the actuarial hazard is the probability that we will not live one more year. The actuary's hazard can tell us the probability of a 100-year-old person dying within the next year. Their hazard does not easily tell us the probability of our living to be 100, however. An annual estimate for the hazard function of centenarians is constructed in Section 11.4.2. The hazard that is used in this chapter is the probability that a subject will experience the event within the next instant of time. For actuaries, that instant is one year; for us, that instant is very small.

Before we go on, it would be useful to look at the actuarial hazard function for our whole lifespan. A great deal of life insurance money is based on the human hazard, so this has been studied for many years and measured with great care. There are also separate estimates of the hazard rate for men and women, different racial groups, and smokers and nonsmokers. In Figure 12.1 we plot the hazard function for the all-combined U.S. population, up to 80 years.[1]

This figure is not entirely useful to us except to emphasize the interpretation of the hazard. The drop in the hazard at the lowest ages illustrate the frailty of small infants. It is not surprising that the hazard rises at older ages as the population increasingly experiences the risks of heart disease, cancer, kidney failure, and other diseases. Most persons seeing this figure are surprised to learn that the minimum occurs around age 10 or 11. The minimum of the hazard corresponds to the age at which humans have the greatest force of vitality (as opposed to mortality) and have the greatest probability of living one more year. Sadly, most of us will view this figure and realize that our prime years have long passed.

[1] See http://www.cdc.gov/nchs/data/nvsr/nvsr54/nvsr54_14.pdf for discussion and details.

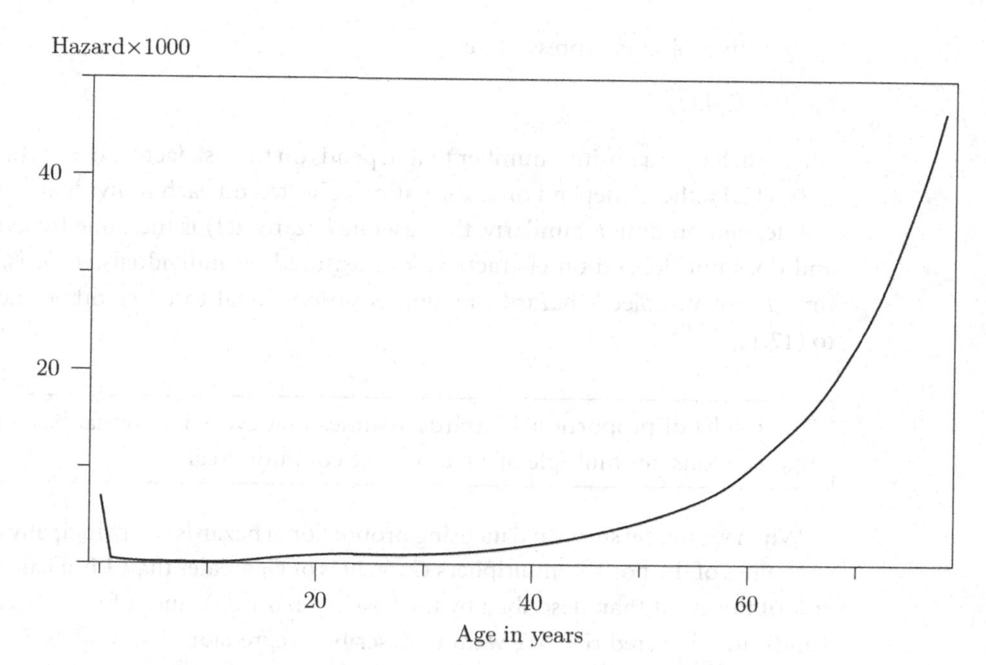

Figure 12.1 **Human lifetime hazard function for the combined 2003 U.S. population.**

The hazard function in this chapter does not use the data in this figure. For the statistical analysis of survival data, we are concerned with selected populations, viewed not over their entire lifetimes, but rather, over a relatively short period of time.

In a single population, we can estimate the hazard function by the Pr[event] in Table 11.2. This is not very useful, because we frequently have several populations we want to compare and, as we see in the following section, want to include covariate effects from additional information collected on each subject.

12.2 The Model of Proportional Hazards Regression

Clearly, having a large value of our hazard function is a bad thing, unless perhaps we are talking about the hazard function for time to winning the lottery. Otherwise, a large hazard function means that there is a greater risk of the event occurring in the next time interval. Larger hazards are associated with even greater imminent risk.

The model of proportional hazards uses this idea. We begin with a *baseline hazard* that models the same underlying risk associated with all subjects in the data. Much as the intercept is common to all observations in a linear regression, the baseline hazard function $h(t)$ is roughly a measure of the average hazard for all subjects at time t.

The variations in individual hazards are expressed as multiples of the baseline $h(t)$. Specifically, the model of *proportional hazards* specifies that the hazard $h_i(t)$

for the ith subject is expressible as

$$h_i(t) = C_i \, h(t) \tag{12.1}$$

where each C_i is a positive number that depends on the risk factors of the ith subject.

In (12.1), the C_i depend on information collected on each individual. The C_i do not depend on time t. Similarly, the baseline hazard $h(t)$ is the same for everybody and does not depend on characteristics measured on individuals. That is, at each time t, every subject's hazard function is proportional to every other's according to (12.1).

> The model of proportional hazards assumes that every individual has a hazard that is a constant multiple of a hazard rate common to all.

When we model survival data using proportional hazards, we principally examine the values of the positive multipliers C_i. Values of C_i greater than 1 indicate a greater risk of the event than described by the baseline hazard. Values of C_i between 0 and 1 indicate a lowered risk. We want to describe a regression that models the value of each individual's C_i.

Proportional hazards regression, sometimes called *Cox regression*,[2] is a way of modeling the multiplier C_i of the hazard function in terms of covariates. The covariates or risk factors are combined in a linear fashion much in the way we have been modeling linear, logistic, or Poisson regression. Proportional hazards regression is performed in SAS using `proc phreg`. This is described in the following section.

In the proportional hazards model, the baseline hazard $h(t)$ acts as an intercept and is the same for every subject. Consequently, we do not usually talk about the baseline hazard. Instead, proportional hazards regression only looks at models of the positive multiplier C_i. Specifically, in proportional hazards regression, we seek to assess the effects of covariate values $x_1, \ldots, x_k$ measured on all subjects and see how these change the multiplier C_i.

Because C_i must be a positive number, we usually assume a log-link and set

$$\log C_i = \beta_1 \, x_1 + \cdots + \beta_k \, x_k \tag{12.2}$$

for regression coefficients $\beta_1, \ldots, \beta_k$ that are estimated by the software.

As an example of the interpretation of this model, if β_1 is positive, then increasing the value of x_1 means an increase in the hazard and a correspondingly shorter survival time or time to event. This is somewhat against our intuition. An increase in the hazard means that the survival is falling faster and survival is shorter. Remember that we are modeling the hazard of survival times and not the survival times themselves. Larger hazards mean shorter survival times.

[2] David R. Cox, a British statistician, published this idea in 1972.

Table 12.1. Output from `phreg` for the AML data.

Analysis of Maximum Likelihood Estimates

Variable	Parameter Estimate	Standard Error	Chi-Square	Pr > ChiSq	Hazard Ratio
group	-0.90422	0.51225	3.1159	0.0775	0.405

Finally, note that there is no intercept in the proportional hazards regression model given at (12.2). An intercept in this model would be the same for all observations and would then be absorbed into the baseline hazard function $h(t)$.

We next show how to fit proportional hazards regression models in SAS.

12.3 Proportional Hazards Regression in SAS

The syntax of `phreg` is similar to that of `lifetest`. We need to specify the name of the time variable and the censoring variable, along with the values associated with censored observations. If we want to repeat the analysis of the AML example using the program in Table 11.3 with proportional hazards regression, add the code

```
proc phreg;
   model surv * cens(0) = group;
   output out=diags xbeta=xb resmart=mart resdev=dev;
run;
```

where `group` is the indicator variable for the two treatments. In the more complicated examples in the exercises of this chapter, you will need to list other variable names as well.

The output from the `phreg` procedure includes a list of estimated regression coefficients for each of the explanatory variables in the `model` statement. Each of these is accompanied by a test of statistical significance similar to those we saw for all other regression models in this book. These test the null hypothesis that the underlying population parameters are zero. For the AML data examined in Section 11.3, this output appears in Table 12.1.

The estimated regression coefficient is negative, indicating that patients with `group` = 1 values have longer times to relapse. There is also an estimated standard error for this regression coefficient and a test of statistical significance. The p-value of .0775 is in between the p-values of the log-rank and Wilcoxon tests we obtained for this data in Section 11.3. The method of proportional hazards regression agrees with those two previous examinations of the data and provides about the same amount of moderate evidence that continued treatment is beneficial for prolonging remission times in AML.

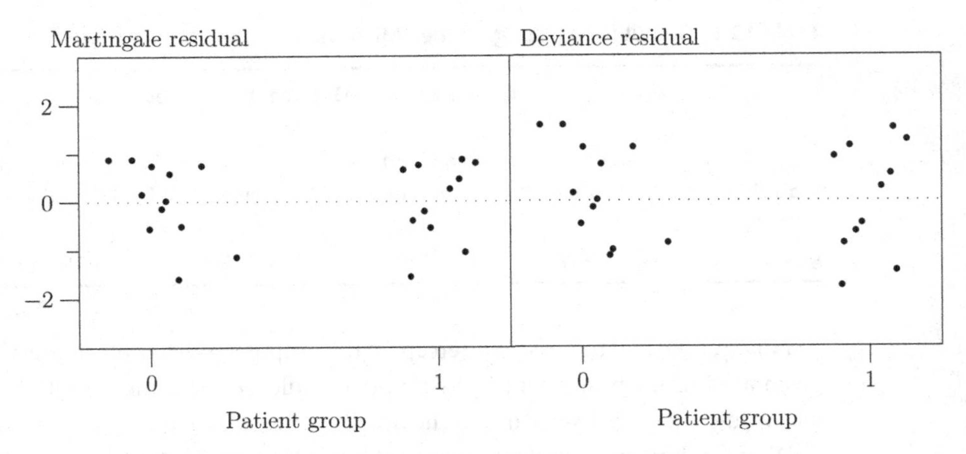

Figure 12.2 Martingale and deviance residuals and jittered treatment group for the AML data.

The hazard ratio in Table 12.1 is calculated as

$$\exp(-0.90422) = 0.405$$

showing that treatment maintained individuals with `group` = 1 values have a hazard that is 0.405 times as large as those with `group` = 0. This lowered hazard for `group` = 1 patients is associated with longer times to relapse.

An important diagnostic for proportional hazards is that the plotted survival curves of different groups do not cross. We see that this is indeed the case for this data in Figure 11.1. If one group has a consistently higher hazard rate, then its survival will always be lower. Similarly, proportional hazards regression may not detect a difference the crossing survival curves in Figure 11.3 is not a valid use of the method.

In addition to the estimated regression coefficients, `proc phreg` provides us two types of residuals. These are the martingale and deviance residuals and are captured in the `output` statement in the example program just given.

We usually plot these residuals against the linear predictor `xbeta`. The linear predictor also appeared in Table 10.4, for example. Recall that the linear predictor is

$$\texttt{xbeta} = \widehat{\beta}_1 x_1 + \widehat{\beta}_2 x_2 + \cdots$$

where $x_1, x_2, \ldots$ are the explanatory variables in the `model` statement. Remember that there is no intercept in proportional hazards regression.

In the case of the AML data, there is only one explanatory variable (treatment group), and this is binary valued. Similarly, the linear predictor in this example will take on only two distinct values and should be jittered in the plot to make these easier to view. There are no extreme residuals, in either of the plots in Figure 12.2, so we conclude that this is a reasonable application of proportional hazards regression.

Table 12.2. The first ten lines of the halibut survival data.

1	209.0	1	30	13	41	8	6.992
2	209.0	1	30	13	44	8	6.992
3	209.0	1	30	13	47	10	6.992
4	209.0	1	30	13	34	10	6.992
5	38.0	1	30	13	40	11	6.992
6	209.0	1	30	13	42	11	6.992
7	140.9	1	30	13	41	12	6.992
8	140.9	1	30	13	30	12	6.992
9	140.1	1	30	1	45	4	4.299
10	208.0	1	30	1	47	5	4.299
	. . .						. . .

Source: Smith *et al.*, Chapter 7 of Lange *et al.* (1984). The full data is available online.

12.4 Exercises

12.1 Why can't we use a linear regression to compare right-censored survival times with covariates?

12.2 Are the hazards proportional if the survival curves cross as in Figure 11.3?

12.4.1 Survival of Halibut

A halibut is a large and tasty fish that is often sought by sportsmen. Halibut travel in large schools that are exploited by commercial fishermen, who can quickly harvest large numbers on hooked lines measuring miles in length. Consequently, halibut fishing must be carefully regulated to prevent the eventual depletion of the stocks. As part of this regulation, these fish populations have been carefully studied in detail.

Here is some halibut trivia. The schools are so large that these can be tracked in satellite images. Halibut have an ear bone with "rings" that allows us to accurately estimate their age just as we would with trees. When young, halibut have one eye on either side of their heads and swim "up and down" or perpendicular to the surface of the water. At about 6 months of age, halibut will begin to swim "flat" with the light-colored side toward the bottom and a much darker side on top. At the time that they make this transition, the eye on the bottom side of the head moves over to the top. The light coloration is for protection from predators looking up toward the surface, and the two eyes on top help to spot smaller prey.

What determines halibut survival once caught? Longer survival translates into fresher fish for the consumer. The dataset contains 294 lines, one for the survival time of each halibut. Only the first ten lines are given in Table 12.2. The whole dataset is available online.[3]

[3] Available online at http://lib.stat.cmu.edu/datasets/csb/ch7.dat.

The following is a list of the information available on each fish:

- Survival time, measured in hours
- Censoring indicator: 1, observed survival time; 0, censored observation
- Time the trawl net was towed along the bottom
- Difference between maximum and minimum depth observed during tow (measured in meters)
- Fork length of halibut (measured in centimeters)
- Handling time (in minutes) between net coming on board vessel and fish being placed in holding tanks
- Logarithm (base e) of total catch of fish in tow

Is there evidence that data from a few catches are pooled together? Similarly, are the survival times listed for individual halibut or a single value for a group of fish?

12.4.2 Stanford Heart Transplant Survival

In the early days of heart transplantation, there was a large epidemiology study to examine the risks and to see if it was all worth while. Subjects were enrolled and randomized to receive a transplant or not. Some subjects who were randomized to receive a transplant died before a donor organ was available. Today we have sophisticated antirejection drugs that prevent recipients' immune systems from attacking the donor organ. At the time of this study, the mismatch score was important in identifying a close match between donor and recipient. Two versions of this data are available online,[4] along with more details and the history of this dataset.

Is there evidence that the effect of age is not monotone? We would expect that the oldest patients would be frail and might not survive the major transplant surgery. The very youngest patients are also vulnerable. A child who needs a heart transplant should be considered to have a different disease than a 60-year-old. That is, the hazard in age might be "U"-shaped.

12.4.3 Primary Biliary Cirrhosis

Primary biliary cirrhosis (PBC) is a disease of the liver characterized by slow loss of bile ducts (bile canaliculi). This results in a buildup of bile, resulting in scarring, fibrosis, cirrhosis, and ultimately liver failure. The disease affects about 1 in 4,000 people, mostly women.

A randomized clinical trial was conducted between 1974 and 1984 at the Mayo Clinic to see if the use of the drug D-penicillamine would be useful in extending life. There were also a large proportion of patients who developed liver toxicity due to the drugs used to treat their disease. As a result, there are two types of end points we can examine in this data: time to toxicity or time to death. Both of these can be modeled as "survival" times.

[4] http://lib.stat.cmu.edu/datasets/stanford.

Table 12.3. List of variables in the PBC study.

```
case number
survival in days
status: 0=censored, 1=censored due to liver toxicity, 2=death
drug: 1=D-penicillamine, 2=placebo
age in days
sex:  0=male, 1=female
presence of asictes: 0=no 1=yes
presence of hepatomegaly: 0=no 1=yes
presence of spiders  0=no 1=yes
edema: 0=no edema; .5=edema present resolved; 1=edema despite therapy
serum bilirubin in mg/dl
serum cholesterol in mg/dl
albumin in gm/dl
urine copper in ug/day
alkaline phosphatase in U/liter
SGOT in U/ml
triglicerides in mg/dl
platelets per cubic ml / 1000
prothrombin time in seconds
histologic stage of disease
```

In the clinical trial, there were 312 patients randomized to the drug; these patients also have the most complete data. An additional 112 cases were not enrolled in the trial. Some data was collected on them, but much of their data is missing, and we should initially concentrate on the 312 who were enrolled in the study.

The data is available online.[5] The website contains a more detailed explanation of the study and provides additional published references to the trial. A complete list of the variables is given in Table 12.3.

Some variables (prothrombin and phosphatase, specifically) are highly significant as explanatory variables of survival. Can you tell whether these are these more indicative of disease progression than of treatment-related outcomes? Specifically, are the values of these variables different in the treated and placebo groups?

Is the rate of censoring different in the two different groups? Was there more censoring due to liver toxicity in the treated group than in the placebo patients? You might use logistic regression to see if censoring due to toxicity was related to any of the other explanatory variables. Was the drug effective in prolonging survival?

12.4.4 Multiple Myeloma

Myeloma is a disease of the immune system in the bone marrow. Presently, it is incurable but symptom-free survival can be achieved with a variety of treatments.

[5] http://lib.stat.cmu.edu/datasets/pbc.

Table 12.4. List of variables in the multiple myeloma dataset.

Survival time, measured in months
Censoring indicator (0=alive, 1=dead)
BUN at time of diagnosis, log scale
Hemoglobin at time of diagnosis
Normal platelets at diagnosis (1=normal, 0=abnormal)
Age, in years, at time of diagnosis
WBC at time of diagnosis, log scale
Fractures at time of diagnosis (0=none, 1=present)
Percent of plasma cells in the bone marrow, PBM, on log scale
Proteinuria: Protein in the urine
Serum calcium at time of diagnosis

Source: Krall, Uthoff, and Harley (1975).

Krall, Uthoff, and Harley (1975) reported on survival data from a study of 65 patients treated with alkylating agents.[6] Of these patients, 48 died during the study and 17 were still alive at the time of the data analysis. The variables given in this dataset are listed in Table 12.4.

Blood urea nitrogen (BUN) is a measure of kidney function. Urea is produced by the liver and cleared from the blood by the kidneys. Hemoglobin (HGB) is an important component of blood involved in transporting gases to be exchanged in the lungs.

Examine the data using proportional hazards models. Notice that BUN is highly significant in explaining survival times. HGB is a little less useful in this role. Are these variables correlated with other explanatory variables? Can you tell whether survival is a general overall decline in health or a function of only these two measures?

There is one extreme outlier using martingale residuals, but this patient is not all that extreme on the deviance residual scale. Identify this patient and see if you can tell why this observation is unusual.

[6] Available online at http://www.jstor.org/stable/2529709.

13

Review of Methods

In the study of statistics, we learn a great many different methods, and it is often unclear which is applicable in a given setting. Half of the problem with data analysis can be traced back to the choice of which method is most appropriate for the data. This chapter provides a review of the methods from the standpoint of the data analyst.

13.1 The Appropriate Method

A number of different situations are presented here, and the reader is encouraged to think about the appropriate statistical method for each. In each of the following questions, briefly explain the best statistical technique to solve the problem and specify the null hypothesis.

13.1 I want to estimate how long it takes for seniors to get back to normal living activities following hip surgery. Does it matter whether the surgery is elective or if it follows an accidental fall and fracture? Some people are climbing ladders within four weeks, but others remain in a wheelchair for the rest of their lives. I also want to investigate the effects of other information including age, sex, Medicaid status, and the need for a home health aide. (What methods should we use? What is the null hypothesis?)

13.2 One of the students tells the following story: Last summer I had a job in a donut factory. Those machines would produce a ton of donuts every day! My job was to run the machine that punched out the holes in the donuts. This worked OK, mostly, but I had to be on the lookout for those few donuts with square holes. The number of these were recorded on a daily basis. I was supposed to throw these out, but I secretly took them home and fed them to my dog. By the end of the summer, my dog got sick from eating too many donuts. I wondered if there was an increase in the number of square-holed donuts as the weather got warmer. Maybe it was worse if the donuts were sugar coated. Glazed donuts were the worst! Definitely. (Method? Null hypothesis?)

13.3 A political scientist studied how long it took for bills to be passed into law by the state and federal legislatures. Different kinds of bills are introduced into debate: for example, funding for roads and schools, changes in taxes, and changes in criminal law. Some bills are quickly passed into law, whereas debate on others continues for years. At the time the political scientist wanted to write an article about the approval process, many bills were pending. Does the length of the approval process depend on what kind of bill is introduced? Does it matter which political party introduces the bill? (What method is appropriate? What is the null hypothesis?)

13.4 Nobody really cares about the color of car tires. One tire manufacturer suspects that darker tires have less grip and take longer to stop on wet pavement. Given data on the shade (measured on a continuous scale) and stopping distance for several brands of tires, how can we test this hypothesis? We tried different tires on different makes and models of cars. (Method? Null hypothesis?)

13.5 Suppose everybody who took a statistics course received a grade of either A or B, without exception. How would we see if grades differed by students' age, sex, major, or number of other courses taken concurrently?

13.6 Most course evaluations are fairly accurate, but there are always a few subjective responses that seem unrelated to the instruction. One professor sometimes gets great evaluations because she wears cool sneakers to class. Another professor sometimes gets poor evaluations because he has a foreign accent. How can we test whether evaluations differ by required or elective courses?

13.7 The number of housing starts is an important economic indicator. People who buy a new house will also spend a lot of money to furnish it. In many parts of the country, most housing construction begins in the spring. If we had data on the (unadjusted) number of housing starts (response variable) for each month over many years, how would we create a "seasonally adjusted" number for each month? Specify the indicator variables that you would create and how you would use these in a linear regression model.

13.8 We want to compare the response rates following the use of two different antibiotics: one is a standard drug, the other is a new competitor. Each patient's response is classified as improved or not. We know that almost all patients will improve even if they are untreated, so a very large clinical trial is needed. As the biostatistician assigned to this project, how are you going to analyze the data? Specifically, what method are you going to use, and what is the null hypothesis?

13.9 In order to study proper diagnostics and drug-prescribing practices, we have data on patients including selected information (compliant with HIPAA, the Health Insurance Portability and Accountability Act) from their health records. Every prescription is classified as being either proper or improper. We want to see if these (proper/improper) rates are different for male versus female patients, for example, and we want to measure the effects of patient's age, comorbidity, type of health insurance, and a lot of other possible covariates. What statistical method do you suggest we use? How would you define your study population?

13.10 Leukemia patients were treated following one of two different medical protocols. They are all now disease-free, but we want to know if their treatment influences the time until their disease recurs. Some patients remain disease-free for the rest of their lives. We also want to take into account the effects of any prior treatments, different ages of the patients, types of health insurance if any, and any comorbidity conditions. (Method? Hypotheses?)

13.11 Hardly anybody contracts rabies these days, yet in Connecticut there are a couple of cases every year. How can we test for a trend in the number of cases over the past 5 years? (Method? Hypotheses?)

13.12 We want to know if older people are more likely to be cat owners. (Everybody is either a cat owner or they aren't. You know which you are!) We decided that "old" means anybody over 25 years old. (Method? Hypotheses?)

13.13 We are in the same situation as in Question 13.12, but we want to use Age as a continuous variable. (Method? Hypothesis?)

13.14 In a case-control study, we first identify a number of individuals with a rare disease and then find a group of otherwise healthy people with similar demographic characteristics such as age, race, and sex.

What statistical method should we use to compare any history of tobacco use among the cases and controls? What are the null and alternative hypotheses for this problem?

Suppose, in the same data, we wanted to compare the level of educational attainment (measured in years) among the cases and controls. What methods should be used? What are the null and alternative hypotheses?

13.15 In a laboratory study, groups of mice were exposed to different doses of a suspected toxin. Write down the linear logistic regression model that expresses the probability of dying (P) in terms of the Dose of exposure.

a. In terms of what you wrote, what is the null hypothesis, and what is the alternative?

b. Suppose the estimated intercept is -3 and the estimated regression slope on Dose is 0.5. Estimate the LD_{50} or Dose that is lethal to 50% of the mice.

13.2 Other Review Questions

13.16 What is the standard deviation? What does it measure? What is the standard error? What does it measure? How do these two measures relate to each other?

13.17 What is meant by the use of the "log link" in Poisson regression? Why is this needed?

13.18 In the lottery winner data from Section 10.1, suppose we fit a model using the following SAS program:

```
proc genmod data=lottery;
  model winners = pop / dist=Poisson;
run;
```

where `winners` is the number of winners and pop is the town population in thousands. What model for the Poisson mean is being fitted?

13.19 Part of the SAS output from the program on the previous question includes the following:

Analysis Of Parameter Estimate

Parameter	Estimate	Standard Error	Wald 95% Confidence Limits		Chi-Square	Pr > ChiSq
Intercept	1.3053	0.1864	0.9400	1.6706	49.04	<.0001
pop	0.0232	0.0056	0.0123	0.0341	17.48	<.0001
Scale	1.0000	0.0000	1.0000	1.0000		

What is the null hypothesis being tested by the chi-squared statistic with a value of 17.48? You can refer to the notation you used on the previous page. Is this test useful in the present context? Why or why not?

Taken by itself, is the intercept useful in the present example? Briefly explain why or why not.

13.20 In logistic regression, what is meant by the "logit"? Why is it needed? How does this differ from the "probit"? Is there anything that you can do using one model that is unavailable to you under the other?

13.21 In the beetle data of Table 8.1, bugs were put in each of six different jars and exposed to different doses of an insecticide. We fit a logistic regression model using the following SAS program:

```
proc logistic;
   model y/n=dose / iplots influence;
run;
```

where n is the number of beetles in each jar and y is the number killed. Write down the model being fitted with this program.

13.22 Part of the SAS output from the program in question 13.21 contains the following:

Analysis of Maximum Likelihood Estimates

Parameter	DF	Estimate	Standard Error	Wald Chi-Square	Pr > ChiSq
Intercept	1	-3.0084	1.0028	9.0002	0.0027
dose	1	2.4348	0.8139	8.9500	0.0028

What null hypothesis is being tested by the chi-squared statistic with a value of 8.95?

13.23 Part of the SAS output of Question 13.21 also contains the following plot of the hat diagonal. The values of this diagnostic are given in the column listed as Value, and the column marked dose is the dose of the insecticide. The hat diagnostic measures influence and leverage. The plot is turned on it side. Explain why the plot is "U"-shaped.

```
                              Hat Matrix Diagonal

   Case                                    (1 unit = 0.04)
  Number        dose       Value         0 2 4 6 8  12  16

     1         1.0800     0.6054        |                 *|
     2         1.1600     0.2621        |       *          |
     3         1.2100     0.1780        |     *            |
     4         1.2600     0.1910        |     *            |
     5         1.3100     0.3060        |        *         |
     6         1.3500     0.4575        |            *     |
```

13.24 Lymphoma patients will usually respond quickly to chemotherapy, but things can go wrong. Sometimes their response takes a long time, and we may not see it by the time we examine the data. Sometimes the patients don't respond at all, and sometimes they die before responding. Summarize all of the kinds of censoring that can occur in this setting when we study the time to response.

13.25 Here are the response times, in weeks, where a "+" indicates a censored time. Draw a Kaplan-Meier survival curve for this data and provide as much detail as possible.

3 3+ 4 6 10+ 12+

13.26 In the previous question, a researcher collected much more data than is presented here. Suppose there were 100 more observations with times shorter than 3 weeks, and all of these observations were censored. How would the addition of this new data change the estimated survival curve?

13.27 In a study of childhood development, we collected data on 6-year-old girls and boys along with their weights. By the end of the data collection process, we noticed that there were a small number of missing values. There were a lot of children with "complete" data, but several children were missing either their sex or their weight values.

What is the best way to estimate a missing weight for a girl or a boy?

In a small number of cases, we recorded the weights but not the sex of the child. What statistical method can we use to estimate the sex of a child from his or her weight?

13.28 In a large clinical trial of cancer, we noticed that some patients responded to the drug and some did not. We want to see if we could characterize these two different types of patients, so we collected data on 500 genes in the laboratory on every subject. We then constructed a total of 500 2×2 tables classifying the numbers of patients who responded (or didn't) and whether or not each of the 500 genes was expressed differently. Every gene was examined in its own 2×2 table. On every 2×2 table, we calculated a chi-squared statistic, and 23 of these were found to be statistically significant at the .05 level. How do we interpret this finding?

13.29 Here are observations from two groups of observations that we want to compare:

Group I: 8 12 97 103
Group II: 19 21 25 27 29 30

Why should we prefer a nonparametric test to the t-test for this data? Why? Perform as much of the Wilcoxon rank-sum test as you can without a calculator or computer.

With this same data, perform as much of the median test as you can. Set it up, but don't perform any calculations.

13.30 All cases of cancer in Connecticut are recorded and reported to federal agencies as part of the national cancer registry SEER program. We examined these lung cancer rates over the past five years and found that New Haven is always worse than the state as a whole. Somebody asked about the p-value. What is the most appropriate thing to do about this?

13.31 Pacemaker batteries are always replaced when they fail, or else every two years, whichever comes first. A manufacturer of a new battery makes claims of a lower failure rate. To test this claim, we enrolled a large number of patients into a randomized, double-blind study. When the patients' batteries were replaced, either the old or the new battery types was used. At the time of our examination of the data, some batteries will have failed, some will have been replaced after their two-year limit, and some may still be functioning normally in patients.

a. Explain how you will treat each of these three different types of data.

b. Describe a robust statistical method for comparing failure rates of the two types of batteries.

c. How can we account for differences in battery failure rates by patient age, sex, body-mass index, and the age of the pacemaker?

13.32 My best friend went to El Salvador and recorded the height and sex of all the third graders in his host village. He came back and performed a linear regression (using `proc reg`) of sex and height, but obtained the unusual residual plot given in Figure 13.1. This is a plot of residual (on the vertical, Y axis) and height (on the horizontal, X axis). He used `proc print` and insists that there is no problem in his `data` step. Can you help him?

13.33 Last summer we went out into the woods and collected a huge number of ticks and recorded the environments in which they were found. The environmental data includes such information as wet or dry areas; sunny or shady; rain or fair

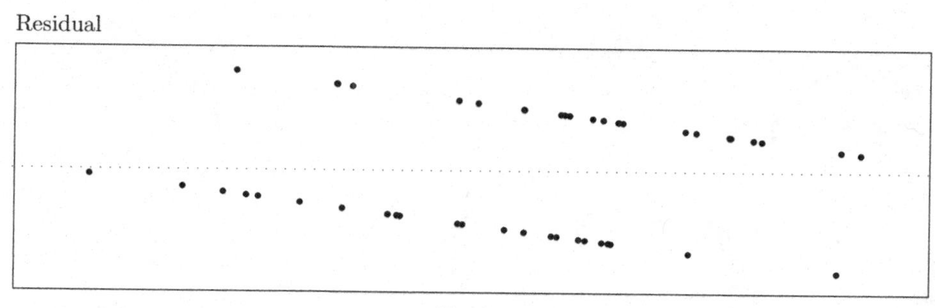

Figure 13.1 What is the problem with these residuals?

weather; and in deep grass or under trees. We spent different amounts of time and effort in each of these settings. Only a small number of these ticks tested positive for Lyme disease. We want to present an advisory to hikers about the risky and safe areas to visit this summer. Describe a statistical analysis to estimate where the infected ticks are likely to occur. Discuss the relative merits of Poisson and logistic regression methodology in this problem.

13.34 We examined families and counted the number of children (under 6) in the household reporting flu symptoms over the past year. We also recorded the number of adults in the home who smoked, the levels of humidity in the home, and the age of the home. Can we treat each family as an independent binomial sample with $N =$ the number of children and the response variable being the count of symptomatic children?

13.35 I am comparing two survival curves. One goes all the way down to zero at the end, and the second curve stops before reaching zero. How do you explain this?

13.36 For each of twelve Asian countries, I performed a linear regression, modeling per-capita health expenditures (Y) in terms of national population (X). China is so much larger than all other nations that I expect something unusual is going to happen. In fact, the slope is negative when I include all of the data, but the slope becomes positive when I fit the model with all countries except China. What is going on here? Draw a picture to illustrate your explanation.

13.37 I got my master's thesis data from a brother-in-law of my sister's roommate in Iowa. "He is such a scatter-brained type that he probably put some decimal places where they don't belong," she said. I suspect that there are some digits reversed, too. I really need to graduate on time, and this is probably the best data available. Is there anything I can do with this? Can you help me? What statistical methods should I be using with this type of data?

Appendix: Statistical Tables

A.1 Normal Distribution

Table A.1 in this Appendix provides the area to the left of x under the standard normal distribution for $x > 0$. This area is illustrated in Figure A.1. Examples of the use of this table are given in Section 2.3.

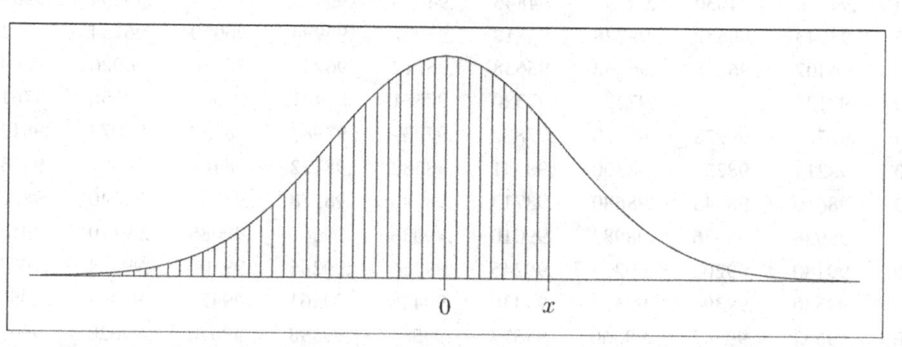

Figure A.1 The area under the standard normal in Table A.1 is to the left of x for positive values of x.

Table A.1. Area under the standard normal curve to the left of x.

	.00	.01	.02	.03	.04	.05	.06	.07	.08	.09
0.00	.50000	.50399	.50798	.51197	.51595	.51994	.52392	.52790	.53188	.53586
0.10	.53983	.54380	.54776	.55172	.55567	.55962	.56356	.56750	.57142	.57535
0.20	.57926	.58317	.58706	.59095	.59483	.59871	.60257	.60642	.61026	.61409
0.30	.61791	.62172	.62552	.62930	.63307	.63683	.64058	.64431	.64803	.65173
0.40	.65542	.65910	.66276	.66640	.67003	.67364	.67724	.68082	.68439	.68793
0.50	.69146	.69497	.69847	.70194	.70540	.70884	.71226	.71566	.71904	.72240
0.60	.72575	.72907	.73237	.73565	.73891	.74215	.74537	.74857	.75175	.75490
0.70	.75804	.76115	.76424	.76730	.77035	.77337	.77637	.77935	.78230	.78524
0.80	.78814	.79103	.79389	.79673	.79955	.80234	.80510	.80785	.81057	.81327
0.90	.81594	.81859	.82121	.82381	.82639	.82894	.83147	.83398	.83646	.83891
1.00	.84134	.84375	.84614	.84850	.85083	.85314	.85543	.85769	.85993	.86214
1.10	.86433	.86650	.86864	.87076	.87286	.87493	.87698	.87900	.88100	.88298
1.20	.88493	.88686	.88877	.89065	.89251	.89435	.89617	.89796	.89973	.90147
1.30	.90320	.90490	.90658	.90824	.90988	.91150	.91309	.91466	.91620	.91774
1.40	.91924	.92073	.92220	.92364	.92507	.92647	.92785	.92922	.93056	.93189
1.50	.93320	.93448	.93574	.93700	.93822	.93943	.94062	.94180	.94295	.94408
1.60	.94520	.94630	.94738	.94845	.94950	.95053	.95154	.95254	.95352	.95449
1.70	.95543	.95637	.95728	.95818	.95907	.95994	.96080	.96164	.96246	.96327
1.80	.96407	.96485	.96562	.96638	.96712	.96784	.96856	.96926	.96995	.97062
1.90	.97128	.97193	.97257	.97320	.97381	.97441	.97500	.97558	.97615	.97670
2.00	.97725	.97778	.97830	.97882	.97932	.97982	.98030	.98077	.98124	.98170
2.10	.98214	.98257	.98300	.98341	.98382	.98422	.98461	.98500	.98537	.98574
2.20	.98610	.98645	.98680	.98713	.98745	.98778	.98809	.98840	.98870	.98899
2.30	.98928	.98956	.98983	.99010	.99036	.99061	.99086	.99110	.99134	.99158
2.40	.99180	.99202	.99224	.99245	.99266	.99286	.99305	.99324	.99343	.99361
2.50	.99380	.99396	.99413	.99430	.99446	.99461	.99477	.99492	.99506	.99520
2.60	.99534	.99547	.99560	.99573	.99585	.99598	.99610	.99620	.99632	.99643
2.70	.99653	.99664	.99674	.99683	.99693	.99702	.99710	.99720	.99728	.99736
2.80	.99744	.99752	.99760	.99767	.99774	.99781	.99788	.99795	.99801	.99807
2.90	.99813	.99820	.99825	.99830	.99836	.99841	.99846	.99851	.99856	.99860
3.00	.99865	.99870	.99874	.99878	.99882	.99886	.99890	.99893	.99896	.99900

A.2 Chi-squared Tables

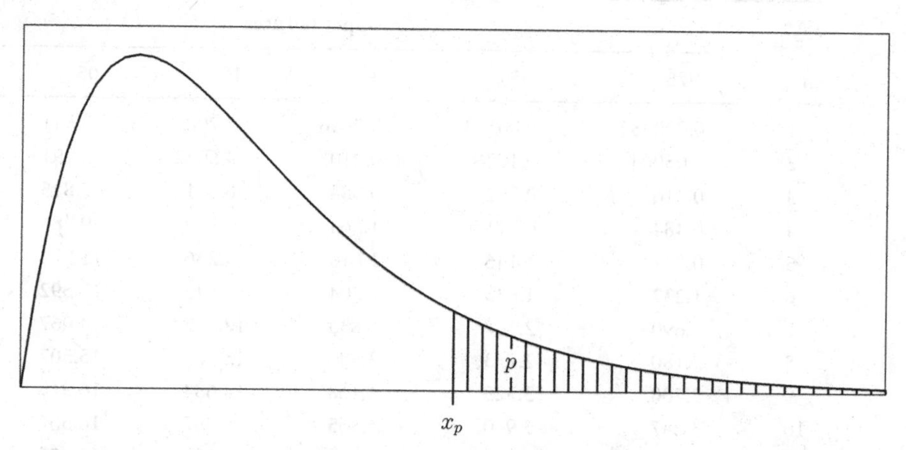

Figure A.2 For specified values of upper tail area p, Table A.2 provides the corresponding quantile x_p.

Table A.2. Quantiles of the chi-squared distribution.

	Upper tail area					
df	.975	.95	.90	.10	.05	.025
1	0.000982	0.00393	0.0158	2.706	3.841	5.024
2	0.05064	0.1026	0.2107	4.6052	5.9915	7.378
3	0.216	0.352	0.584	6.251	7.815	9.348
4	0.484	0.711	1.064	7.779	9.488	11.143
5	0.831	1.146	1.610	9.236	11.071	12.833
6	1.237	1.635	2.204	10.645	12.592	14.449
7	1.690	2.167	2.833	12.017	14.067	16.013
8	2.180	2.733	3.490	13.362	15.507	17.535
9	2.700	3.325	4.168	14.684	16.919	19.023
10	3.247	3.940	4.865	15.987	18.307	20.483
11	3.816	4.575	5.578	17.275	19.675	21.920
12	4.404	5.226	6.304	18.549	21.026	23.337
13	5.009	5.892	7.042	19.812	22.362	24.736
14	5.629	6.571	7.790	21.064	23.685	26.119
15	6.262	7.261	8.547	22.307	24.996	27.488
16	6.908	7.962	9.312	23.542	26.296	28.845
17	7.564	8.672	10.085	24.769	27.587	30.191
18	8.231	9.390	10.865	25.989	28.868	31.526
19	8.907	10.117	11.651	27.204	30.144	32.852
20	9.591	10.851	12.443	28.412	31.41	34.17
21	10.28	11.59	13.24	29.62	32.67	35.48
22	10.98	12.34	14.04	30.81	33.92	36.78
23	11.69	13.09	14.85	32.01	35.17	38.08
24	12.40	13.85	15.66	33.20	36.42	39.36
25	13.12	14.61	16.47	34.38	37.65	40.65
26	13.84	15.38	17.29	35.56	38.89	41.92
27	14.57	16.15	18.11	36.74	40.11	43.19
28	15.31	16.93	18.94	37.92	41.34	44.46
29	16.05	17.71	19.77	39.09	42.56	45.72
30	16.79	18.49	20.60	40.26	43.77	46.98
60	40.48	43.19	46.46	74.40	79.08	83.30
90	65.65	69.13	73.29	107.6	113.2	118.1
120	91.57	95.70	100.6	140.2	146.6	152.2
150	118.0	122.7	128.3	172.6	179.6	185.8

References

Abbruzzese JL *et al.* (1996). Phase I clinical and plasma and cellular pharmacological study of topotecan with and without granulocyte colony-stimulating factor. *Clinical Cancer Research* **2**: 1489–97.

Agresti A (1990). *Categorical Data Analysis.* New York: Wiley.

Andrews DF and Herzberg AM (1985). *Data.* New York: Springer-Verlag.

Anscombe FJ (1973). Graphs in statistical analysis, *American Statistician,* **27**: 17–21.

Bates DM and Watts DG (1988). *Nonlinear Regression Analysis and Its Applications.* New York: Wiley.

Brown BW (1980). Prediction analysis for binary data. In *Biostatistics Casebook.* R. G. Miller, B. Efron, B. W. Brown, and L. E. Moses (editors), p. 318. New York: Wiley.

Cody RP and Smith JK (2006). *Applied Statistics and the SAS Programming Language*, fifth edition. Upper Saddle River, NJ: Pearson Prentice Hall.

Davidian M and Giltinan DM (1995). *Nonlinear Models for Repeated Measurement Data.* Boca Raton, FL: Chapman & Hall.

Delwiche LD and Slaughter SJ (1998). *The Little SAS Book,* second edition. Cary, NC: SAS Institute.

Dobson AJ (2002). *An Introduction to Generalized Linear Models,* second edition. Boca Raton, FL: Chapman & Hall.

Efron B (1978). Regression and ANOVA with zero-one data: Measures of residual variation. *Journal of the American Statistical Association* **73**: 113–21.

Embury SH, Elias L, Heller PH, *et al.* (1977). Remission maintenance therapy in acute myelogenous leukemia. *Western Journal of Medicine* **126**: 267–72.

Farmer JH, Kodell RL, Greenman DL, and Shaw GW (1979). Dose and time response models for the incidence of bladder and liver neoplasms in mice fed 2-acetylaminofluorene continuously. *Journal of Environmental Pathology and Toxicology* **3**: 55–68.

Fleming T, O'Fallon JR, O'Brien PD, and Harrington DP (1980). Modified Kolmogorov-Smirnov test procedures with application to arbitrarily right-censored data. *Biometrics* **36**: 607–25.

Frisby JP and Clatworthy, JL (1975). Learning to see complex random-dot stereograms. *Perception* **4**: 173–8.

Friedland L, Joffe M, Moore D, *et al.* (1992). Effect of educational program on compliance with glove use in a pediatric emergency department. *American Journal of Diseases of Childhood* **146**: 1355–8.

Freund RJ, and Littell RC (2000). *SAS System for Regression*, third edition. New York: Wiley.

Glovsky L and Rigrodsky S (1964). A developmental analysis of mentally deficient children with early histories of aphasis. *Training School Bulletin* **61**: 76–96.

Henderson HV and Velleman PF (1981). Building multiple regression models interactively. *Biometrics* **37**: 391–411.

Hosmer DW Jr. and Lemeshow S (2000). *Applied Logistic Regression*, second edition. New York: Wiley.

Innes, JRM, Ulland BM, Valerio MG, Petrucelli L, Fishbein L, Hart ER, Pallotta AJ, Bates RR, Falk HL, Gart JJ, Klein, M, Mitchell I, and Peters J. (1969). Bioassay of pesticides and industrial chemicals for tumorigenicity in mice: A preliminary note. *Journal of the National Cancer Institute* **42**: 1101–14.

Johnson, MP, and Raven, PH (1973). Species number and endemism: The Galápagos Archipelago revisited. *Science* **179:** 893–5.

Kannisto V (1988). On the survival of centenarians and the span of life. *Population Studies* **42**: 389–406.

Kaplan EL and Meier P (1958). Nonparametric estimation from incomplete observations. *Journal of the American Statistical Association* **53**: 457–81.

Koziol JA, Maxwell DA, Fukushima M, Colmerauer MEM, and Pilch YH (1981). A distribution-free test for tumor-growth curve analysis with application to an animal tumor immunotherapy experiment. *Biometrics* **37**: 383–90.

Krall JM, Uthoff VA, and Harley JB (1975). A step-up procedure for selecting variables associated with survival. *Biometrics* **31**: 49–57.

Lange N, Ryan L, Billard L, Brillinger D, Conquest L, and Greenhouse J (1984). *Case Studies in Biometry*. New York: Wiley. The datasets and their descriptions are available online at http://lib.stat.cmu.edu/datasets/csb/

Lee JAH, Hitosugi M, and Peterson GR (1973). Rise in mortality from tumors of the testis in Japan, 1947–70. *Journal of the National Cancer Institute* **51:** 1485–90.

Leviton A, Fenton T, Kuban KCK, and Pagano M (1991). Labor and delivery characteristics and the risk of germinal matrix hemorrhage in low birth weight infants. *Journal of Child Neurology* **6**: 35–40.

Littell R, Stroup WW, and Freund R (2002). *SAS for Linear Models*, fourth edition. New York: Wiley/SAS.

Mosteller F and Tukey JW (1977). *Data Analysis and Regression. A Second Course in Statistics*. Reading, MA: Addison-Wesley.

Pagano M and Gauvreau K (2000). *Principles of Biostatistics*, second edition. Pacific Grove, CA: Duxbury.

Plackett RL (1981). *The Analysis of Categorical Data*, second edition. London: Charles Griffin.

Stuckler D, King LP, and Basu S (2008). International Monetary Fund programs and tuberculosis outcomes in post-communist countries. *PLOS Medicine*. Available online. doi:10.1371/journal.pmed.0050143.

Teasdale N, Bard C, LaRue J, and Fleury M (1993). On the cognitive penetrability of posture control. *Experimental Aging Research* **19**: 1–13.

van Wattum PJ, Chappell PB, Zelterman D, Scahill LD, and Lecktman JF (2000). Patterns of response to acute naloxone infusion in Tourette's syndrome. *Movement Disorders* **15**: 1252–4.

Wheler J, Tsimberidou AM, Hong D, Naing A, Jackson T, Liu S, Feng L, and Kurzrock R (2009). Survival of patients in a Phase I clinic. *Cancer* **115**: 1091–9.

Zelterman D (1992). A statistical distribution with an unbounded hazard function and its application to a theory from demography. *Biometrics* **48**: 807–18.

Selected Solutions and Hints

1.4 Pink eye is an infection and can often be traced to swimming in unclean water or contact with chlorine in the water.

2.3 a. We expect 2, and the standard deviation is $8 \times 0.25 \times (1 - 0.25) = 1.225$.

b. The probability that all eight are cold-free is $.75^8$. The probability that three or more have a cold is

$$\begin{aligned}\Pr[3 \text{ or more}] &= 1 - \Pr[2 \text{ or fewer}] \\ &= 1 - (.25^8) - (8 \times .25^7 \times .75) - (28 \times .25^6 \times .75^2)\end{aligned}$$

c. Is the health status of the children independent?

2.4 a. Alternative hypotheses that are further away from the null hypothesis have greater power. Intuitively, it is easy to tell whether the null or alternative hypothesis is true when these are very different.

b. The alternative that is furthest from the null hypothesis has the greatest power, but such alternatives are rarely useful to us. If such a large difference existed and was visible, then it would already be well known.

c. As the sample size increases, we are able to test hypotheses that are closer together and more subtle differences can be detected.

2.6 The probability of a kangaroo flush, or any other five-card hand for that matter, is

$$1 \Big/ \binom{52}{5} = \frac{5 \times 4 \times 3 \times 2 \times 1}{52 \times 51 \times 50 \times 49 \times 48} = 3.85 \times 10^{-7}.$$

2.9 c. Are infections independent events?

3.3 a. Two infants who differ by 1 cm in length should differ in average weight by about 61.65 g.

b. The estimated intercept would correspond to the estimated weight of an infant with zero length.

3.6 This is a map of residuals. Notice that Washington and Texas, which may have large or small amounts of rain, are receiving normal amounts according to this map.

4.1 The variance is not constant. It is increasing with more recent years. The residuals are also correlated: Profitable years are also followed by other profitable years. Similarly, unprofitable years are likely followed by more of the same.

4.2 Three points can achieve a correlation of +1 or −1 if they all fall on a straight line with nonzero slope.

4.3 Adding a constant to all values does not change the correlation. Neither does multiplying by a positive number. Multiplying by a negative number reverses the sign of the correlation coefficient.

4.4 The complete ANOVA is as follows:

Source	df	Sum of squares	Mean square	F-value
Model	1	32.0	32.0	4.0
Error	20	160.0	8.0	
Total	21	192.0		

5.1 The model with as many parameters as observations will have 0 df for error. It will also have a perfect fit and $R^2 = 1$. Such a model is useless because it offers no simplification of the original data.

6.5 This is an example of regression to the mean.

6.6 The four assumptions are
1. The errors in each of the groups are independent
2. The errors in each group have the same variances
3. All errors in all groups have zero means
4. The errors in each group have normal distributions

6.8 If consumption is measured on a linear scale, we have

$$\text{Price} = \alpha + \beta\, C,$$

where C is the per-person average daily consumption. If C increases by one unit, then the estimated price increases by β dollars.
When consumption is measured on a log scale, the model is

$$\text{Price} = \alpha + \beta\, \log(C).$$

If we double consumption, then

$$\begin{aligned}\text{Price} &= \alpha + \beta\, \log(2C)\\ &= \alpha + \beta\, \log(C) + \beta\, \log(2)\end{aligned}$$

shows that the estimated price increases by $\beta\, \log(2)$.

8.2 Recall that $\log(x) = -\log(1/x)$. Then

$$\log\left(\frac{p}{1-p}\right) = -\log\left(\frac{1-p}{p}\right),$$

so that we only have to reverse the signs of the fitted regression coefficients in the computer output.

13.1 Survival analysis is appropriate. The outcome is time to recovery, defined as a certain level of ambulatory independence. Some wheelchair-bound individuals never recover and should be considered censored. We can use proportional hazards regression to model the effects of covariates such as age, sex, and the need for a home health aide. The null hypothesis is that none of these has any effect on time to recovery.

13.2 This is an example of the Poisson model. Square holes are rare, but a large number of donuts are produced. We can perform a Poisson regression to see if the temperature or coating resulted in different numbers of defective donuts. The null hypothesis is that these have no effect on the number of defective donuts.

13.3 This is an example of survival analysis with right censoring. We know when the bill is introduced (left end point) and the day it passes (right end point) or whether it is still pending legislative approval (censored). Proportional hazards regression can be used to see if the type of bill or the party that sponsored it is useful in explaining how long it took to pass. The null hypothesis is that these explanatory variables are not useful.

13.4 Linear regression might be useful here. Stopping distance is always positive but never censored. We can model the effects of pavement conditions, make and model of car, and color. The null hypothesis is that none if these factors influences stopping distance.

13.5 If everybody received either an A or a B, then these binary-valued outcomes should be modeled using logistic regression. The null hypothesis is that sex, age, major, and other courses have no relationship to the grade in the statistics course.

13.6 When we hear that the data has a lot of noise, we should use nonparametric methods. The rank-sum or median test can compare evaluations from required or elective course students. The null hypothesis is that these should be about the same.

13.7 In this linear regression we might use twelve indicator variables – one for each month. If that gets too confusing, we might use four indicators for each of the four seasons. The null hypothesis is that housing starts are the same year-round.

13.8 We might use logistic regression because all of the responses are either improved status or not. Because almost all of the patients recover, the trial is large and the probability of failure is so small we might also use Poisson regression. The null hypothesis in either of these regressions is that there is no difference in the failure rate for the two different drugs.

13.9 Every record is either proper or improper. These binary-valued outcomes should be modeled using logistic regression. The null hypothesis is that the patient's sex, age, comorbidity, and type of health insurance have no effect on the likelihood of the an improper use of their HIPAA information.

13.10 We can use survival analysis here to model the time until relapse. Patients who have not relapsed at the time of the statistical analysis are considered censored. The null hypothesis in proportional hazards regression is that these covariates have no effect on the relapse time.

13.11 There are many people at risk for rabies, but the chances of contracting it are very small. The Poisson regression is appropriate here. The null hypothesis is no trend.

13.12 This is a 2×2 table of frequencies. We count the number of people who are either old or young and are either cat owners or not. We might use the chi-squared or exact test to see if age is related to ownership. The null hypothesis is that these are independent of each other.

13.13 If age is measured on a continuous scale, then we should use logistic regression to model the binary-valued outcome of cat ownership or not. The null hypothesis is that age does not matter.

13.14 Every individual is either a case or a control. If tobacco use is also binary valued, then we can analyze these data using a chi-squared test for this 2×2 table of frequencies. The null hypothesis is that the risk of disease is not related to tobacco use. We can also use logistic regression to compare education levels in the case-control data. The null hypothesis is that education level is independent of the risk of disease.

13.15 The linear logistic model of the probability P of dying is

$$\text{logit}(P) = \alpha + \beta \text{ Dose} \tag{S.1}$$

where

$$\text{logit}(P) = \log\left(\frac{P}{1-P}\right).$$

a. The null hypothesis is $\beta = 0$, and the alternative is that β is different from zero.

b. When $P = .5$, then

$$\text{logit}(P) = \log(.5/.5) = \log(1) = 0.$$

If $\alpha = -3$ and $\beta = .5$, then solving for Dose in (S.1) gives us Dose $= 6$ as the estimated LD_{50}.

13.35 The survival curve goes all the way to zero if the longest-surviving individual has his or her event. The survival curve will stop before reaching zero if the longest-surviving individual is censored.

13.37 Unreliable data with known outliers such as these are good candidates for nonparametric methods.

Index